Compendium of Abridged ESC Guidelines 2008

Wolters Kluwer Health | Lippincott Williams & Wilkins

Disclaimer: The ESC Guidelines represent the views of the ESC and were arrived at after careful consideration of the available evidence at the time they were written. Health professionals are encouraged to take them fully into account when exercising their clinical judgment. The guidelines do not, however, override the individual responsibility of health professionals to make appropriate decisions in the circumstances of the individual patients, in consultation with that patient, and where appropriate and necessary the patient's guardian or carer. It is also the health professional's responsibility to verify the rules and regulations applicable to drugs and devices at the time of prescription.

ESC Staff involved in the publication of this document:

Keith H. McGregor, Scientific Director
Veronica Dean, Head of Practice Guidelines Department
Catherine Després, Research Analyst, Practice Guidelines Department

Contact e-mail: guidelines@escardio.org

Published by Lippincott Williams & Wilkins

250 Waterloo Road
London
SE1 8RD
UK
Bridie Reilly, Supplements Manager
E-mail: bridie.reilly@wolterskluwer.com

Typeset by Thomson Digital
Indexed by Dr Laurence Errington
Printed by Page Brothers, UK

ISBN: 978-0-7817-6421-6

ESC Committee for Practice Guidelines (CPG 2006–2008)

Alec Vahanian (Chairperson) France

John Camm, United Kingdom
Raffaele De Caterina, Italy
Veronica Dean, France
Kenneth Dickstein, Norway
Gerasimos Filippatos, Greece
Christian Funck-Brentano, France
Irene Hellemans, The Netherlands
Steen Dalby Kristensen, Denmark
Keith McGregor, France
Udo Sechtem, Germany
Sigmund Silber, Germany
Michal Tendera, Poland
Petr Widimsky, Czech Republic
José Luis Zamorano Gomez, Spain

Address for correspondence:

Practice Guidelines Department
2035 Route des Colles
Les Templiers – BP 179
06903 Sophia Antipolis Cedex
France
E-mail : guidelines@escardio.org

CONTENTS

Section V: Myocardial Disease 101

Section VI: Pericardial Disease 109

Section VII: Congenital Heart Disease 125

Section XII: Arrhythmias 217

Section XIII: Myocardial Infraction 291

Preface

In recent years there has been an increasing tendency towards optimization of medical practice through the application of Evidence Based Medicine. One of the consequences of this approach is an enormous increase in the number of clinical trials thus creating an environment in which keeping abreast of clinical advances, even within a single medical subspecialty, is an extremely demanding task. In this setting, clinicians have become increasingly reliant on clinical practice guidelines to help them decide on the diagnostic procedures and treatment options, which are most appropriate for the management of their patients.

The ESC is committed to reduce the burden of cardiovascular diseases in Europe and therefore considers that the development of Practice Guidelines is a strategic step to achieve this goal.

The production of ESC Practice Guidelines is coordinated by the Committee for Practice Guidelines (CPG). This committee is the body responsible for the nomination of the Task Forces, which are appointed to produce the different guidelines. The Committee selects the Task Force members ensuring the recruitment of leading scientific experts in each field and the participation of representatives from ESC Working Groups and ESC Associations.

The approval process of the documents includes the validation of each scientific statement by expert reviewers and ESC Board Members. In this respect, the recommendations included in the Guidelines reflect the official position of the European Society of Cardiology. ESC Guidelines are produced with the goal of covering all major topics defined in the ESC Core Syllabus.

All ESC Guidelines documents are posted on the ESC web site (http://www.escardio.org/guidelines/). The executive summaries of these guidelines are published in the European Heart Journal and are linked to an accredited Continuous Medical Education programme that allows physicians to earn CME credits online to show that they have achieved the learning objectives set for each published guideline.

The ESC Guidelines are endorsed, translated and adopted by most of the ESC National Societies. The implementation of the Guidelines is ensured through an active partnership between the ESC and its Working Groups, Associations, Councils and National Societies.

The ESC Pocket Guidelines are a concise summary of the fundamental recommendations made in the parent guidelines documents. These pocket guidelines are highly appreciated by medical professionals and have become an important guidelines dissemination tool. In view of the utility of these documents and the strong demand for a compilation of all of the available pocket guidelines, the Committee for Practice Guidelines commissioned the production of this ESC Guidelines Compendium 2008.

It is our hope and that of the Committees for Practice Guidelines 2006-2008 and 2008-2010, that this new tool will be of help to clinicians to follow the most recent recommendations in the practice of our rapidly evolving field of medicine.

Alec Vahanian; MD, FRCP
Chairperson of the
ESC Committee For Practice Guidelines
2006-2008 and 2008-2010

Foreword

It is with great pleasure that the European Society of Cardiology offers the ESC Guidelines Compendium, a compilation of all current ESC Pocket Guidelines titles, to its members.

ESC Pocket Guidelines have been published as individual booklets for a few years but as the list of titles has now grown, it became apparent that a compilation of all of the titles would be very useful to healthcare professionals as a resource to assist in clinical decision making at the point of care.

The 2007 edition of the ESC Guidelines compendium has been so successful that we are delighted to now produce the 2008 compendium which of course includes pocket guidelines published since the last edition.

By definition, pocket guidelines can provide only the most important recommendations extracted from extensive and scientifically well grounded full text guidelines. In some cases the clinician may still need to go back to these source documents in order to make a proper diagnostic or therapeutic decision.

We hope that you will find the ESC Guidelines Compendium a useful new tool in your practice and that it will help you to achieve the mission to reduce the burden of cardiovascular disease in Europe.

Kim Fox
President of the European Society of Cardiology
(2006-2008)

Roberto Ferrari
President of the European Society of Cardiology
(2008-2010)

Guidelines Overview: Review of 2008

Guidelines and Expert consensus documents aim to present management recommendations based on all of the relevant evidence on a particular subject. This is done in order to help physicians select the best possible management strategies for the individual patient suffering from a specific condition, taking into account the impact on outcome and also the risk:benefit ratio of a particular diagnostic or therapeutic procedure. Numerous studies have demonstrated that patient outcomes improve when guideline recommendations, based on the rigorous assessment of evidence based research, are applied in clinical practice.

A great number of Guidelines and Expert Consensus Documents have been issued in recent years by the European Society of Cardiology (ESC) and also by other organisations or related societies. The profusion of documents can put at stake the authority and credibility of guidelines, particularly if discrepancies appear between different documents on the same issue, as this can lead to confusion in the mind of physicians. In order to avoid these pitfalls, the ESC and other organisations have issued recommendations for formulating and issuing Guidelines and Expert Consensus Documents. The ESC recommendations for guideline production can be found on the ESC website [http://www.escardio.org]. It is beyond the scope of this preamble to recall all but the basic rules.

In brief, the ESC appoints experts in the field to carry out a comprehensive review of the literature, with a view to making a critical evaluation of the use of diagnostic and therapeutic procedures, and assessing the risk:benefit ratio of the therapies recommended for management and/or prevention of a given condition. Estimates of expected health outcomes are included, where data exists. The strength of evidence for or against particular procedures or treatments is weighed, according to predefined scales for grading recommendations and levels of evidence, as outlined below.

The Task Force members of the writing panels, as well as the document reviewers, are asked to provide disclosure statements of all relationships they may have which might be perceived as real or potential conflicts of interest. These disclosure forms are kept on file at the European Heart House, headquarters of the ESC, and can be made available by written request to the ESC President. Any changes in conflicts of interest that arise during the writing period must be notified to the ESC.

Guidelines and recommendations are presented in formats that are easy to interpret. They should help physicians to make clinical decisions in their daily routine practice, by describing the range of generally acceptable approaches to diagnosis and treatment. However, the ultimate judgement regarding the care of an individual patient must be made by the physician in charge of his/her care.

The ESC Committee for Practice Guidelines (CPG) supervises and coordinates the preparation of new Guidelines and Expert Consensus Documents produced by Task Forces, expert groups or consensus panels. The Committee is also responsible for the endorsement of these Guidelines and Expert Consensus Documents or statements.

Once the document has been finalised and approved by all the experts involved in the Task Force, it is submitted to outside specialists for review. In some cases, the document can be presented to a panel of key opinion leaders in Europe, specialists in the relevant condition at hand, for discussion and critical review. If necessary, the document is revised once more, and finally approved by the CPG and selected members of the Board of the ESC and subsequently published.

After publication, dissemination of the message is of paramount importance. Publication of executive summaries, the production of pocket-sized and PDA-downloadable versions of the recommendations are helpful. However, surveys have shown that the intended end-users are often not aware of the existence of guidelines or simply don't put them into practice. Implementation programmes are thus necessary and form an important component of the dissemination of knowledge. Meetings are organised by the ESC, and directed towards its member National Societies and key opinion leaders in Europe. Implementation meetings can also be undertaken at a national level, once the guidelines have been endorsed by the ESC member societies and translated into the local language as required.

The task of writing Guidelines or Expert Consensus documentation not only involves the integration of the most recent research, but also the creation of educational tools and implementation programmes for the recommendations. The cyclical nature of clinical research, writing of guidelines and implementing them into clinical practice can then only be completed if surveys and registries are organised to verify that actual clinical practice is in keeping with what is recommended by the guidelines. Such surveys and registries also make it possible to check the impact of strict implementation of the guidelines on patient outcome.

Classes of Recommendations	Definition
Class I	**Evidence and/or general agreement that a given treatment or procedure is beneficial, useful, effective.**
Class II	**Conflicting evidence and/or a divergence of opinion about the usefulness /efficacy of the given treatment or procedure.**
Class IIa	**Weight of evidence/opinion is in favour of usefulness/efficacy.**
Class IIb	**Usefulness/efficacy is less well established by evidence/opinion.**
Class III	**Evidence or general agreement that the given treatment or procedure is not useful/ effective, and in some cases may be harmful.**

Level of Evidence A	**Data derived from multiple randomized clinical trials or meta-analyses.**
Level of Evidence B	**Data derived from a single randomized clinical trial or large non-randomized studies.**
Level of Evidence C	**Consensus of opinion of the experts and/or small studies, retrospective studies, registries.**

Section I:
Prevention of Cardiovascular Disease

1. Cardiovascular Disease Prevention in Clinical Practice

Chapter 1

Cardiovascular Disease Prevention in Clinical Practice*

2007

Chairperson:
Professor Ian Graham (ESC)
Department of Cardiology
The Adelaide and Meath Hospital
Tallaght, Dublin 24
Ireland
Tel.: +35 (3) 1 414 4105
Fax: +35 (3) 1 414 3052
E-mail: ian.graham@amnch.ie

Task Force Members:
1. Dan Atar, Oslo, Norway (ESC)
2. Knut Borch-Johnsen, Gentofte, Denmark (EASD/IDF-Europe)
3. Gudrun Boysen, Copenhagen, Denmark (EUSI)
4. Gunilla Burell, Uppsala, Sweden (ISBM)
5. Renata Cifkova, Praha, Czech Republic (ESH)
6. Jean Dallongeville, Lille, France (ESC)
7. Guy De Backer, Gent, Belgium (ESC)
8. Shah Ebrahim, London, England (ESC/Center for Evidence Based Medicine)
9. Bjørn Gjelsvik, Oslo, Norway (ESGP/FM/Wonca)
10. Christoph Herrmann-Lingen, Gottingen, Germany (ISBM)
11. Arno W. Hoes, Utrecht, The Netherlands (ESGP/FM/Wonca)
12. Steve Humphries, London, England (ESC)
13. Mike Knapton, London, England (EHN)
14. Joep Perk, Oskarshamn, Sweden (EACPR)
15. Silvia G. Priori, Pavia, Italy (ESC)
16. Kalevi Pyorala, Kuopio, Finland (ESC)
17. Zeljko Reiner, Zagreb, Croatia (EAS)
18. Luis Ruilope, Madrid, Spain (ESC)
19. Susana Sans-Menendez, Barcelona, Spain (ESC)
20. Wilma Scholte Op Reimer, Rotterdam, The Netherlands
21. Peter Weissberg, London, England (EHN)
22. David Wood, London, England (ESC)
23. John Yarnell, Belfast, Northern Ireland (EACPR)
24. Jose Luis Zamorano, Madrid, Spain (ESC/CPG)

Other experts who contributed to parts of the guidelines:
1. Marie-Therese Cooney, Dublin, Ireland
2. Alexandra Dudina, Dublin, Ireland
3. Tony Fitzgerald, Dublin, Ireland
4. Edmond Walma, Schoonhoven, The Netherlands (ESGP/FM/Wonca)

Societies:
European Association for the Study of Diabetes (EASD); International Diabetes Federation Europe (IDF-Europe); European Atherosclerosis Society (EAS); European Heart Network (EHN); European Society of Hypertension (ESH); European Society of Cardiology (ESC); European Society of General Practice/Family Medicine (ESGP/FM/Wonca); European Stroke Initiative (EUSI); International Society of Behavioral Medicine (ISBM); European Association for Cardiovascular Prevention & Rehabilitation (EACPR)

ESC Staff:
1. Keith McGregor, Sophia Antipolis, France
2. Veronica Dean, Sophia Antipolis, France
4. Catherine Després, Sophia Antipolis, France

The European Heart Health Charter and the Guidelines on Cardiovascular Disease Prevention

- The European Heart Health Charter advocates the development and implementation of comprehensive health strategies, measures and policies at European, national, regional and local level that promote cardiovascular health and prevent cardiovascular disease.
- These guidelines aim to assist physicians and other health professionals to fulfil their role in this endeavour, particularly with regard to achieving effective preventive measures in day-to-day clinical practice.

* Adapted from the ESC Guidelines on the Fourth Joint European Societies' Task Force on cardiovascular disease prevention in clinical practice. Executive Summary (European Heart Journal 2007 - doi:10.1093/eurheartj/ehm316) and full text European Journal of Cardiovascular Prevention and Rehabilitation 2007;4(Suppl. 2).

Summary Flow Chart

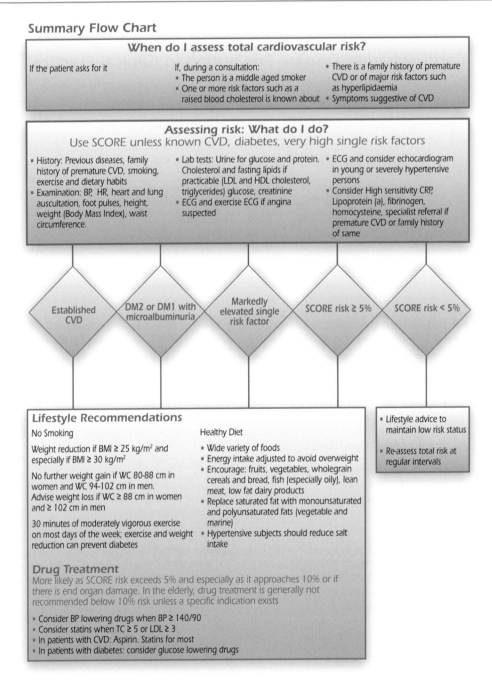

When do I assess total cardiovascular risk?

If the patient asks for it

If, during a consultation:
- The person is a middle aged smoker
- One or more risk factors such as a raised blood cholesterol is known about
- There is a family history of premature CVD or of major risk factors such as hyperlipidaemia
- Symptoms suggestive of CVD

Assessing risk: What do I do?

Use SCORE unless known CVD, diabetes, very high single risk factors

- History: Previous diseases, family history of premature CVD, smoking, exercise and dietary habits
- Examination: BP, HR, heart and lung auscultation, foot pulses, height, weight (Body Mass Index), waist circumference.
- Lab tests: Urine for glucose and protein. Cholesterol and fasting lipids if practicable (LDL and HDL cholesterol, triglycerides) glucose, creatinine
- ECG and exercise ECG if angina suspected
- ECG and consider echocardiogram in young or severely hypertensive persons
- Consider High sensitivity CRP, Lipoprotein (a), fibrinogen, homocysteine, specialist referral if premature CVD or family history of same

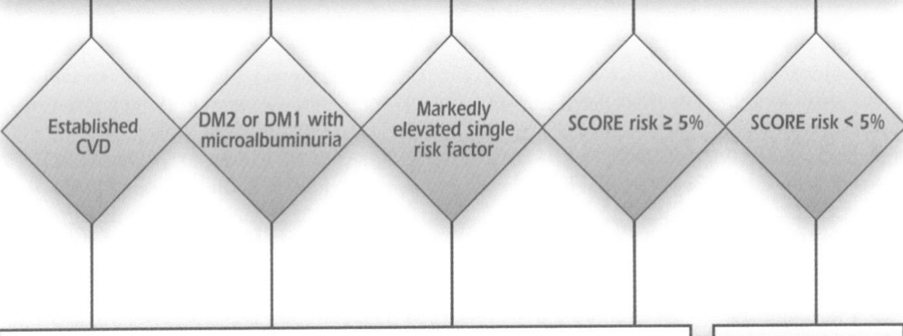

Lifestyle Recommendations

No Smoking

Weight reduction if BMI ≥ 25 kg/m^2 and especially if BMI ≥ 30 kg/m^2

No further weight gain if WC 80-88 cm in women and WC 94-102 cm in men. Advise weight loss if WC ≥ 88 cm in women and ≥ 102 cm in men

30 minutes of moderately vigorous exercise on most days of the week; exercise and weight reduction can prevent diabetes

Healthy Diet
- Wide variety of foods
- Energy intake adjusted to avoid overweight
- Encourage: fruits, vegetables, wholegrain cereals and bread, fish (especially oily), lean meat, low fat dairy products
- Replace saturated fat with monounsaturated and polyunsaturated fats (vegetable and marine)
- Hypertensive subjects should reduce salt intake

Drug Treatment

More likely as SCORE risk exceeds 5% and especially as it approaches 10% or if there is end organ damage. In the elderly, drug treatment is generally not recommended below 10% risk unless a specific indication exists

- Consider BP lowering drugs when BP ≥ 140/90
- Consider statins when TC ≥ 5 or LDL ≥ 3
- In patients with CVD: Aspirin. Statins for most
- In patients with diabetes: consider glucose lowering drugs

- Lifestyle advice to maintain low risk status
- Re-assess total risk at regular intervals

- They reflect the consensus arising from a multi-disciplinary partnership between the major European professional bodies represented.

Why develop a preventive strategy in clinical practice?

- Cardiovascular disease (CVD) is the major cause of premature death in Europe. It is an important cause of disability and contributes substantially to the escalating costs of health care.
- The underlying atherosclerosis develops insidiously over many years and is usually advanced by the time that symptoms occur.
- Death from CVD often occurs suddenly and before medical care is available, so that many therapeutic interventions are either inapplicable or palliative.
- The mass occurrence of CVD relates strongly to lifestyles and to modifiable physiological and biochemical factors.
- Risk factor modifications have been shown to reduce CVD mortality and morbidity, particularly in high risk subjects.

What are the objectives of these guidelines?

- To help health professionals to reduce the occurrence of coronary heart disease, stroke and peripheral artery disease and their complications.
- To achieve this by providing practical and accessible advice with regard to the rationale for prevention, priorities, objectives, risk assessment and management through lifestyle measures and selective drug usage.
- To encourage the development of national guidance through the formation of multi-disciplinary national guideline and implementation partnerships that are compatible with local, political, social, economic and medical circumstances.

People who stay healthy tend to have certain characteristics:

	0 3 5 140 5 3 0
0	No tobacco
3	Walk 3 km daily, or 30 mins any moderate activity
5	Portions of fruit and vegetables a day
140	Blood pressure less than 140 systolic
5	Total blood cholesterol < 5mmol/L
3	LDL cholesterol < 3 mmol/L
0	Avoidance of overweight and diabetes

What are the priorities for CVD prevention in clinical practice?

Patients with established atherosclerotic CVD.

Asymptomatic individuals who are at increased risk of CVD because of:

Multiple risk factors resulting in raised total CVD risk (≥ **5% 10 year risk of CVD death**)

Diabetes type 2 & type 1 with microalbuminuria

Markedly increased single risk factors especially if associated with end organ damage

Close relatives of subjects with premature atherosclerotic CVD or of those at particularly high risk.

What are the objectives of CVD prevention?

1. **To assist those at low risk of CVD to maintain this state lifelong, & to help those at higher increased total CVD risk to reduce it.**

2. **To achieve the characteristics of people who tend to stay healthy:**
   - No smoking
   - Healthy food choices
   - Physical activity: 30 min. of moderate activity a day
   - BMI < 25 Kg/m^2 and avoidance of central obesity
   - BP < 140/90 mmHg
   - Total cholesterol < 5 mmol/L (~ 190 mg/dL)
   - LDL cholesterol < 3 mmol/L (~ 115 mg/dL)
   - Blood glucose < 6 mmo/L (~ 110 mg/dL)

3. **To achieve more rigorous risk factor control in high risk subjects, especially those with established CVD or diabetes:**
   - Blood pressure under 130/80 mmHg if feasible
   - Total cholesterol < 4.5 mmol/L (~ 175 mg/dL) with an option of < 4 mmol/L (~ 155 mg/dL) if feasible
   - LDL- cholesterol < 2.5 mmol/L (~ 100 mg/dL) with an option of < 2 mmol/L (~ 80 mg/dL) if feasible
   - Fasting blood glucose < 6 mmol/L (~ 110 mg/dL) and HbA_{1c} < 6.5% if feasible

4. **To consider cardioprotective drug therapy in these high risk subjects especially those with established atherosclerotic CVD.**

When do I assess cardiovascular risk?

- If the patient asks for it.
- If, during a consultation:
  - The person is a middle aged smoker
  - There is obesity, especially abdominal
  - One or more risk factors such as blood pressure, lipids or glucose is raised
  - There is a family history of premature CVD or of other risk factors
  - There are symptoms suggestive of CVD. If confirmed, risk factors should be assessed but use of the SCORE chart is not necessary as the person is already at high risk

Why do the Guidelines stress the assessment of total CVD risk?

- Multiple risk factors usually contribute to the atherosclerosis that causes CVD.
- These risk factors interact, sometimes multiplicatively.
- Thus the aim should be to reduce total risk; if a target cannot be reached with one risk factor, total risk can still be reduced by trying harder with others.

How do I assess CVD risk quickly and easily?

- Those with:
  - known CVD
  - type 2 diabetes or type 1 diabetes with microalbuminuria,
  - very high levels of individual risk factors

are automatically at INCREASED CARDIOVASCULAR RISK and need management to all risk factors.

- For all other people, the SCORE risk charts can be used to estimate total risk: this is critically important because many people have mildly raised levels of several risk factors that, in combination, can result in unexpectedly high levels of total cardiovascular risk.

Assessing cardiovascular risk: What are the components?

- History: Previous CVD or related diseases, family history of premature CVD, smoking, exercise and dietary habits, social and educational status.
- Examination: BP, heart rate, heart and lung auscultation, foot pulses, height, weight (Body Mass Index), waist circumference. Fundoscopy in severe hypertension.
- Lab test: Urine for glucose and protein, microalbuminuria in diabetics. Cholesterol and if practicable, fasting lipids (LDL and HDL cholesterol, triglycerides) glucose, creatinine.
- ECG and exercise ECG if angina suspected.
- ECG and consider echocardiogram in hypertensive persons.
- Premature or aggressive CVD, especially with a family history of premature CVD: Consider High sensitivity CRP, Lipoprotein (a), fibrinogen, homocysteine and, if feasible, specialist referral.

How do I use the SCORE charts to assess CVD risk in asymptomatic persons?

1. Use the low risk chart in Belgium*, France, Greece*, Italy, Luxembourg, Spain*, Switzerland and Portugal; use the high risk chart in other countries of Europe.
   *Updated, re-calibrated charts are now available for Belgium, Germany, Greece, The Netherlands, Spain, Sweden and Poland.

2. Find the cell nearest to the person's age, cholesterol and BP values, bearing in mind that risk will be higher as the person approaches the next age, cholesterol or BP category.

3. Check the qualifiers.

4. Establish the total 10 year risk for fatal CVD.

Note that a low total cardiovascular risk in a young person may conceal a high relative risk; this may be explained to the person by using the relative risk chart. As the person ages, a high relative risk will translate into a high total risk. More intensive lifestyle advice will be needed in such persons.

Risk estimation using SCORE: Qualifiers

- The charts should be used in the light of the clinician's knowledge and judgement, especially with regard to local conditions.
- As with all risk estimation systems, risk will be over estimated in countries with a falling CVD mortality rate, and under estimated if it is rising.
- At any given age, risk appears lower for women than men. This is misleading since, ultimately, more women than men die from CVD. Inspection of the charts shows that their risk is merely deferred by 10 years.
- Risk may be higher than indicated in the chart in:
  - Sedentary or obese subjects, especially those with central obesity
  - Those with a strong family history of premature CVD
  - The socially deprived
  - Subjects with diabetes- risk may be 5 fold higher in women with diabetes and 3 fold higher in men with diabetes compared to those without diabetes
  - Those with low HDL cholesterol or high triglycerides
  - Asymptomatic subjects with evidence of pre-clinical atherosclerosis, for example a reduced ankle-brachial index or on imaging such as carotid ultrasonography or CT scanning

10 year risk of fatal CVD in high risk regions of Europe

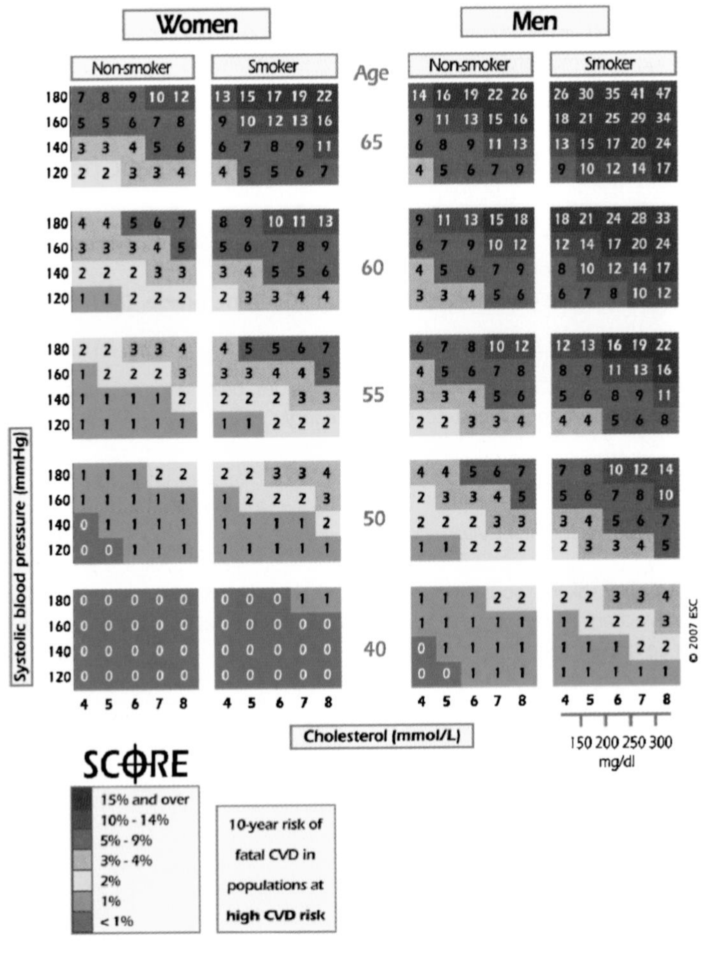

10 year risk of fatal CVD in low risk regions of Europe

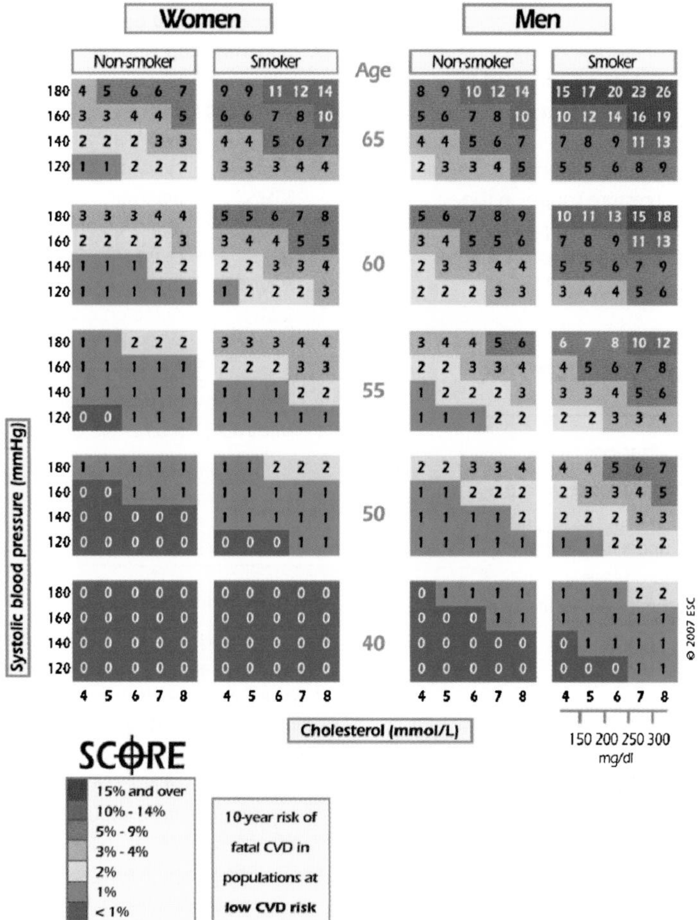

Age	Systolic blood pressure (mmHg)	Women Non-smoker 4	5	6	7	8	Women Smoker 4	5	6	7	8	Men Non-smoker 4	5	6	7	8	Men Smoker 4	5	6	7	8
65	180	4	5	6	6	7	9	9	11	12	14	8	9	10	12	14	15	17	20	23	26
	160	3	3	4	4	5	6	6	7	8	10	5	6	7	8	10	10	12	14	16	19
	140	2	2	2	3	3	4	4	5	6	7	4	4	5	6	7	7	8	9	11	13
	120	1	1	2	2	2	3	3	3	4	4	2	3	3	4	5	5	5	6	8	9
60	180	3	3	3	4	4	5	5	6	7	8	5	6	7	8	9	10	11	13	15	18
	160	2	2	2	2	3	3	4	4	5	5	3	4	5	5	6	7	8	9	11	13
	140	1	1	1	2	2	2	2	3	3	4	2	3	3	4	4	5	5	6	7	9
	120	1	1	1	1	1	1	2	2	2	3	2	2	2	3	3	3	4	4	5	6
55	180	1	1	2	2	2	3	3	3	4	4	3	4	4	5	6	6	7	8	10	12
	160	1	1	1	1	1	2	2	2	3	3	2	2	3	3	4	4	5	6	7	8
	140	1	1	1	1	1	1	1	1	2	2	1	2	2	2	3	3	3	4	5	6
	120	0	0	1	1	1	1	1	1	1	1	1	1	1	2	2	2	2	3	3	4
50	180	1	1	1	1	1	1	1	2	2	2	2	2	3	3	4	4	4	5	6	7
	160	0	0	1	1	1	1	1	1	1	1	1	1	2	2	2	2	3	3	4	5
	140	0	0	0	0	0	1	1	1	1	1	1	1	1	1	2	2	2	2	3	3
	120	0	0	0	0	0	0	0	0	1	1	1	1	1	1	1	1	1	2	2	2
40	180	0	0	0	0	0	0	0	0	0	0	0	1	1	1	1	1	1	1	2	2
	160	0	0	0	0	0	0	0	0	0	0	0	0	0	1	1	1	1	1	1	1
	140	0	0	0	0	0	0	0	0	0	0	0	0	0	0	0	0	1	1	1	1
	120	0	0	0	0	0	0	0	0	0	0	0	0	0	0	0	0	0	0	1	1

Relative Risk Chart

This chart may be used to show younger people at low total risk that, relative to others in their age group, their risk may be many times higher than necessary. This may help to motivate decisions about avoidance of smoking, healthy nutrition and exercise, as well as flagging those who may become candidates for medication.

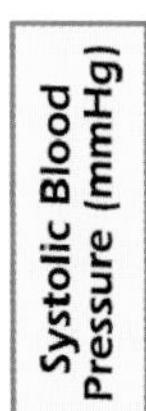

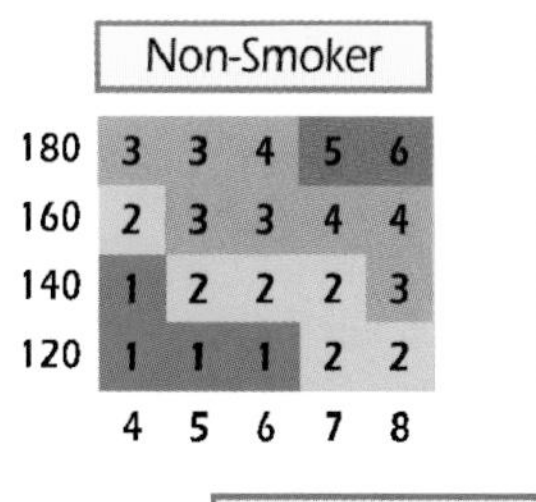

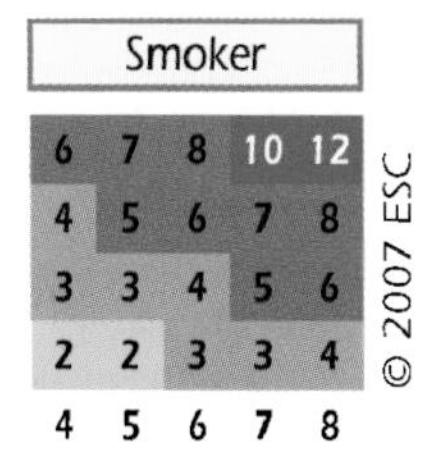

Systolic Blood Pressure (mmHg)	Non-Smoker 4	5	6	7	8	Smoker 4	5	6	7	8
180	3	3	4	5	6	6	7	8	10	12
160	2	3	3	4	4	4	5	6	7	8
140	1	2	2	2	3	3	3	4	5	6
120	1	1	1	2	2	2	2	3	3	4

How do I manage the components of total CVD risk?

- The patient and the doctor agree that a risk assessment is indicated, and the patient is informed that the result may lead to suggestions regarding life style change and the possibility of life long medication.
- There are time and resources to discuss and follow up advice and treatment.
- The doctor should be aware of and respect the patients own values and choices.

Total risk CVD management: A key message

- Management of the individual components of risk such as smoking, diet, exercise, blood pressure and lipids impacts on total cardiovascular risk.
- Thus, if perfect control of a risk factor is difficult (for example, blood pressure control in the elderly), total risk can still be reduced by reducing other risk factors such as smoking or blood cholesterol.

Managing total cardiovascular risk

Tips to help behaviour change

- Develop a sympathetic alliance with the patient.
- Ensure the patient understands the relationship between lifestyle and disease.
- Use this to gain commitment to lifestyle change.
- Involve the patient in identifying the risk factors to change.
- Explore potential barriers to change.
- Help design a lifestyle change plan.
- Be realistic and encouraging- "ANY increase in exercise is good and can be built on".
- Reinforce the patient's efforts to change.
- Monitor progress through follow-up contacts.
- Involve other health care staff wherever possible.

Why do people find it hard to change their life?

- **Socio-economic status:** Low SES, including low educational level and low income, impedes the ability to adopt lifestyle change.
- **Social isolation:** People living alone are more likely to have unhealthy lifestyles.
- **Stress:** Stress at work and at home makes it more difficult for people to adopt and sustain a healthy lifestyle.
- **Negative emotions:** Depression, anxiety and hostility impede lifestyle change.
- **Complex or confusing advice.**

Increased physician awareness of these factors facilitates empathy, counselling and the provision of sympathetic, simple and explicit advice.

Smoking

All smokers should be professionally encouraged to permanently stop smoking all forms of tobacco.

The 5 A's can help:

A - ASK: systematically identify all smokers at every opportunity.

A - ASSESS: determine the person's degree of addiction and his/her readiness to cease smoking.

A - ADVISE: Unequivocally urge all smokers to quit.

A - ASSIST: Agree on a smoking cessation strategy including behavioural. counselling, nicotine replacement therapy and/or pharmacological intervention.

A - ARRANGE: a schedule of follow-up visits.

Healthy food choices

All individuals should be advised about food choices that are associated with lower CVD risk. High risk persons should receive specialist dietary advice if feasible. General recommendations should suit the local culture:

- A wide variety of foods should be eaten.
- Energy intake should be adjusted to avoid overweight.
- Encourage: Fruits, vegetables, wholegrain cereals and bread, fish (especially oily), lean meat, low fat dairy products.
- Replace saturated fat with the above foods and with monounsaturated and polyunsaturated fats from vegetable and marine sources to reduce total fat to < 30% of energy, of which less than 1/3 is saturated.
- Reduce salt intake if blood pressure is raised by avoiding table salt and salt in cooking, and by choosing fresh or frozen unsalted foods. Many processed and prepared foods, including bread, are high in salt.

Physical activity

- Stress that positive health benefits occur with almost any increase in activity; small amounts of exercise have an additive effect; exercise opportunities exist in the workplace, for example by using stairs instead of the lift.
- Try to find leisure activities that are positively enjoyable.
- 30 minutes of moderately vigorous exercise on most days of the week will reduce risk and increase fitness.
- Exercising with family or friends tends to improve motivation.
- Added benefits include a sense of well being, weight reduction and better self esteem.
- Continued physician encouragement and support may help in the long term.

Body weight

- Increasing body weight is associated with increased total and CVD mortality and morbidity, mediated in part through increases in blood pressure and blood cholesterol, reduced HDL cholesterol and an increased likelihood of diabetes.
- Weight reduction is recommended for obese people (BMI ≥ 30 kg/m^2) and should be considered for those who are overweight (BMI ≥ 25 and < 30 kg/m^2).
- Men with a waist circumference of 94-102 cm and women with a waist circumference of 80-88 cm are advised not to increase their weight. Men above 102 cm and women above 88 cm are advised to lose weight.
- Restriction of total calorie intake and regular physical exercise are the cornerstones of weight control. It is likely that improvements in central fat metabolism occur with exercise even before weight reduction occurs.

Blood pressure

In ALL cases, look for and manage all risk factors. Those with established CVD, diabetes or renal disease are at markedly increased risk and a BP of < 130/80 is desirable if feasible. For all other people, check SCORE risk. Those with target organ damage are managed as "increased risk".

SCORE CVD risk	Normal <130/85	High N 130-139/ 85-89	Grade 1 140-159/ 90-99	Grade 2 160-179/ 100-109	Grade 3 ≥ 180/110
Low < 1%	Lifestyle advice	Lifestyle advice	Lifestyle advice	Drug Rx if persists	Drug Rx
Mod 1-4%	Lifestyle advice	Lifestyle advice	+ consider drug Rx	Drug Rx if persists	Drug Rx
Increased 5-9%	Lifestyle advice	+ consider drug Rx	+ consider drug Rx	Drug Rx	Drug Rx
Markedly increased ≥ 10%	Lifestyle advice	+ consider drug Rx	Drug Rx	Drug Rx	Drug Rx

Lipids

In ALL cases, look for and manage all risk factors. Those with established CVD, diabetes type 2 or type 1 with microalbuminuria or with severe hyper-lipidaemia are already at high risk. For all other people, the SCORE charts can be used to estimate total risk.

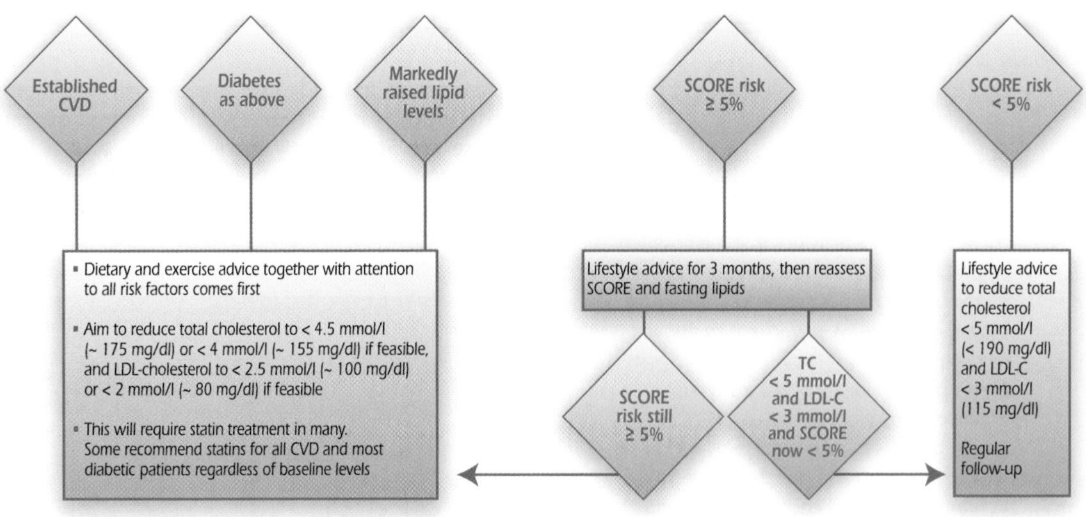

Treatment goals are not defined for HDL cholesterol and triglycerides but HDL-C < 1.0 mmol/L (40 mg/dL) for men and < 1.2 mmol/L (45 mg/dL) for women and fasting triglycerides of > 1.7 mmol/L (150 mg/dL) are markers of increased cardiovascular risk.

Treatment targets in patients with type 2 diabetes		
	Unit	**Target**
HbA_{1c} (aligned DCCT)	HbA_{1c} (%)	≤ 6.5 if feasible
Plasma glucose	Fasting/pre-prandial mmol/L (mg/dL)	< 6.0 (110) if feasible
	Post-prandial mmol/L (mg/dL)	< 7.5 (135) if feasible
Blood pressure	mmHg	≤ 130/80
Total cholesterol	mmol/L (mg/dL) mmol/L (mg/dL)	< 4.5 (175) < 4.0 (155) if feasible
LDL cholesterol	mmol/L (mg/dL) mmol/L (mg/dL)	< 2.5 (100) < 2.0 (80) if feasible

The metabolic syndrome

- The term "metabolic syndrome" refers to the combination of several factors that tend to cluster together- central obesity, hypertension, low HDL-cholesterol, raised triglycerides and raised blood sugar- to increase risk of diabetes and CVD.
- This implies that, if one component is identified, a systematic search for the others is indicated, together with an active approach to managing all of these risk factors.
- Physical activity and weight control can radically reduce the risk of developing diabetes in those with the metabolic syndrome.

Renal impairment and cardiovascular risk

- Risk of CVD rises progressively from microalbuminuria with preserved GFR to end stage renal disease, when it is 20-30x that of general population.
- Applies to apparently healthy people and those with hypertension, CVD and heart failure.
- Associated with high blood pressure, hyperlipidaemia, metabolic syndrome, uric acid, homocysteine, anaemia.
- Particularly vigorous risk factor control needed.

When to prescribe cardio-protective drugs in addition to those used to treat blood pressure, lipids and diabetes?

- Aspirin for virtually all with established CVD, and in persons at > 10% SCORE risk once blood pressure has been controlled.
- Beta-blockers after myocardial infarction and, in carefully titrated doses, in those with heart failure.
- ACE-inhibitors in those with left ventricular dysfunction and in diabetic subjects with hypertension or nephropathy.
- Anti-coagulants in those at increased risk of thrombo-embolic events, particularly atrial fibrillation.

Why screen close relatives?

- Close relatives of patients with premature CVD and persons who belong to families with inherited dyslipidaemias such as familial hypercholesterolaemia are at increased risk of developing CVD and should be examined for all cardiovascular risk factors.

What would make the practice of CVD prevention easier?

- Simple, clear, credible guidelines.
- Sufficient time.
- Positively helpful government policies (defined prevention strategy with resources, incentives including remuneration for prevention as well as treatment).
- Educational policies that facilitate patient adherence to advice.

Section II: Hypertension

1. The Management of Arterial Hypertension

Chapter 1

The Management of Arterial Hypertension* 2007

Co-chairperson:
Giuseppe Mancia (ESH)
Ospedale San Gerardo
Universita Milano-Bicocca
Via Pergolesi, 33
20052 Monza Milano
Italy
Tel.: +39 0 39 233 33 57
Fax: +39 0 39 32 22 74
E-mail: giuseppe.mancia@unimib.it

Co-chairperson:
Guy De Backer (ESC)
University Hospital
Ghent University
De Pintelaan 185
9000 Gent
Belgium
Tel.: +32 9 240 36 27
Fax: +32 9 240 49 94
E-mail: guy.debacker@ugent.be

Task Force Members:
1. Renata Cifkova, Prague, Czech Republic
2. Anna Dominiczak, Glasgow, UK
3. Robert Fagard, Leuven, Belgium
4. Giuseppe Germanó, Roma, Italy
5. Guido Grassi, Monza, Italy
6. Anthony M. Heagerty, Manchester, UK
7. Sverre E. Kjeldsen, Oslo, Norway
8. Stephane Laurent, Paris, France
9. Krzysztof Narkiewicz, Gdansk, Poland
10. Luis Ruilope, Madrid, Spain
11. Andrzej Rynkiewicz, Gdansk, Poland
12. Roland E. Schmieder, Erlangen, Germany
13. Harry A.J. Struijker Boudier, Maastricht, the Netherlands
14. Alberto Zanchetti, Milan, Italy

ESC Staff:
1. Keith McGregor, Sophia Antipolis, France
2. Veronica Dean, Sophia Antipolis, France
3. Catherine Després, Sophia Antipolis, France

Special thanks to Jose L. Rodicio Diaz for his contribution.

1. Arterial hypertension

Definition and classification

Blood pressure has a unimodal distribution in the population as well as a continuous relationship with CV risk.

For practical reasons the term "hypertension" is used in daily practice and patients are categorized as shown in Table 1. However the real threshold for defining "hypertension" must be considered as flexible, being high or low based on the total CV risk of each individual.

Table 1: Definitions and Classification of blood pressure (BP) levels (mmHg)

Category	Systolic		Diastolic
Optimal	< 120	and	< 80
Normal	120–129	and/or	80–84
High normal	130–139	and/or	85–89
Grade 1 hypertension	140–159	and/or	90–99
Grade 2 hypertension	160–179	and/or	100–109
Grade 3 hypertension	≥ 180	and/or	≥ 110
Isolated systolic hypertension	≥ 140	and	< 90

Isolated systolic hypertension should be graded (1,2,3) according to systolic blood pressure values in the ranges indicated, provided that diastolic values are < 90 mmHg.

* Adapted from the 2007 Guidelines for the Management of Arterial Hypertension (European Heart Journal 2007;28:1462-1536)

2. Total cardiovascular (CV) risk

- All patients should be classified not only in relation to the grades of hypertension but also in terms of the total CV risk resulting from the coexistence of different risk factors, organ damage and disease.

- Decisions on treatment strategies (initiation of drug treatment, BP threshold and target for treatment, use of combination treatment, need of a statin and other non-antihypertensive drugs) all importantly depend on the initial level of risk.

- There are several methods by which total CV risk can be assessed, all with advantages and limitations. Categorization of total risk as low, moderate, high, and very high added risk has the merit of simplicity and can therefore be recommended. The term 'added risk' refers to the risk additional to the average one.

- Total risk is usually expressed as the absolute risk of having a CV event within 10 years. Because of its heavy dependence on age, in young patients absolute total CV risk can be low even in the presence of high BP with additional risk factors. If insufficiently treated, however, this condition may lead to a partly irreversible high risk condition years later. In younger subjects treatment decisions should better be guided by quantification of relative risk, i.e. the increase in risk in relation to average risk in the population.

- Using rigid cut-offs of absolute risk (e.g. > 20% within 10 years) in order to decide on treatment is discouraged.

3. Stratification of total CV risk

In the Figure 1 total CV risk is stratified in four categories. Low, moderate, high and very high risks refer to 10 year risk of a fatal or non-fatal CV event. The term "added" indicates that in all categories risk is greater than average. The dashed line indicates how the definition of hypertension (and thus the decision about the initiation of treatment) is flexible, i.e. may be variable depending on the level of total CV risk.

Figure 1: Stratification of CV risk in four categories of added risk

	Blood Pressure (mmHg)				
Other risk factors, OD or disease	Normal SBP 120-129 or DBP 80-84	High Normal SBP 130-139 or DBP 85-89	Grade 1 HT SBP 140-159 or DBP 90-99	Grade 2 HT SBP 160-179 or DBP 100-109	Grade 3 HT SBP ≥ 180 or DBP ≥ 110
No other risk factors	Average risk	Average risk	Low added risk	Moderate added risk	High added risk
1-2 risk factors	Low added risk	Low added risk	Moderate added risk	Moderate added risk	Very high added risk
3 or more risk factors MS, OD or Diabetes	Moderate added risk	High added risk	High added risk	High added risk	Very High added risk
Established CV or renal disease	Very high added risk	Very high added risk	Very high added risk	Very high added risk	Very high added risk

SBP = systolic blood pressure; DBP = diastolic blood pressure; CV = cardiovascular; HT = hypertension; OD = subclinical organ damage; MS = metabolic syndrome

4. Clinical variables that should be used to stratify total CV risk

Risk factors	Subclinical Organ Damage
• Systolic and diastolic BP levels • Levels of pulse pressure (in the elderly) • Age (M > 55 years; W > 65 years) • Smoking • Dyslipidaemia - TC > 5.0 mmol/L (190 mg/dL) or: - LDL-C > 3.0 mmol/L (115 mg/dL) or: - HDL-C: M < 1.0 mmol/L (40mg/dL), W < 1.2 mmol/L (46 mg/dL) or: - TG > 1.7 mmol/L (150 mg/dL) • Fasting plasma glucose 5.6-6.9 mmol/L (102-125 mg/dL) • Abnormal glucose tolerance test • Abdominal obesity (Waist circumference > 102 cm (M), > 88 cm (W)) • Family history of premature CV disease (M at age < 55 years; W at age < 65 years)	• Electrocardiographic LVH (Sokolow-Lyon > 38 mm; Cornell > 2440 mm/ms) or: • Echocardiographic LVH* (LVMI M ≥ 125 g/m^2, W ≥ 110 g/m^2) • Carotid wall thickening (IMT > 0.9 mm) or plaque • Carotid-femoral pulse wave velocity > 12 m/sec • Ankle/Brachial BP index < 0.9 • Slight increase in plasma creatinine: M: 115-133 μmol/L (1.3-1.5 mg/dL); W: 107-124 μmol/L (1.2-1.4 mg/dL) • Low estimated glomerular filtration rate** (< 60 ml/min/1.73m^2) or creatine clearance*** (< 60 ml/min) • Microalbuminuria 30-300 mg/24h or albumin-creatinine ratio: ≥ 22 (M); or ≥ 31 (W) mg/g creatinine
Diabetes Mellitus	**Established CV or renal disease**
• Fasting plasma glucose ≥ 7.0 mmol/L (126 mg/dL) on repeated measurement or: • Postload plasma glucose > 11.0 mmol/L (198 mg/dL) Note: the cluster of three out of 5 risk factors among abdominal obesity, altered fasting plasma glucose, BP ≥ 130/85 mmHg, low HDL - cholesterol and high TG (as defined above) indicates the presence of metabolic syndrome.	• Cerebrovascular disease: ischaemic stroke; cerebral haemorrhage; transient ischaemic attack • Heart disease: myocardial infarction; angina; coronary revascularization; heart failure • Renal disease: diabetic nephropathy; renal impairment (serum creatinine M > 133; W > 124 μmol/L); proteinuria (> 300 mg/24h) • Peripheral artery disease • Advanced retinopathy: haemorrhages or exudates, papilloedema

M = men; W = women; CV = cardiovascular disease; IMT = intima-media thickness; BP = blood pressure; TG = triglycerides; C = cholesterol; * = Risk maximal for concentric LVH (left ventricular hypertrophy); ** = MDRD formula; *** = Cockroft Gault formula; increased LVMI (left ventricular mass index) with a wallthickness/rasius ratio ≥ 0.42

5. Diagnostic evaluation

AIMS

- Establishing BP values
- Identifying secondary causes of hypertension
- Searching for
  a) other risk factors;
  b) subclinical organ damage;
  c) concomitant diseases;
  d) accompanying CV and renal complications.

PROCEDURES

- repeated BP measurements
- family and clinical history
- physical examination
- laboratory and instrumental investigations

6. Blood pressure (BP) measurement

When measuring BP, care should be taken to:

- Allow the patients to sit quietly for several minutes;
- Take at least two measurements spaced by 1-2 minutes;
- Use a standard bladder (12-13 cm long and 35 cm wide) but have a larger bladder available for fat arms and a smaller one for thin arms and children;
- Have the cuff at the level of the heart, whatever the position of the patient;
- Deflate the cuff at a speed of 2 mmHg/s;
- Use phase I and V (disappearance) Korotkoff sounds to identify SBP and DBP, respectively;
- Measure BP in both arms at first visit to detect possible differences due to peripheral vascular disease. In this instance, take the higher value as the reference one;
- Measure BP 1 and 5 min after assumption of the standing position in elderly subjects, diabetic patients, and when postural hypotension may be frequent or suspected;
- Measure heart rate by pulse palpation (at least 30 sec).

7. Ambulatory and home BP measurements

AMBULATORY BP

- Although office BP should be used as the reference, ambulatory BP may improve prediction of CV risk in untreated and treated patients.
- 24-h ambulatory BP monitoring should be considered, in particular, when
  - considerable variability of office BP is found
  - high office BP is measured in subjects otherwise at low total CV risk
  - there is a marked discrepancy between BP values measured in the office and at home
  - resistance to drug treatment is suspected
  - hypotensive episodes are suspected, particularly in elderly and diabetic patients
  - sleep apnoea is suspected
  - office BP is elevated in pregnant women and pre-eclampsia is suspected

Normal values for 24 hour average BP are lower than for office BP, i.e. < 125-130 mmHg systolic and < 80 mmHg diastolic. Normal values of daytime BP are < 130-135 mmHg systolic and < 85 mmHg diastolic.

HOME BP

- Self-measurement of BP at home is of clinical value. Home BP measurements should be encouraged in order to:
  - provide more information on the BP lowering effect of treatment at trough, and thus on therapeutic coverage throughout the dose-to-dose time interval
  - improve patient's adherence to treatment regimens
  - understand technical reliability/environmental conditions of ambulatory BP data

- Self-measurement of BP at home should be discouraged whenever:
  - it causes anxiety to the patient
  - it induces self-modification of the treatment regimen
- Normal values for home BP are lower than for office BP, i.e. < 130-135 mmHg systolic and < 85 mmHg diastolic

PARTICULAR CONDITIONS

Isolated office hypertension (White coat hypertension)

Office BP persistently ≥ 140/90 mmHg
Normal daytime ambulatory (< 130-135/85 mmHg) or home (< 130-135/85 mmHg) BP

In these subjects CV risk is less than in individuals with raised office and ambulatory or home BP but may be slightly greater than that of individuals with in and outof-office normotension

Isolated ambulatory hypertension (Masked hypertension)

Office BP persistently normal (< 140/90 mmHg)
Elevated ambulatory (≥ 125-130/80 mmHg) or home (≥ 130-135/85 mmHg) BP

In these subjects CV risk is close to that of individuals with in and out-of-office hypertension

8. Diagnostic evaluation: medical history and physical examination

Family and clinical history	
1.	Duration and previous level of high BP
2.	Indications of secondary hypertension
3.	Risk factors
4.	Symptoms of organ damage
5.	Previous antihypertensive therapy (efficacy, adverse events)
6.	Personal, family, environmental factors
Physical examinations	
1.	Signs suggesting secondary hypertension
2.	Signs of organ damage
3.	Evidence of visceral obesity

9. Laboratory investigation

ROUTINE TESTS

- Fasting plasma glucose
- Serum total cholesterol
- Serum LDL-cholesterol
- Serum HDL-cholesterol
- Fasting serum triglycerides
- Serum potassium
- Serum uric acid
- Serum creatinine
- Estimated creatinine clearance (Cockroft-Gault formula) or glomerular filtration rate (MDRD formula)
- Haemoglobin and haematocrit
- Urinalysis (complemented by microalbuminuria dipstick test and microscopic examination)
- Electrocardiogram

RECOMMENDED TESTS

- Echocardiogram
- Carotid ultrasound
- Quantitative proteinuria (if dipstick test positive)
- Ankle-brachial BP Index
- Fundoscopy
- Glucose tolerance test (if fasting plasma glucose > 5.6 mmol/L (100 mg/dL)
- Home and 24h ambulatory BP monitoring
- Pulse wave velocity measurement (where available)

EXTENDED EVALUATION (domain of the specialist)

- Further search for cerebral, cardiac, renal and vascular damage. Mandatory in complicated hypertension.
- Search for secondary hypertension when suggested by history, physical examination or routine tests: measurement of renin, aldosterone, corticosteroids, catecholamines in plasma and/or urine; arteriographies; renal and adrenal ultrasound; computer-assisted tomography; magnetic resonance imaging.

10. Searching for subclinical organ damage

Due to the importance of subclinical organ damage as an intermediate stage in the continuum of vascular disease and as a determinant of total CV risk, signs of organ involvement should be sought carefully by appropriate techniques:

HEART

Electrocardiography should be part of all routine assessment of subjects with high BP in order to detect left ventricular hypertrophy, patterns of "strain", ischaemia and arrhythmias. Echocardiography is recommended when a more sensitive method of detection of left ventricular hypertrophy is considered useful as well as assessment of left ventricular systolic function. Geometric patterns can be defined echocardiographically, of which concentric hypertrophy carries the worse prognosis. Diastolic dysfunction can be evaluated by transmitral Doppler.

BLOOD VESSELS

Ultrasound scanning of the extracranial carotid arteries is recommended when detection of vascular hypertrophy or asymptomatic atherosclerosis is deemed useful. Large artery stiffening (leading to isolated systolic hypertension in the elderly) can be measured by pulse wave velocity. It might be more widely recommended if its availability were greater. A low ankle-brachial BP index signals advanced peripheral artery disease.

KIDNEY

Diagnosis of hypertension-related renal damage is based on a reduced renal function or an elevated urinary excretion of albumin. Estimation from serum creatinine of glomerular filtration rate (MDRD formula, requiring age, gender, race) or creatinine clearance (Cockroft-Gault formula, requiring also body weight) should be routine procedure. Urinary protein should be sought in all hypertensives by dipstick. In dipstick negative patients low grade albuminuria (microalbumniuria) should be determined in spot urine and related to urinary creatinine excretion.

FUNDOSCOPY

Examination of eye grounds is recommended in severe hypertensives only. Mild retinal changes are largely non-specific except in young patients. Haemorrhages, exudates and papilloedema, only present in severe hypertension, are associated with increased CV risk.

BRAIN

Silent brain infarcts, lacunar infarctions, microbleeds and white matter lesions are not infrequent among hypertensives, and can be detected by MRI or CT. Availability and costs do not allow indiscriminate use of these techniques. In elderly hypertensives, cognitive tests may help to detect initial brain deterioration.

Table 2 summarizes availability, prognostic value and cost of procedures to detect subclinical organ damage.

Table 2: Availability, Prognostic Value and Cost of some markers of organ damage (scored from 1 to 4 pluses)

Markers	CV predicitive value	Availability	Cost
Electrocardiography	++	++++	+
Echocardiography	+++	+++	++
Carotid Intima-Media Thickness	+++	+++	++
Arterial stiffness (Pulse wave velocity)	+++	+	++
Ankle-Brachial index	++	++	+
Coronary calcium content	+	+	++++
Cardiac/Vascular tissue composition	?	+	++
Circulatory collagen markers	?	+	++
Endothelial dysfunction	++	+	+++
Cerebral lacunae/ White matter lesions	?	++	++++
Est. Glomerular Filtration Rate or Creatinine Clearance	+++	++++	+
Microalbuminuria	+++	++++	+

11. Evidence on the benefit of antihypertensive treatment

- Placebo controlled trials have provided uncontroversial evidence that BP lowering reduces fatal and non-fatal cardiovascular events. Beneficial effects have been found when treatment is initiated with a thiazide diuretic, a β-blocker, a calcium antagonist, an ACE-inhibitor or an angiotensin receptor blocker.

- Trials comparing different antihypertensive drugs have not been able to conclusively demonstrate that for the same reduction in BP different antihypertensive drugs (or drug combinations) reduce to different degree CV events. These trials (and their meta-analysis and meta-regressions) underline the crucial role of BP lowering in reducing all kinds of CV events, i.e. stroke, myocardial infarction and heart failure, independently of the agents used.

- BP-independent effects related to use of specific drugs have been reported for cause-specific events, e.g. stroke, heart failure and coronary events, but these effects are smaller than the dominant effect of BP lowering.

- BP-independent effects attributable to specific drugs have been more consistently shown for events that occur earlier in the continuum of CV disease, e.g. protection against subclinical organ damage and prevention of high risk conditions such as diabetes, renal failure and atrial fibrillation.

12. Initiation of BP lowering therapy

- Initiation of BP lowering therapy should be decided on two criteria:

  1. The level of SBP and DBP

  2. The level of total CV risk

  - This is detailed in Figure 2 which considers treatment based on lifestyle changes and antihypertensive drugs with, in addition, recommendations on the time delay to be used for assessing the BP lowering effects.

Figure 2: Initiation of antihypertensive treatment

	Blood Pressure (mmHg)				
Other risk factors, OD or disease	Normal SBP 120-129 or DBP 80-84	High Normal SBP 130-139 or DBP 85-89	Grade 1 HT SBP 140-159 or DBP 90-99	Grade 2 HT SBP 160-179 or DBP 100-109	Grade 3 HT SBP ≥ 180 or DBP ≥ 110
No other risk factors	No BP intervention	No BP intervention	Lifestyle changes for several months then drug treatment if BP uncontrolled	Lifestyle changes for several weeks then drug treatment if BP uncontrolled	Lifestyle changes + immediate drug treatment
1-2 risk factors	Lifestyle changes	Lifestyle changes	Lifestyle changes for several weeks then drug treatment if BP uncontrolled	Lifestyle changes for several weeks then drug treatment if BP uncontrolled	Lifestyle changes + immediate drug treatment
≥ 3 risk factors, MS or OD	Lifestyle changes	Lifestyle changes and consider drug treatment	Lifestyle changes + drug treatment	Lifestyle changes + drug treatment	Lifestyle changes + immediate drug treatment
Diabetes	Lifestyle changes	Lifestyle changes + drug treatment	Lifestyle changes + drug treatment	Lifestyle changes + drug treatment	Lifestyle changes + immediate drug treatment
Established CV or renal disease	Lifestyle changes + immediate drug treatment	Lifestyle changes + immediate drug treatment	Lifestyle changes + immediate drug treatment	Lifestyle changes + immediate drug treatment	Lifestyle changes + immediate drug treatment

The following points should be emphasized:

- Drug treatment should be initiated promptly in grade 3 hypertension as well as in grade 1 and 2 when total CV risk is high or very high.

- In grade 1 or 2 hypertensives with moderate total CV risk drug treatment may be delayed for several weeks and in grade 1 hypertensives without any other risk factor for several months. However, even in these patients lack of BP control after a suitable period should lead to initiation of drug treatment.

- When initial BP is in the high normal range the decision on drug intervention heavily depends on the level of risk. In the case of diabetes, history of cerebrovascular, coronary or peripheral artery disease, the recommendation to start BP lowering drugs is justified by the results of controlled trials. Subjects with BP in the high normal range in whom total CV risk is high because of a subclinical organ damage should be advised to implement intense lifestyle measures. In these subjects BP should be closely monitored and drug treatment considered in the presence of a worsening of the clinical condition.

13. Goals of treatment

- In hypertensive patients, the primary goal of treatment is to achieve maximum reduction in the long-term total risk of CV disease.

- This requires treatment of the raised BP per se as well as of all associated reversible risk factors.

- BP should be reduced to at least below 140/90 mmHg (systolic/diastolic), and to lower values, if tolerated, in all hypertensive patients.

- Target BP should be at least < 130/80 mmHg in patients with diabetes and in high or very high risk patients, such as those with associated clinical conditions (stroke, myocardial infarction, renal dysfunction, proteinuria).

- Despite use of combination treatment, reducing systolic BP to < 140 mmHg may be difficult and more so if the target is a reduction to < 130 mmHg. Additional difficulties should be expected in elderly, in patients with diabetes, and in general, in patients with CV damage.

- In order to more easily achieve goal BP, antihypertensive treatment should be initiated before significant CV damage develops.

14. Lifestyle changes

- Lifestyle measures should be instituted, whenever appropriate, in all patients, including those who require drug treatment. The purpose is to lower BP, to control other risk factors and to reduce the number or the doses of antihypertensive drugs.

- Lifestyle measures are also advisable in subjects with high normal BP and additional risk factors to reduce the risk of developing hypertension.

- The lifestyle measures that are widely recognized to lower BP and/or CV risk, and that should be considered are:

  - smoking cessation
  - weight reduction (and weight stabilization)
  - reduction of excessive alcohol intake
  - physical exercise
  - reduction of salt intake
  - increase in fruit and vegetable intake and decrease in saturated and total fat intake

- Lifestyle recommendations should not be given as lip service but instituted with adequate behavioural and expert support, and reinforced periodically.

- Because long-term compliance with lifestyle measures is low and the BP response highly variable, patients under non-pharmacological treatment should be followed-up closely to start drug treatment when needed and in a timely fashion.

15. Choice of antihypertensive drugs

- The main benefits of antihypertensive therapy are due to lowering of BP *per se*

- Five major classes of antihypertensive agents – thiazide diuretics, calcium antagonists, ACE-inhibitors, angiotensin receptor blockers and β-blockers – are suitable for the initiation and maintenance of antihypertensive treatment, alone or in combination. β-blockers, especially in combination with a thiazide diuretic, should not be used in patients with the metabolic syndrome or at high risk of incident diabetes.

- In many patients more than one drugs is needed, so emphasis on identification of the first class of drug to be used is often futile. Nevertheless, there are conditions for which there is evidence in favour of some drugs versus others either as initial treatment or as part of a combination.

- The choice of a specific drug or a drug combination, and the avoidance of others should take into account the following:

  1. The previous favourable or unfavourable experience of the individual patient with a given class of compounds.
  2. The effect of drugs on CV risk factors in relation to the CV risk profile of the individual patient.
  3. The presence of subclinical organ damage, clinical CV disease, renal disease or diabetes, which may be more favourably treated by some drugs than others.
  4. The presence of other disorders that may limit the use of particular classes of antihypertensive drugs.
  5. The possibilities of interactions with drugs used for other conditions.
  6. The cost of drugs, either to the individual patient or to the health provider. However, cost considerations should never predominate over efficacy, tolerability, and protection of the individual patient.

- Continuing attention should be given to side-effects of drugs, because they are the most important cause of non-compliance. Drugs are not equal in terms of adverse effects, particularly in individual patients.

- The BP lowering effect should last 24 hours. This can be checked by office or home BP measurements at trough or by ambulatory BP monitoring.

- Drugs which exert their antihypertensive effect over 24 hours with a once-a-day administration should be preferred because a simple treatment schedule favours compliance.

16. Conditions favouring the use of some antihypertensive drugs versus others

SUBCLINICAL ORGAN DAMAGE	
LVH	ACEI, CA, ARB
Asymptomatic atherosclerosis	CA, ACEI
Microalbuminuria	ACEI, ARB
Renal dysfunction	ACEI, ARB
CLINICAL EVENT	
Previous stroke	any BP lowering agent
Previous MI	BB, ACEI, ARB
Angina pectoris	BB, CA
Heart failure	diuretics, BB, ACEI, ARB, anti-aldosterone agents
Atrial fibrillation	
Recurrent	ARB, ACEI
Permanent	BB, non-dihydropiridine CA
Tachyarrhythmias	BB
ESRD/proteinuria	ACEI, ARB, loop diuretics
Peripheral artery disease	CA
LV dysfunction	ACEI
CONDITION	
ISH (elderly)	diuretics, CA
Metabolic syndrome	ACEI, ARB, CA
Diabetes mellitus	ACEI, ARB
Pregnancy	CA, methyldopa, BB
Black people	diuretics, CA
Glaucoma	BB
ACEI induced cough	ARB

LVH = left ventricular hypertrophy; ISH = Isolated systolic hypertension; ESRD = renal failure; ACEI = ACE-inhibitors; ARB = angiotensin receptor blockers; CA = calcium antagonists; BB = beta-blockers

17. Contra-indications to use certain antihypertensive drugs

	Compelling contra-indications	Possible contra-indications
Thiazide diuretics	Gout	- Metabolic syndrome - Glucose intolerance - Pregnancy
Beta-blockers	Asthma A-V block (grade 2 or 3)	- Peripheral artery disease - Metabolic syndrome - Glucose intolerance - Athletes and physically active patients - Chronic obstructive pulmonary disease
Calcium antagonists (dihydropiridines)		- Tachyarrhythmias - Heart failure
Calcium antagonists (verapamil, diltiazem)	A-V block (grade 2 or 3) Heart failure	
ACE-inhibitors	Pregnancy Angioneurotic oedema Hyperkalaemia Bilate ral renal artery stenosis	
Angiotensin receptor blockers	Pregnancy Hyperkalaemia Bilateral renal artery stenosis	
Diuretics (antialdosterone	Renal failure Hyperkalaemia	

18. Monotherapy versus combination therapy

- Regardless of the drug employed, monotherapy allows to achieve BP target in only a limited number of hypertensive patients.

- Use of more than one agent is necessary to achieve target BP in the majority of patients. A vast array of effective and well tolerated combinations is available.

- Initial treatment can make use of monotherapy or combination of two drugs at low doses with a subsequent increase in drug doses or number, if needed.

- Monotherapy could be the initial treatment for mild BP elevation with low or moderate total CV risk. A combination of two drugs at low doses should be preferred as the first step in treatment when the initial BP is in the grade 2 or 3 or total CV risk is high or very high with mild BP elevation.

- Fixed combinations of two drugs can simplify the treatment schedule and favour compliance.

Monotherapy versus combination therapy strategies

Choose between

Mild BP elevation
Low/moderate CV risk
Conventional BP target

Marked BP elevation
high/very high CV risk
Lower BP target

Single agent at low dose

Two-drug combination at low dose

If goal BP not achieved

Previous agent at full dose

Switch to different agent at low dose

Previous combination at full dose

Add a third drug at low dose

If goal BP not achieved

Two-to three-drug combination at full dose

Full dose monotherapy

Two-three drug combination at full dose

- In several patients BP control is not achieved by two drugs, and a combination of three of more drugs is required.

- In uncomplicated hypertensives and in the elderly, antihypertensive therapy should normally be initiated gradually. In higher risk hypertensives, goal BP should be achieved more promptly, which favours initial combination therapy and quicker adjustment of doses.

19. Possible combinations between some classes of antihypertensive drugs

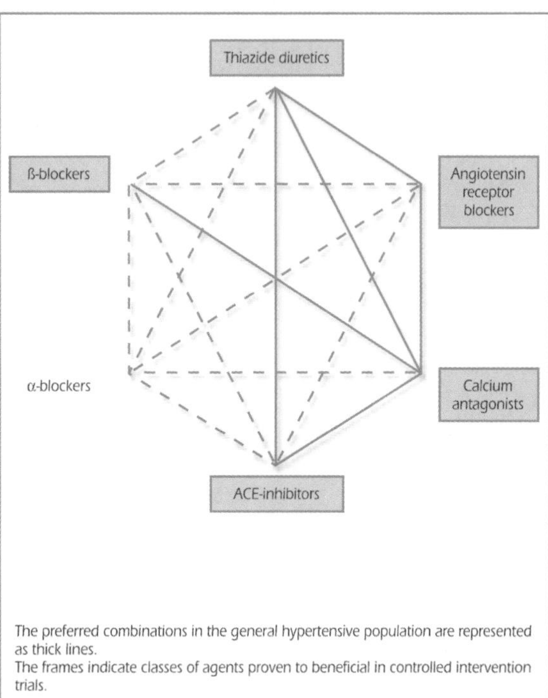

The preferred combinations in the general hypertensive population are represented as thick lines.
The frames indicate classes of agents proven to beneficial in controlled intervention trials.

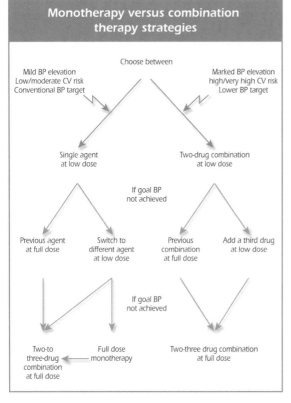

20. Antihypertensive treatment in special groups

Antihypertensive treatment may differ from the one recommended in the general hypertensive population, in special groups of patients or in specific clinical conditions. The specific requirements under these circumstances are detailed below.

20.1. Elderly patients

- Drug treatment can be initiated with thiazide diuretics, calcium antagonists, angiotensin receptor blockers, ACE-inhibitors, and β-blockers, in line with general guidelines. Trials specifically addressing treatment of isolated systolic hypertension have shown the benefit of thiazides and calcium antagonists but subanalysis of other trials also show efficacy of angiotensin receptor blockers.

- Initial doses and subsequent dose titration should be more gradual because of a greater chance of undesirable effects, especially in very old and frail subjects.

- BP goal is the same as in younger patients, i.e. < 140/90 mmHg or below, if tolerated. Many elderly patients need two or more drugs to control blood pressure and reductions to < 140 mmHg systolic may be difficult to obtain.

- Drug treatment should be tailored to the risk factors, target organ damage and associated cardiovascular and non-cardiovascular conditions that are frequent in the elderly. Because of the increased risk of postural hypotension, BP should always be measured also in the erect posture.

- In subjects aged 80 years and over, evidence for benefits of antihypertensive treatment is as yet inconclusive. However, there is no reason for interrupting a successful and well tolerated therapy when a patient reaches 80 years of age.

20.2. Diabetic patients

- Where applicable, intense non-pharmacological measures should be encouraged in all patients with diabetes, with particular attention to weight loss and reduction of salt intake in type 2 diabetes.

- Goal BP should be < 130/80 mmHg and anti-hypertensive drug treatment may be started already when BP is in the high normal range.

- To lower BP, all effective and well tolerated drugs can be used. A combination of two or more drugs is frequently needed.

- Available evidence indicates that lowering BP also exerts a protective effect on appearance and progression of renal damage. Some additional protection can be obtained by the use of a blocker of the renin-angiotensin system (either an angiotensin receptor blocker or an ACE-inhibitor).

- A blocker of the renin-angiotensin system should be a regular component of combination treatment and the one preferred when monotherapy is sufficient.

- Microalbuminuria should prompt the use of antihypertensive drug treatment also when initial BP is in the high normal range. Blockers of the reninangiotensin system have a pronounced antiproteinuric effect and their use should be preferred.

- Treatment strategies should consider an intervention against all CV risk factors, including a statin.

- Because of the greater chance of postural hypotension, BP should also be measured in the erect posture.

20.3. Patients with renal dysfunction

- Renal dysfunction and failure are associated with a very high risk of CV events.

- Protection against progression of renal dysfunction has two main requirements: a) strict blood pressure control (< 130/80 mmHg and even lower if proteinuria is > 1g/day); b) lowering proteinuria to values as near to normal as possible.

- To achieve the BP goal, combination therapy of several antihypertensive agents (including loop diuretics) is usually required.

- To reduce proteinuria, an angiotensin receptor blocker, an ACE-inhibitor or a combination of both are required.

- There is controversial evidence as to whether blockade of the renin–angiotensin system has a specific beneficial role in preventing or retarding nephrosclerosis in non-diabetic non-proteinuric hypertensives, except perhaps in Afro-American individuals. However, inclusion of one of these agents in the combination therapy required by these patients appears well founded.

- An integrated therapeutic intervention (anti-hypertensive, statin and antiplatelet therapy) has to be frequently considered in patients with renal damage because, under these circumstances, CV risk is extremely high.

20.4. Patients with cerebrovascular disease

- In patients with a history of stroke or transient ischaemic attacks, antihypertensive treatment markedly reduces the incidence of stroke recurrence and also lowers the associated high risk of cardiac events.

- Antihypertensive treatment is beneficial in hypertensive patients as well as in subjects with

BP in the high normal range. BP goal should be < 130/80 mmHg

- Because evidence from trials suggests that the benefit largely depends on BP lowering per se, all available drugs and rational combinations can be used. Trial data have been mostly obtained with ACE-inhibitors and angiotensin receptor blockers, in association with or on the top of diuretic and conventional treatment, but more evidence is needed before their specific cerebrovascular protective properties are established.

- There is at present no evidence that BP lowering has a beneficial effect in acute stroke but more research is under way. Until more evidence is obtained antihypertensive treatment should start when post-stroke clinical conditions are stable, usually several days after the event. Additional research in this is necessary because cognitive dysfunction is present in about 15% and dementia in 5% of subjects aged ≥ 65 years.

- In observational studies, cognitive decline and incidence of dementia have a positive relationship with BP values. There is some evidence that both can be somewhat delayed by antihypertensive treatment.

20.5. Patients with coronary heart disease and heart failure

- In patients surviving a myocardial infarction, early administration of β-blockers, ACE-inhibitors or angiotensin receptor blockers reduces the incidence of recurrent myocardial infarction and death. These beneficial effects can be ascribed to the specific protective properties of these drugs but possibly also to the associated small BP reduction.

- Antihypertensive treatment is also beneficial in hypertensive patients with chronic coronary heart disease. The benefit can be obtained with different drugs and drug combinations (including calcium antagonists) and appears to be related to the degree of BP reduction. A beneficial effect has been demonstrated also when initial BP is < 140/90 mmHg and for achieved BP around 130/80 mmHg or less.

- A history of hypertension is common while a raised BP is relatively rare in patients with congestive heart failure. In these patients, treatment can make use of thiazide and loop diuretics, as well as of β-blockers, ACE-inhibitors, angiotensin receptor blockers and antialdosterone drugs on top of diuretics. Calcium antagonists should be avoided unless needed to control BP or anginal symptoms.

- Diastolic heart failure is common in patients with a history of hypertension and has an adverse prognosis. There is at present no evidence on the superiority of specific antihypertensive drugs.

20.6. Patients with atrial fibrillation

- Hypertension is the most important risk factor for atrial fibrillation. Atrial fibrillation markedly increases the risk of CV morbidity and mortality, particularly of embolic stroke.

- Increased left ventricular mass and left atrium enlargement are independent determinants of atrial fibrillation, and require intense antihypertensive therapy.

- Strict blood pressure control is required in patients under anticoagulant treatment to avoid intracerebral and extracerebral bleeding.

- Less new onset and recurrent atrial fibrillation has been reported in hypertensive patients treated with angiotensin receptor blockers.

- In permanent atrial fibrillation, β-blockers and non-dihydropyridine calcium antagonists (verapamil, diltiazem) help controlling ventricular rate.

21. Hypertension in women

TREATMENT

Response to antihypertensive agents and beneficial effects of BP lowering appear to be similar in women and in men. However, ACE-inhibitors and angiotensin receptor blockers should be avoided in pregnant and women planning pregnancy because of potential teratogenic effects during pregnancy.

ORAL CONTRACEPTIVES

Even oral contraceptives with low oestrogen content are associated with an increased risk of hypertension, stroke and myocardial infarction. The progestogenonly pill is a contraceptive option for women with high BP, but their influence on cardiovascular outcomes has been insufficiently investigated.

HORMONE REPLACEMENT THERAPY

The only benefit of this therapy is a decreased incidence of bone fractures and colon cancer, accompanied, however, by increased risk of coronary events, stroke, thromboembolism, breast cancer, gallbladder disease and dementia. This therapy is not recommended for cardioprotection in postmenopausal women.

HYPERTENSION IN PREGNANCY

- Hypertensive disorders in pregnancy, particularly pre-eclampsia, may adversely affect neonatal and maternal outcomes.

- Non-pharmacological management (including close supervision and restriction of activities) should be considered for pregnant women with SBP 140-149 mmHg or DBP 90-95 mmHg. In the presence of gestational hypertension (with or without proteinuria) drug treatment is indicated at BP levels > 140/90 mmHg. SBP levels ≥ 170 or DBP ≥ 110 mmHg should be considered an emergency requiring hospitalization.

- In non-severe hypertension, oral methyldopa, labetalol, calcium antagonists and (less frequently) β-blockers are drugs of choice.

- In pre-eclampsia with pulmonary oedema, nitroglycerine is the drug of choice. Diuretic therapy is inappropriate because plasma volume is reduced.

- As emergency, intravenous labetalol, oral methyldopa and oral nifedipine are indicated. Intravenous hydralazine is no longer the drug of choice because of an excess of perinatal adverse effects. Intravenous infusion of sodium nitroprusside is useful in hypertensive crises, but prolonged administration should be avoided.

- Calcium supplementation, fish oil and low dose aspirin are not recommended. However, low dose aspirin may be used prophylactically in women with a history of early onset pre-eclampsia.

22. The metabolic syndrome

- The metabolic syndrome is characterized by the variable combination of visceral obesity and alterations in glucose metabolism, lipid metabolism and BP. It has a high prevalence in the middle age and elderly population.

- Subjects with the metabolic syndrome also have a higher prevalence of microalbuminuria, left ventricular hypertrophy and arterial stiffness than those without metabolic syndrome. Their CV risk is high and the chance of developing diabetes markedly increased.

- In patients with metabolic syndrome diagnostic procedures should include a more in-depth assessment of subclinical organ damage. Measuring ambulatory and home BP is also desirable.

- In all individuals with metabolic syndrome intense lifestyle measures should be adopted. When there is hypertension drug treatment should start with a drug unlikely to facilitate onset to diabetes. Therefore a blocker of the reninangiotensin system should be used and followed, if needed, by the addition of a calcium antagonist or a low-dose thiazide diuretic. It appears desirable to bring BP to the normal range.

- Lack of evidence from specific clinical trials prevents firm recommendations on use of antihypertensive drugs in all metabolic syndrome subjects with a high normal BP. There is some evidence that blocking the renin-angiotensin system may also delay incident hypertension.

- Statins and antidiabetic drugs should be given in the presence of dyslipidemia and diabetes, respectively. Insulin sensitizers have been shown to markedly reduce new onset diabetes, but their advantages and disadvantages in the presence of impaired fasting glucose or glucose intolerance as a metabolic syndrome component remain to be demonstrated.

23. Resistant hypertension

DEFINITION:

BP ≥ 140/90 mmHg despite treatment with at least three drugs (including a diuretic) in adequate doses and after exclusion of spurious hypertension such as isolated office hypertension and failure to use large cuffs on large arms.

CAUSES:

- Poor adherence to therapeutic plan;

- Failure to modify lifestyle including:

  weight gain

  heavy alcohol intake (NB: binge drinking);

- Continued intake of drugs that raise blood pressure (liquorice, cocaine, glucocorticoids, non-steroid anti-inflammatory drugs, etc.);

- Obstructive sleep apnea;

- Unsuspected secondary cause;
- Irreversible or limited reversibility of organ damage;
- Volume overload due to: inadequate diuretic therapy progressive renal insufficiency high sodium intake hyperaldosteronism

TREATMENT

- Adequate investigation of causes
- If necessary, use of more than three drugs, including an aldosterone antagonist

24. Hypertensive emergencies

Hypertensive Emergencies
• Hypertensive encephalopathy • Hypertensive left ventricular failure • Hypertension with myocardial infarction • Hypertension with unstable angina • Hypertension and dissection of the aorta • Severe hypertension associated with subarachnoid haemorrhage or cerebrovascular accident • Crisis associated with phaeochromocytoma • Use of recreational drugs such as amphetamines, LSD, cocaine or ecstasy • Hypertension perioperatively • Severe pre-eclampsia or eclampsia

25. Treatment of associated risk factors

LIPID LOWERING AGENTS

- All hypertensive patients with established CV disease or with type 2 diabetes should be considered for statin therapy aiming at serum total and LDL cholesterol levels of, respectively, < 4.5 mmol/L (175 mg/dL) and < 2.5 mmol/L (100 mg/dL), and lower, if possible.
- Hypertensive patients without overt CV disease but with high CV risk (≥ 20% risk of events in 10 years) should also be considered for statin treatment even if their baseline total and LDL serum cholesterol levels are not elevated.

ANTIPLATELET THERAPY

- Antiplatelet therapy, in particular low-dose aspirin, should be prescribed to hypertensive patients with previous CV events, provided that there is no excessive risk of bleeding.
- Low-dose aspirin should also be considered in hypertensive patients without a history of CV disease if older than 50 years and with a moderate increase in serum creatinine or with a high CV risk. In all these conditions, the benefit-to-risk ratio of this intervention (reduction in myocardial infarction greater than the risk of bleeding) has been proven favourable.
- To minimize the risk of haemorrhagic stroke, antiplatelet treatment should be started after achievement of BP control.

GLYCAEMIC CONTROL

- Effective glycaemic control is of great importance in patients with hypertension and diabetes.
- In these patients dietary and drug treatment of diabetes should aim at lowering plasma fasting glucose to values 6 mmol/L (108 mg/dL) and at a glycated haemoglobin of < 6.5%.

26. Patients' follow-up

- Effective and timely titration to BP control requires frequent visits in order to timely modify the treatment regimen in relation to BP changes and the appearance of side-effects.
- Once the target BP has been reached, the frequency of visits can be considerably reduced. However, excessively wide intervals between visits are not advisable because they interfere with a good doctor-patient relationship, which is crucial for patient's compliance.
- Patients at low risk or with grade 1 hypertension may be seen every 6 months and regular home BP measurements may further extend this interval. Visits should be more frequent in high or very high risk patients. This is the case also in patients under non-pharmacological treatment alone due to the variable antihypertensive response and the low compliance to this intervention.
- Follow-up visits should aim at maintaining control of all reversible risk factors as well as at checking the status of organ damage. Because treatment-induced changes in left ventricular mass and carotid artery wall thickness are slow, there is no reason to perform these examinations at less than 1 year intervals.
- Treatment of hypertension should be continued for life because in correctly diagnosed patients cessation of treatment is usually followed by

return to the hypertensive state. Cautious downward titration of the existing treatment may be attempted in low risk patients after long-term BP control, particularly if non- pharmacological treatment can be successfully implemented.

27. How to improve compliance with blood pressure lowering therapy

- Inform the patient of the risk of hypertension and the benefit of effective treatment.
- Provide clear written and oral instructions about treatment.
- Tailor the treatment regimen to patient's lifestyle and needs.
- Simplify treatment by reducing, if possible, the number of daily medicaments.
- Involve the patient's partner or family in information on disease and treatment plans.
- Make use of self measurement of BP at home and of behavioural strategies such as reminder systems.
- Pay great attention to side-effects (even if subtle) and be prepared to timely change drug doses or types, if needed.
- Dialogue with patient regarding adherence and be informed of his/her problems.
- Provide reliable support system and affordable prices.
- Arrange a schedule of follow-up visits.

Section III:
Diabetic Heart Disease

1. Diabetes, Pre-diabetes and Cardiovascular Diseases

Chapter 1

Diabetes, Pre-diabetes and Cardiovascular Diseases*

2007

Co-chairperson:
Lars Rydén
Representing ESC
Department of Cardiology
Karolinska University
Hospital Solna
SE-171 76 Stockholm, Sweden
Phone: + 46 (8) 5177 2171
Fax: + 46 (8) 34 49 64
E-mail: lars.ryden@ki.se

Co-chairperson:
Eberhard Standl
Representing EASD
Diabetes Research Institute at GSF
D-85764 Neuherberg, Germany
Phone: + 49 (89) 3081 733
Fax: + 49 (89) 3187 2971
E-mail: eberhard.standl@lrz.uni-muenchen.de

Task Force Members:
1. Malgorzata Bartnik, Poland
2. Greet Van den Berghe, Belgium
3. John Betteridge, UK
4. Menko-Jan de Boer, The Netherlands
5. Francesco Cosentino, Italy
6. Bengt Jönsson, Sweden
7. Markku Laakso, Finland
8. Klas Malmberg, Sweden
9. Silvia Priori, Italy
10. Jan Östergren, Sweden
11. Jaakko Tuomilehto, Finland
12. Inga Thrainsdottir, Iceland

ESC Staff:
1. Keith McGregor, Sophia Antipolis, France
2. Veronica Dean, Sophia Antipolis, France
3. Catherine Després, Sophia Antipolis, France

1. Preamble

The ESC Committee for Practice Guidelines (CPG) supervises and coordinates the preparation of new Guidelines and Expert Consensus Documents produced by Task Forces, expert groups, or consensus panels. The chosen experts in these writing panels are asked to provide disclosure statements of all relationships they may have, which might be perceived as real or potential conflicts of interest. These disclosure forms are kept on file at the European Heart House, headquarters of the ESC. The Committee is also responsible for the endorsement of these Guidelines and Expert Consensus Documents or statements.

Guidelines and Expert Consensus documents aim to present patients management recommendations based on all of the relevant evidence on a particular subject in order to help physicians to select the best possible management strategies for the individual patient, suffering from a specific condition, taking into account not only the impact on outcome, but also the risk benefit ratio of a particular diagnostic or therapeutic procedure.

The Task Force has classified and ranked the usefulness or efficacy of the recommended procedures and/or treatments and their levels of evidence as indicated in the tables overleaf.

*Adapted from the ESC Guidelines on Diabetes, Pre-diabetes, and Cardiovascular Diseases, Executive Summary (European Heart Journal (2007); 28: 88-136) and Full Text (European Heart Journal 2007;9 (Suppl. C):1-74 and http://www.easd.org)

Classes of Recommendations

Class I	Evidence and/or general agreement that a given diagnostic procedure/treatment is beneficial, useful and effective.
Class II	Conflicting evidence and/or a divergence of opinion about the usefulness/efficacy of the treatment or procedure.
Class IIa	Weight of evidence/opinion is in favour of usefulness/efficacy.
Class IIb	Usefulness/efficacy is less well established by evidence/opinion.
Class III	Evidence or general agreement that the treatment or procedure is not useful/effective and, in some cases, may be harmful.

Levels of Evidence

Level of Evidence A	Data derived from multiple randomized clinical trials or meta-analyses
Level of Evidence B	Data derived from a single randomized trial or large non-randomized studies
Level of Evidence C	Consensus of opinion of the experts and/or small studies, retrospective studies, registries

2. Introduction

Diabetes and cardiovascular diseases (CVD) often appear as two sides of a coin. Diabetes mellitus (DM) has been rated as an equivalent of coronary heart disease, and conversely, many patients with established coronary heart disease suffer from diabetes or its pre-states. Thus, it is high time that diabetologists and cardiologists join their forces to improve the quality management in diagnosis and care for the millions of patients who have coexisting cardiovascular and metabolic diseases.

An algorithm (Figure 1) has been developed to help discover the alternate cardiovascular diseases in patients with diabetes, and vice versa, the metabolic diseases in patients with coronary heart disease, setting the basis for appropriate joint therapy. The cardio-diabetological approach not only is of utmost importance for the sake of patient management, but is also instrumental for further progress in the fields of cardiology, diabetology and prevention. Treatment targets for life style counselling, glycemic control, blood pressure and blood lipids are discussed in different chapters. To give the reader a comprehensive overview they are summarised in Table 1.

Figure 1. Investigational algorithm for patients with coronary artery disease (CAD) and diabetes mellitus (DM)

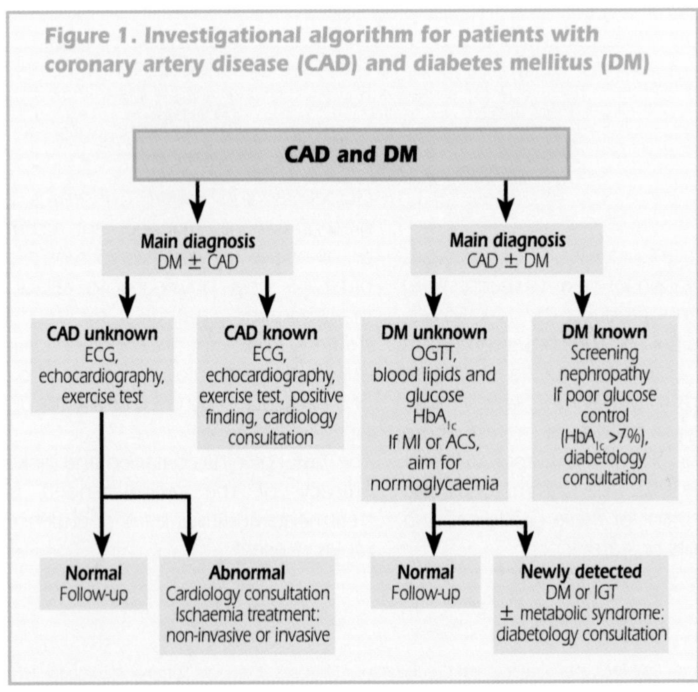

Table 1. Recommended treatment targets for patients with diabetes and CAD

	Variable	Treatment target
Blood pressure	Systolic/diastolic (mm Hg)	< 130/80
	In case of renal impairment or proteinuria > 1 g/24 h	< 125/75
Glycaemic control	HbA_{1c} (%)*	≤ 6.5
	Glucose (venous plasma; mmol/L) mg/dL	
	Fasting	< 6.0 (108)
	Post-prandial (peak)	
	Type 1 diabetes	7.5 -9.0 (135-160)
	Type 2 diabetes	< 7.5 (135)
Lipid profile (mmol/L) (mg/dL)	Total cholesterol	< 4.5 (175)
	LDL cholesterol	≤ 1.8 (70)
	HDL cholesterol	
	Men	> 1.0 (40)
	Women	> 1.2 (46)
	Triglycerides**	< 1.7 (150)
	Total/HDL cholesterol**	< 3
Life style counselling	Smoking cessation	Obligatory
	Regular physical activity (min/day)	> 30-45
	Weight control BMI (kg/m^2)	< 25
	In case of overweight, weight reduction (%)	10
	Waist circumference (optimum; ethnic specific; cm)	
	Men (European)	< 94
	Women (European)	< 80
	Dietary habits	
	Salt intake (g/day)	< 6
	Fibre intake	> 30 g per day
	Liquid mono- and disaccharides	avoid
	Fat intake (% of dietary energy)	≤ 30-35
	Saturated	< 10
	Trans-fat	< 2
	Polyunsaturated n-6	4-8
	Polyunsaturated n-3	2 g/day of linolenic acid and 200 mg/day of very long chain fatty acids

* DCCT-Standardized for recalculation formula for some national standards in Europe. ** Not recommended for guiding treatment, but recommended for metabolic/risk assessment.

3. Definition, classification, and screening of diabetes and pre-diabetic glucose abnormalities

Recommendation	Class	Level
The definition and diagnostic classification of diabetes and its pre-states should be based on the level of the subsequent risk of cardiovascular complications.	I	B
Early stages of hyperglycaemia and asymptomatic type 2 diabetes are best diagnosed by an oral glucose tolerance test (OGTT) that gives both fasting and 2 h post-load glucose values.	I	B
Primary screening for the potential type 2 diabetes can be done most efficiently by using a non-invasive risk score, combined with a diagnostic OGTT in people with high score values.	I	A

Definition and classification

Diabetes mellitus is a metabolic disorder characterised by chronic hyperglycaemia with disturbances of carbohydrate, fat and protein metabolism resulting from defects of insulin secretion, insulin action, or a combination of both. Type 1 diabetes is due to a lack of endogenous pancreatic insulin production while the increase in blood glucose in type 2 diabetes results from more complex processes.

Traditionally, diabetes was diagnosed based on symptoms due to hyperglycaemia, but during the last decades emphasis has been placed on the need to identify diabetes and other forms of glucose abnormalities in asymptomatic subjects.

Diabetes mellitus is associated with development of long-term organ damage including retinopathy, nephropathy, neuropathy and autonomic dysfunction. Patients with diabetes are at a particularly high risk for cardiovascular, cerebrovascular and peripheral artery disease.

Four main aetiology categories of diabetes have been identified as diabetes type 1, type 2, other specific types such as Maturity-Onset Diabetes in the Young (MODY) or secondary to other conditions or diseases e.g. surgery and gestational diabetes.

The current classification criteria (Table 2) have been issued by World Health Organisation (WHO) and American Diabetes Association (ADA). The WHO recommendations for glucometabolic classification are based on measuring both fasting and two hour post-load glucose concentrations and recommend that a standardised 75 g

Table 2. Criteria used for glucometabolic classification from WHO (1999 and 2006) and ADA (1997 and 2003)

Glucometabolic category	Source	Classification criteria Venous plasma glucose mmol/L (mg/dL)
Normal glucose regulation (NGR)	WHO	FPG < 6.1 (110) + 2 h PG < 7.8 (140)
	ADA (1997)	FPG < 6.1 (110)
	ADA (2003)	FPG < 5.6 (100)
Impaired fasting glucose (IFG)	WHO	FPG ≥ 6.1 (110) and < 7.0 (126) + 2 h PG < 7.8 (140)
	ADA (1997)	FPG ≥ 6.1 (110) and < 7.0 (126)
	ADA (2003)	FPG ≥ 5.6 (110) and < 7.0 (126)
Impaired glucose tolerance (IGT)	WHO	FPG < 7.0 (126) + 2 h PG ≥ 7.8 and < 11.1 (200)
Impaired glucose homeostasis (IGH)	WHO	IFG or IGT
Diabetes mellitus (DM)	WHO	FPG ≥ 7.0 (126) or 2 h PG ≥ 11.1 (200)
	ADA (1997)	FPG ≥ 7.0 (126)
	ADA (2003)	FPG ≥ 7.0 (126)

FPG = fasting plasma glucose; 2-h PG=two-hour post-load plasma glucose (1 mmol/L = 18 mg/dL).

IGT can only be diagnosed by OGTT. OGTT is performed in the morning, after 8–14 h fast; one blood sample is taken before and one 120 min after intake of 75 g glucose dissolved in 250–300 mL water for 5 min (timing is from the beginning of the drink).

Figure 2. Fasting and post-load glucose levels identify different individuals with asymptomatic diabetes. FPG, fasting plasma glucose; 2hPG, 2 h post-load plasma glucose (adapted from the DECODE Study Group).

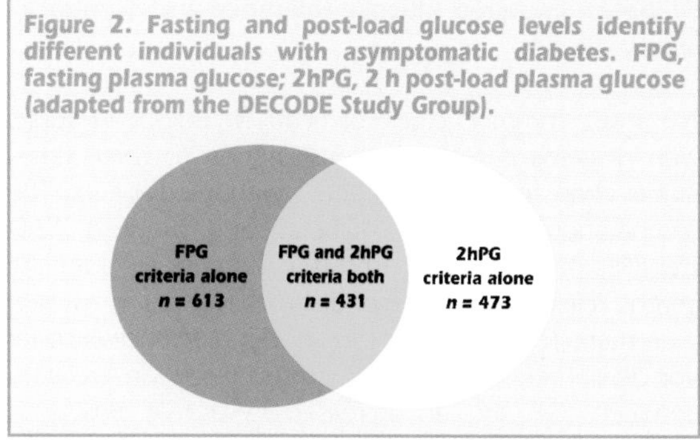

oral glucose tolerance test (OGTT) should be performed in the absence of overt hyperglycaemia.

The use of an OGTT for glucometabolic classification is recommended. As shown in Figure 2 FPG and 2 h post-load PG may identify the same individuals but they do often not coincide.

Glycated haemoglobin (HbA_{1c}) is a useful measure of metabolic control and the efficacy of glucose lowering treatment in people with diabetes. It represents a mean value of blood glucose during the preceding six to eight weeks (life span of erythrocytes). HbA_{1c} is not recommended as a diagnostic test for diabetes. It is insensitive in the low range and a normal value does not exclude diabetes or impaired glucose tolerance.

Detection of people at high risk for diabetes

The approaches for early detection are for:

1) measuring blood glucose to determine prevalent impaired glucose homeostasis;

2) using demographic, clinical characteristics and previous laboratory tests to determine the likelihood of future incident diabetes;

3) collecting questionnaire based information on aetiological factors for type 2 diabetes.

The two latter are cost-efficient screening tools. Option two is suited for certain groups with pre-existing cardiovascular disease and women who have had gestational diabetes while the third option is better suited for the general population.

Glycaemic testing (OGTT) is always necessary as a secondary step to accurately define impaired glucose homeostasis. Glucometabolic abnormalities are common in patients with CVD and an OGTT should be carried out in them.

Figure 3. FINnish Diabetes Risk SCore (FINDRISC) to assess the 10 year risk of type 2 diabetes in adults. Available at www.diabetes.fi/english

Type 2 diabetes risk assessment form

Circle the right alternative and add up your points.

1. Age
0 p. Under 45 years
2 p. 45-54 years
3 p. 55-64 years
4 p. Over 64 years

2. Body mass Index
0 p. Lower than 25 kg/m²
1 p. 25-30 kg/m²
3 p. Higher than 30 kg/m²

3. Waist circumference measured below the ribs (usually at the level of the navel)

	MEN	WOMEN
0 p.	Less than 94 cm	Less than 80 cm
3 p.	94-102 cm	80-88 cm
4 p.	More than 102 cm	More than 88 cm

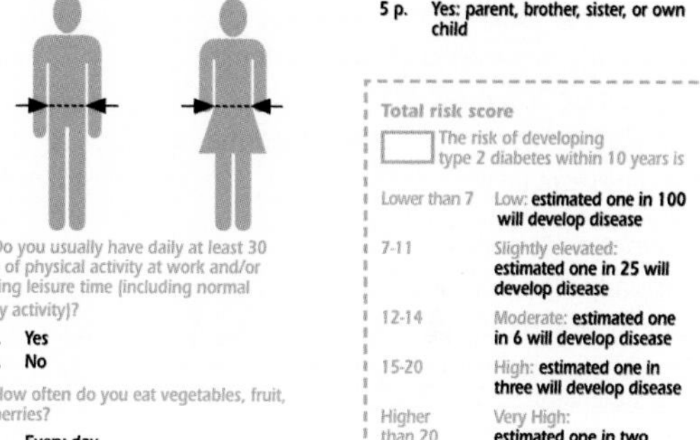

4. Do you usually have daily at least 30 min of physical activity at work and/or during leisure time (including normal daily activity)?
0 p. Yes
2 p. No

5. How often do you eat vegetables, fruit, or berries?
0 p. Every day
1 p. Not every day

6. Have you ever taken anti-hypertensive medication regularly?
0 p. No
2 p. Yes

7. Have you ever been found to have high blood glucose (e.g. in a health examination, during an illness, during pregnancy)?
0 p. No
5 p. Yes

8. Have any of the members of your immediate family of other relatives been diagnosed with diabetes (type 1 or type 2)?
0 p. No
3 p. Yes: grandparent, aunt, uncle, or first cousin (but no own parent, brother, sister or child)
5 p. Yes: parent, brother, sister, or own child

Total risk score

The risk of developing type 2 diabetes within 10 years is

Lower than 7	Low: estimated one in 100 will develop disease
7-11	Slightly elevated: estimated one in 25 will develop disease
12-14	Moderate: estimated one in 6 will develop disease
15-20	High: estimated one in three will develop disease
Higher than 20	Very High: estimated one in two will develop disease

Test designed by Professor Jaakko Tuomilehto. Department of Public Health, University of Helsinki, and Dr Jaana Lindstrôm, MFS, National Public Health Institute.

In the general population the appropriate strategy is to start with risk assessment as the primary screening tool combined with subsequent glucose testing (OGTT) of individuals identified to be at a high risk. An example of such screening tool is shown in Figure 3.

4. Epidemiology of diabetes, IGH, and cardiovascular risk

Recommendation	Class	Level
The relationship between hyperglycaemia and CVD should be seen as a continuum. For each 1% increase of HbA_{1c}, there is a defined increased risk for CVD.	I	A
The risk of CVD for people with overt diabetes is increased by two to three times for men and three to five times for women compared with people without diabetes.	I	A
Information on post-prandial (post-load) glucose provides better information about the future risk for CVD than fasting glucose, and elevated post-prandial (post-load) glucose also predicts increased cardiovascular risk in subjects with normal fasting glucose levels.	I	A
Glucometabolic perturbations carry a particularly high risk for cardiovascular morbidity and mortality in women, who in this respect need special attention.	IIa	B

Prevalence of diabetes in relation to age

The age-specific prevalence of diabetes rises with age in both men and women (Figure 4). The lifetime risk of diabetes in European people has been estimated to 30-40%. Approximately half of those affected are unaware of their condition. Among middle aged Europeans the prevalence of impaired glucose tolerance is about 15% increasing to 35-40% in the elderly.

Figure 4. Age-and gender-specific prevalence of diabetes in 13 European population - based cohorts included in the DECODE study.

DMF, diabetes determined by FPG ≥ 7.0 mmol/L and 2 h plasma glucose < 11.1 mmol/L; DMP, diabetes determined by 2 h plasma glucose ≥ 11.1 mmol/L and FPG < 7.0 mmol/L; DMF and DMP, diabetes determined by FPG ≥ 7.0 mmol/L and 2 h plasma glucose ≥ 11.1 mmol/L; known diabetes, previously diagnosed diabetes.
*P < 0.05 and **P < 0.001 for the difference in prevalence between men and women, respectively.

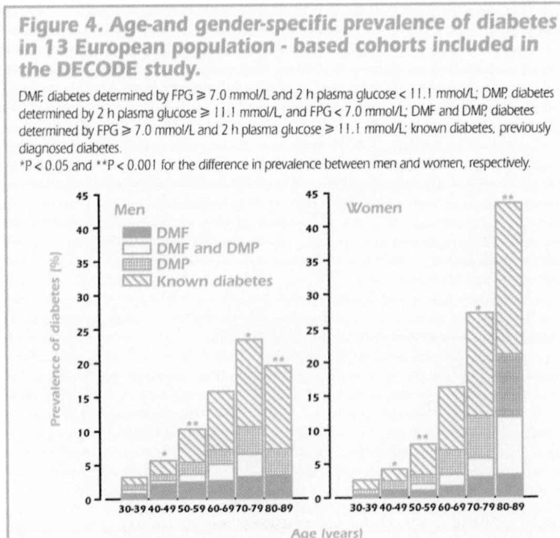

Diabetes, impaired glucose tolerance and coronary artery disease

The most common cause of death in European adults with diabetes is CAD. Their risk is two to three times higher than that among people without diabetes. The combination of type 2 diabetes and previous CAD identifies patients with particularly high risk for coronary deaths. The relative effect of diabetes is larger in women than men. The reason for this gender difference is so far not clear. There is also convincing evidence for a relation between IGT and an increased CAD risk. Following adjustment for major cardiovascular risk factors, mortality and cardiovascular morbidity is predicted by elevated 2-hour post-load plasma glucose, however, not by fasting glucose. Thus hyperglycaemia in itself is very important for the increased risk. Although some evidence points in this direction it remains to be proven if lowering of high post-load glucose will reduce this risk. Studies are underway and a meta-analysis of seven long-term studies using acarbose is promising, but data are scarce.

The risk for cerebrovascular morbidity and mortality is also magnified by diabetes while considerably less is known about the frequency of asymptomatic diabetes and impaired glucose tolerance in patients with stroke.

5. Identification of subjects at high risk for CVD or diabetes

Recommendation	Class	Level
The metabolic syndrome identifies people at a higher risk of CVD than the general population, although it may not provide a better or even equally good prediction of cardiovascular risk than scores based on the major cardiovascular risk factors (blood pressure, smoking, and serum cholesterol).	II	B
Several cardiovascular risk assessment tools exist and they can be applied to both non-diabetic and diabetic subjects.	I	A
An assessment of predicted type 2 diabetes risk should be part of the routine health care using the risk assessment tools available.	II	A
Patients without known diabetes but with established CVD should be investigated with an OGTT.	I	B
People at high risk for type 2 diabetes should receive appropriate lifestyle counselling and, if needed, pharmacological therapy to reduce or delay their risk of developing diabetes. This may also decrease their risk to develop CVD.	I	A
Diabetic patients should be advised to be physically active in order to decrease their cardiovascular risk.	I	A

The metabolic syndrome

There has been an interest in the clustering factors, each one associated with increased risk for CVD, to what has become known as the "metabolic syndrome". It is debated whether such clustering represents a disease entity in its own, but it helps identifying individuals at high risk for cardiovascular disease and type 2 diabetes. Currently there are several definitions. The most recent has been issued by the International Federation of Diabetes (Table 3). The pathogenesis of the metabolic syndrome and its components is complex and not well understood. However, central obesity and insulin resistance are important causative factors. Abdominal circumference is the clinical screening factor for the metabolic syndrome, much more associated with metabolic risk than body mass index.

Table 3. International Diabetes Federation: Metabolic Syndrome Definition

Central Obesity (defined as waist circumference ≥ 94 cm for Europid men and ≥ 80 cm for Europid women, with ethnicity specific values for other groups)
plus any two of the following four factors:

- **Raised TG level:** ≥ 1.7 mmol/L (150 mg/dL), **or specific treatment for this lipid abnormality.**
- **Reduced HDL cholesterol:** < 1.03 mmol/L (40 mg/dL) in males and < 1.29 mmol/L (50 mg/dL) in females, **or specific treatment for this lipid abnormality**.
- **Raised blood pressure:** systolic BP ≥ 130 or diastolic BP ≥ 85 mmHg, **or treatment of previously diagnosed hypertension.**
- **Raised fasting plasma glucose (FPG)** ≥ 5.6 mmol/L (100 mg/dL), **or previously diagnosed type 2 diabetes.**

If above 5.6 mmol/L or 100 mg/dL, OGTT is strongly recommended but is not necessary to define presence of the syndrome.

Various risk charts or scores have been developed to assess the risk for non-fatal or fatal cardiovascular events within a given time frame in individuals without a previous cardiovascular diagnosis. The European Heart Score (1) takes CVD risk into account. It does, however, only include traditional risk factors while diabetes has not yet been taken into account. FINDRISC (Figure 3) predicts the risk for developing type 2 diabetes with great accuracy, including asymptomatic diabetes and abnormal glucose tolerance and in addition the incidence of myocardial infarction and stroke.

Preventing progression to diabetes

The development of type 2 diabetes is preceded by altered metabolic states, including glucose intolerance and insulin resistance, and normally present years before overt type 2 diabetes. Although not all patients with such abnormalities progress to diabetes, their risk of developing the disease is significantly enhanced. A poor diet and a sedentary lifestyle have a major impact on this risk. Effective lifestyle interventions (Table 4) can prevent or at least delay the progression to type 2 diabetes in such individuals.

If life style interaction fails, pharmacological therapy may be used as an alternative. The following compounds are of proven value: acarbose, metformin and rosiglitazone. When metformin was compared with life-style interaction the number needed to treat to save one case of diabetes was 50% lower with lifestyle than metformin. The combined use of these two measures does not improve preventive efficacy.

Table 4. Summary of findings in some lifestyle intervention studies aiming at preventing type 2 diabetes in people with impaired glucose tolerance.

Study	Cohort size	Mean BMI (kg/m2)	Duration (years)	RRR (%)	ARR (%)	NNT
Malmö	217	26.6	5	63	18	28
DPS	523	31.0	3	58	12	22
DPP	2161*	34.0	3	58	15	21
Da Qing	500	25.8	6	46	27	25

RRR=Relative risk reduction; ARR=absolute risk reduction/1000 person-years; NNT=numbers needed to treat to prevent one case of diabetes over 12 months.

* Combined numbers for placebo and diet and exercise groups.

6. Treatment to reduce cardiovascular risk

Recommendation	Class	Level
Structured patient education improves metabolic and blood pressure control.	I	A
Non-pharmacological life style therapy improves metabolic control.	I	A
Self-monitoring improves glycaemic control.	I	A
Near normoglycaemic control (HbA_{1c} ≤ 6.5%*). reduces microvascular complications. reduces macrovascular complications.	 I I	 A A
Intensified insulin therapy in type 1 diabetes reduces morbidity and mortality.	I	A
Early escalation of therapy towards predefined treatment targets improves a composite of morbidity and mortality in type 2 diabetes.	IIa	B
Early initiation of insulin should be considered in patients with type 2 diabetes failing glucose target.	IIb	C
Metformin is recommended as first line drug in overweight type 2 diabetes.	IIa	B

* Diabetes Control and Complication Trial-standardized.

Lifestyle and comprehensive management

Non-pharmacological therapy as outlined in Table 1 is essential for a successful glucose lowering regimen especially at early stages of diabetes. Life style measures are at least as effective as any glucose lowering drug therapy, which yields a mean HbA_{1c} decrease of 1.0-1.5% in placebo controlled randomized studies.

Glycaemic control

Treatment aiming at lowering haemoglobin HbA_{1c} towards the normal range is associated with a reduction of microvascular and neuropathic complications in people with type 1 and type 2 diabetes. A 1.0% lower HbA_{1c} seems associated with a 25% decline in the risk of microvascular complications with a rather low absolute risk at HbA_{1c} levels below 7.5%.

Microvascular complications at the kidney and eye level, warrant meticulous therapeutic measures, including adequate control of blood pressure with the use of ACE-inhibitors and/or angiotensin II receptor blockers. Accordingly screening for microalbuminuria and retinopathy is mandatory on an annual basis. The relation between macrovascular disease and hyperglycaemia is less clear than the relation to microangiopathy, however, rather suggestive.

In type 1 diabetes, the gold standard is insulin therapy based on appropriate nutrition and blood glucose self-monitoring, aiming at HbA_{1c} below 7%. The risk for hypoglycaemic episodes needs to be titrated against this goal and severe episodes should be few. In type 2 diabetes, a common pharmacologic treatment approach is less well accepted. Some aspects on the choice of drug are given in Table 5 and recommended treatment targets in Table 1.

Combination therapy including early escalation to insulin, if oral drugs in appropriate doses and combinations fail, is advocated to maximize efficacy and minimize side-effects. A medium dose of an oral agent yields about 80% of the glucose-lowering effect, minimizing potential side-effects (Tables 6 and 7).

Table 5. Suggested policy for the selection of glucose-lowering therapy according to the glucometabolic situation

Glucometabolic situation	Policy
Post-prandial hyperglycaemia	Alpha-glucosidase inhibitors, short-acting sulphonylureas, glinides, short-acting regular insulin, or insulin analogs
Fasting hyperglycaemia	Biguanides, long acting sulphonylureas, glitazones, long-acting insulin or insulin analogs
Insulin resistance	Biguanides, glitazones, alpha-glucosidase inhibitors
Insulin deficiency	Sulphonylureas, glinides, insulin

Table 6. Mean efficacy of pharmacological treatment options in patients with type 2 diabetes

Pharmacological agent	Mean lowering of initial HbA1c (%)
Alpha-glucosidase inhibitors	0.5–1.0
Biguanides	1.0–1.5
Glinides	0.5–1.5
Glitazones	1.0–1.5
Insulin	1.0–2.0
Sulphonylurea derivatives	1.0–1.5

Table 7. Potential downsides of pharmacological treatment modalities in patients with type 2 diabetes

Potential problems*	Avoid or reconsider
Unwanted weight gain	Sulphonylureas, glinides, glitazones, insulin
Gastrointestinal symptoms	Biguanides, alpha-glucosidase inhibitors
Hypoglycaemia	Sulphonylureas, glinides, insulin
Impaired kidney function	Biguanides, sulphonylureas
Impaired liver function	Glinides, glitazones, biguanides, alpha-glucosidase inhibitors
Impaired cardio-pulmonary function	Biguanides, glitazones

* Oedema or lipid disorders may need further considerations

Dyslipidaemia

Recommendation	Class	Level
Elevated LDL and low HDL cholesterol are important risk factors for CVD in people with diabetes.	I	A
Statins are first-line agents for lowering LDL cholesterol in diabetic patients.	I	A
In diabetic patients with CVD, statin therapy should be initiated regardless of baseline LDL cholesterol, with a treatment target of < 1.8–2.0 mmol/L (< 70–77 mg/dL).	I	B
Statin therapy should be considered in adult patients with type 2 diabetes, without CVD, if total cholesterol > 3.5 mmol/L (> 135 mg/dL), with a treatment targeting an LDL cholesterol reduction of 30–40%.	IIb	B
Given the high lifetime risk of CVD, it is suggested that all type 1 patients over the age of 40 years should be considered for statin therapy. In patients 18–39 years (either type 1 or type 2), statin therapy should be considered when other risk factors are present, e.g. nephropathy, poor glycaemic control, retinopathy, hypertension, hypercholesterolaemia, features of the metabolic syndrome, or family history of premature vascular disease.	IIb	C
In diabetic patients with hypertriglyceridaemia > 2 mmol/L (177 mg/dL) remaining after having reached the LDL cholesterol target with statins, statin therapy should be increased to reduce the secondary target of non-HDL cholesterol. In some cases, combination therapy with the addition of ezetimibe, nicotinic acid, or fibrates may be considered.	IIb	B

Dyslipidaemia and vascular risk

Dyslipidaemia is part of the metabolic syndrome and the pre-diabetic state. It persists despite instigation of hypoglycaemic therapy and requires specific therapy with life style interaction and drugs. Typically in type 2 diabetes there is moderate hypertriglyceridaemia, low high density lipoprotein (HDL) cholesterol and abnormal post-prandial lipidaemia. Total and low density lipoprotein (LDL) cholesterol levels are similar to those in subjects without

Table 8. Subgroups of patients with DM in the major secondary prevention trials with statins and the proportionate risk reduction in patients with and without diabetes

Variables			Proportion of events (%)		Relative risk reduction (%)	
Trial	Type of event	Treatment	Diabetes present		Type of patients	
			No	Yes	All	Diabetes
4S Diabetes n = 202	CHD death or non-fatal MI	Simvastatin Placebo	19 27	23 45	32	55
4S Reanalysis Diabetes n = 483	CHD death or non-fatal MI	Simvastatin Placebo	19 26	24 38	32	42
HPS Diabetes n = 3050	Major coronary event, stroke, or revascularization	Simvastatin Placebo	20 25	31 36	24	18
CARE Diabetes n = 586	CHD death or non-fatal MI	Pravastatin Placebo	12 15	19 23	23	25
LIPID Diabetes n = 782	CHD death, non-fatal MI, revascularization	Pravastatin Placebo	19 25	29 37	24	19
LIPS Diabetes n = 202	CHD death, non-fatal MI, revascularization	Fluvastatin Placebo	21 25	22 38	22	47
GREACE Diabetes n = 313	CHD death, non-fatal MI, UAP, CHF, revascularization, stroke	Atorvastatin Standard care	12 25	13 30	51 -	58 -

diabetes, however, LDL particles are small and dense, which relates to increased atherogenicity.

Statins

Statins, whether used for primary or secondary prevention, show similar benefits in reducing cardiovascular events in patients with and without diabetes. Since the absolute risk is higher in patients with diabetes the number needed to treat becomes lower (Table 8). There is strong support for aggressive LDL cholesterol lowering in this patient category as detailed in Table 1. Evidence favors the use of statins for primary prevention in diabetic patients with a total cholesterol > 3.5 mmol/L (> 135 mg/dL), targeting a LDL reduction of 30-40% from the actual one.

Fibrates

Less information is available on the benefits of fibrates. Given this information gap the guidelines are less specific with regard to targets for HDL cholesterol and triglycerides. They do, however, recognize low HDL cholesterol (< 1 mmol/L (39 mg/dL) in men and < 1.2 mmol/L (46 mg/dL) in women) and fasting triglycerides > 1.7 mmol/L (151 mg/dL) as markers of increased vascular risk.

If triglycerides remain > 2.0 mmol/L (> 177 mg/dL) after having reached the LDL cholesterol target with statins, a secondary treatment target of non-HDL cholesterol (total cholesterol minus HDL cholesterol) is suggested with a goal 0.8 mmol/L (31 mg/dL) higher that the identified LDL cholesterol goal. This may require the addition of ezetimibe, fibrates or nicotinic acid.

Blood pressure

Recommendation	Class	Level
In patients with diabetes and hypertension, the recommended target for blood pressure control is <130/80 mm Hg.	I	B
The cardiovascular risk in patients with diabetes and hypertension is substantially enhanced. The risk can be effectively reduced by blood pressure-lowering treatment.	I	A
The diabetic patient usually requires a combination of several anti-hypertensive drugs for satisfactory blood pressure control.	I	A
The diabetic patient should be prescribed a renin–angiotensin–system inhibitor as part of the blood pressure-lowering treatment.	I	A
Screening for microalbuminuria and adequate blood pressure-lowering therapy including the use of ACE-inhibitors and angiotensin receptor II blockers improves micro-and macrovascular morbidity in type 1 and type 2 diabetes.	I	A

Blood pressure control needs to be meticulous in diabetic patients as indicated in Table 1. Such treatment strategy is associated with a lower incidence of cardiovascular complications. Life style changes are usually insufficient and most patients need a combination of blood pressure lowering drugs. The beneficial effects of diuretics are as well documented as, those of beta-blockers, calcium channel blockers and ACE-inhibitors and angiotensin II receptor blockers. Blockade of the renin-angiotensin-aldosterone system is of particular value in the diabetic patient. ACE-inhibitors and angiotensin II receptor blockers are the preferred therapies for delaying microalbuminuria/proteinuria and renal impairment.

7. Management of cardiovascular disease

Coronary artery disease

Recommendation	Class	Level
Early risk stratification should be part of the evaluation of the diabetic patient after ACS.	IIa	C
Treatment targets, as listed in Table 1, should be outlined and applied in each diabetic patient following an ACS.	IIa	C
Patients with acute MI and diabetes should be considered for thrombolytic therapy on the same grounds as their non-diabetic counterparts.	IIa	A
Whenever possible, patients with diabetes and ACS should be offered early angiography and mechanical revascularization.	IIa	B
Beta-blockers reduce morbidity and mortality in patients with diabetes and ACS.	IIa	B
Aspirin should be given for the same indications and in similar dosages to diabetic and non-diabetic patients.	IIa	B
Adenosine diphosphate (ADP) receptor dependent platelet aggregation inhibitor (clopidogrel) may be considered in diabetic patients with ACS in addition to aspirin.	IIa	C
The addition of an ACE-inhibitor to other therapies reduces the risk for cardiovascular events in patients with diabetes and established CVD.	I	A
Diabetic patients with acute MI benefit from tight glucometabolic control. This may be accomplished by different treatment strategies.	IIa	B

Patients with acute coronary syndromes (ACS) and concomitant diabetes mellitus are at high risk for complications. Their absolute mortality is high, 7-18% at 30 days and 15-34% after one year, and the adjusted relative risk for mortality ranging from 1.3 to 5.4, is somewhat higher in women than men underlining the profound role of the glucometabolic derangement. Registry studies reveal that diabetic patients are not as well treated as non-diabetic patients with regard to evidence-based therapy and coronary interventions. One reason may be that, due to autonomic neuropathy, silent ischaemia or atypical symptoms are common in the diabetic patient. Another reason is that diabetes is experienced as a relative contra-indication to some treatment modalities. Nevertheless, evidence-based coronary care treatment, including early coronary angiography and, if possible, revascularization, is at least as effective in the diabetic patient as in the non-diabetic patient without indications for increased numbers of side-effects. Thus, they should be given meticulous attention according to existing management guidelines for patients with acute coronary syndromes.

Available treatment options meant to preserve and optimize myocardial function, achieve stabilisation of vulnerable plaques, prevent recurrent events by controlling prothrombotic activity and counteract progression of atherosclerotic lesions are summarised in Table 9.

Table 9. Treatment options based on accumulated evidence

Revascularization
Anti-ischaemic medication
Anti-platelet agents
Anti-thrombin agents
Secondary prevention by means of
- Lifestyle habits including food and physical activity
- Smoking cessation
- Blocking the renin–angiotensin system
- Blood pressure control
- Lipid-lowering medication

Blood glucose control
- Acute if needed by means of insulin infusion
- Long term as demanded

Specific treatment

Thrombolytic drugs and coronary interventions are as efficient in patients with as those without diabetes. Due to a significantly higher absolute risk the relative benefits are substantially larger in diabetic than in non diabetic patients.

Oral *beta-blockers* are, in the absence of contra-indications, recommended for all diabetic patients with acute coronary syndromes.

Acetylsalicylic acid (ASA) reduces mortality and morbidity in patients with CAD. It has been claimed, but not verified, that ASA is less efficient in diabetic patients and that they need particularly high doses of ASA.

Clopidogrel may be considered in addition to ASA.

ACE-inhibitors protect diabetic patients from future events and should be considered in particular if the patient is hypertensive or has sign of renal impairment.

Glucose control by means of insulin should be immediately initiated in diabetic patients admitted for acute myocardial infarctions with significantly elevated blood glucose levels in order to reach normoglycaemia as soon as possible. Patients admitted with relatively normal glucose levels may be handled with oral glucose lowering agents. Strict glucose control should be continued based on life style counseling and supplemented with oral glucose lowering agents and/or insulin. Importantly long-term control has to be followed closely with glucose levels targeted as normal as possible (see also elsewhere in these guidelines).

Risk assessment and secondary prevention

A comprehensive risk assessment (Table 10) will help identify specific threats and outline goals for long-term management aiming at the prevention of further events and progression to irreversible myocardial damage in patients with acute coronary events.

Table 10. Risk assessment of patients with diabetes and acute coronary syndromes

Variable	Examination tools
Peripheral, renal and cerebrovascular disease	Case history, clinical examination
Traditional risk factors	
Eating and exercise habit	Case history
Smoking	Case history
Blood lipids	Blood chemistry
Blood pressure	Record (including ankle)
Previous or ongoing diseases Autonomic dysfunction Hypotension Heart failure Arrhythmias Ischaemic heart disease	Case history and clinical examination supplemented by special examinations as indicated (exercise testing, holter monitoring, echo-doppler examination, magnetic resonance imaging, myocardial scintigraphy, ST-segment monitoring, stress echo)

Recommendations for secondary prevention are the same for patients with as those without diabetes. For an equal treatment induced proportionate risk reduction, the number of patients needed to treat to save one life or prevent one defined end-point, is lower among diabetic patients due to their higher absolute risk.

Important treatment targets are usually more ambitious for those with than those without diabetes, as outlined in Table 1.

In general it seems that many diabetic patients presently are less well controlled than they deserve and great efforts should be made to improve the situation for this group of patients at a high cardiovascular risk.

Diabetes and coronary revascularization

Recommendation	Class	Level
Treatment decisions regarding revascularization in patients with diabetes should favour coronary artery bypass surgery over percutaneous intervention.	IIa	A
Glycoprotein IIb/IIIa inhibitors are indicated in elective PCI in a diabetic patient.	I	B
When PCI with stent implantation is performed in a diabetic patient, drug-eluting stents (DES) should be used.	IIa	B
Mechanical reperfusion by means of primary PCI is the revascularization mode of choice in a diabetic patient with acute MI.	I	A

Patients with diabetes have a higher mortality and morbidity after bypass surgery (CABG) compared with non-diabetics. This is also seen in patients undergoing percutaneous coronary interventions (PCI). The influence of glucometabolic control on the outcome after revascularisation is still unclear. Patients who require insulin have more adverse events, but this may be related to longer diabetes duration or more advanced diabetes affecting the morbidity or perhaps by so far unknown variables.

Surgery vs. percutaneous intervention

The effectiveness of PCI and CABG has been compared in randomised controlled trials. Originally major concerns were raised when a post-hoc subgroup analysis of patients with diabetes and multivessel disease, demonstrated a less favourable prognosis after PCI than after CABG. Other studies (Table 11), including those applying coronary stenting (Table 12) could, however, not confirm the negative outcome with PCI. In BARI the survival difference was linked to diabetic patients who received at least one arterial internal mammary graft.

Table 11. Trials addressing diabetes and revascularization for multivessel disease

Trial	Patients (n)	Follow-up (years)	Mortality (%) CABG	PCI	p-value
BARI	353	7	23.6	44.3	<0.001
CABRI	124	4	12.5	22.6	ns
EAST	59	8	24.5	39.9	ns
BARI registry	339	5	14.9	14.4	ns

Drug Eluting Stents have been hailed to improve the outcome of PCI in the diabetic patient. A recent meta-analysis comparing drug eluting stents to bare metal stents in diabetic subpopulations revealed that drug eluting stents were associated with a 80% relative risk reduction for restenosis during the first year of follow-up. However, trials comparing drug eluting stents with CABG are still needed to determine the optimal revascularization strategy.

Table 12. Revascularization in diabetes patients with multivessel disease in the stent-era

Trial	Patients (n)	Follow up (years)	Mortality (%) CABG	PCI	Repeat revascularization (%) CABG	PCI	Mortality p value
ARTS	208	3	4.2	7.1	8.4	41.1	0.39
SoS	150	1	0.8	2.5			ns
AWESOME	144	5	34	26			0.27

Adjunctive therapy

Glycoprotein IIb/IIIa inhibitors improve the outcome after PCI when administered during the procedure in diabetic patients. Moreover adenosine diphosphate receptor antagonists like clopidogrel prevent early as well as late thrombotic complications after stent implantation, particularly in patients with diabetes.

Revascularization and reperfusion in MI

An analysis of diabetic patients included in randomized trials demonstrated a survival benefit for those treated with primary percutaneous coronary interventions over those with thrombolytic treatment.

8. Heart failure and diabetes

Recommendation	Class	Level
ACE-inhibitors are recommended as first-line therapy in diabetic patients with reduced left ventricular dysfunction with or without symptoms of heart failure.	I	C
Angiotensin-II receptor blockers have similar effects in heart failure as ACE-inhibitors and can be used as an alternative or even as added treatment to ACE-inhibitors.	I	C
BBs in the form of metoprolol, bisoprolol, and carvedilol are recommended as first-line therapy in diabetic patients with heart failure.	I	C
Diuretics, in particular loop diuretics, are important for symptomatic treatment of diabetic patients with fluid overload owing to heart failure.	IIa	C
Aldosterone antagonists may be added to ACE-inhibitors, BBs, and diuretics in diabetic patients with severe heart failure.	IIb	C

There is a strong association between diabetes and heart failure and this combination has a deleterious prognosis. Few if any clinical trials on heart failure treatment have specifically addressed diabetic patients. Thus, information on treatment efficacy of various drugs is based on diabetic subgroups in various heart failure trials. Most data favour a similar efficacy in patients with and without diabetes, which means that the relative benefit is higher in the latter patient category who have a higher absolute risk. As outlined in European guidelines for heart failure (2) management should be based on diuretics, ACE-inhibitors and beta-blockers. Moreover it has been assumed that meticulous metabolic control should be beneficial in heart failure patients with diabetes.

9. Arrhythmias, atrial fibrillation and sudden cardiac death

Atrial fibrillation

Recommendation	Class	Level
Aspirin and anticoagulant use as recommended for patients with atrial fibrillation should be rigorously applied in diabetic patients with atrial fibrillation to prevent stroke.	I	C
Chronic oral anticoagulant therapy in a dose adjusted to achieve a target international normalized ratio (INR) of 2–3 should be considered in all patients with atrial fibrillation and diabetes, unless contra-indicated.	IIa	C
Control of glycaemia even in the pre-diabetic stage is important to prevent the development of the alterations that predispose to sudden cardiac death.	I	C
Microvascular disease and nephropathy are indicators of increased risk of sudden cardiac death in diabetic patients.	IIa	B

Diabetes seems to favour the occurrence of atrial fibrillation although the underlying mechanisms remain to be elucidated. In the guidelines on atrial fibrillation from the American College of Cardiology/American Heart Association/European Society of Cardiology (3), diabetes is classified as a moderate risk factor together with age > 75 years, hypertension, heart failure and a left ventricular ejection fraction < 35%. In patients with permanent or paroxysmal atrial fibrillation, who already had a stroke or a transient ischaemic attack, anticoagulant therapy with an INR between 2.0 and 3.0 is indicated. Also patients with more than one moderate risk factor for thrombo-embolism, whereof diabetes is one, should receive anticoagulant therapy. Recommendation for antithrombotic therapy in the presence of only one moderate risk factor is aspirin 81-325 mg daily or anticoagulant therapy. Aspirin in a dose of 325 mg is indicated as an alternative in patients with contra-indications to oral anticoagulation.

Sudden Cardiac Death

The incidence of cardiac arrhythmias, including ventricular fibrillation and sudden death is enhanced in the diabetic patient. Ischaemic heart disease, direct metabolic alterations, ion channel abnormalities and autonomic dysfunction may all contribute to create the substrate for sudden cardiac death. Recent evidence favours the concept that the risk relates to the glucose level, present already at the stage of impaired glucose tolerance. The identification of independent predictors of sudden cardiac death in diabetic patients has not yet progressed to a stage where it is possible to devise a risk stratification scheme for the prevention of such deaths. Microvascular disease and nephropathy may, however, be indicators of an increased risk.

10. Peripheral and cerebrovascular disease

Peripheral vascular disease

Recommendation	Class	Level
All patients with type 2 diabetes and CVD are recommended treatment with low-dose aspirin.	IIa	B
In diabetic patients with peripheral vascular disease, treatment with clopidogrel or low molecular weight heparin may be considered in certain cases.	IIb	B
Patients with critical limb ischaemia should, if possible, undergo revascularization procedures.	I	B
An alternative treatment for patients with critical limb ischaemia, not suited for revascularization, is prostacyclin infusion.	I	A

Subjects with diabetes have a two to four-fold increase in the incidence of peripheral vascular disease and an abnormal ankle-brachial blood pressure index is present in approximately 15% of such patients.

Diagnosis

Symptoms of leg ischaemia in diabetic patients may be atypical and vague due to peripheral neuropathy. Rather than experience typical pain in the legs the patient may suffer from leg fatigue or only inability to walk at a normal pace. Physical examination is of critical importance for the diagnosis (Table 13).

A valuable tool for early detection of peripheral artery disease is to measure the ankle-brachial blood pressure index. This is defined as the ratio between the arterial pressure at the ankle level and in the brachial artery with the highest pressure (Figure 5). Measurement is made in the supine position after 5 minutes of rest. The ankle-brachial blood pressure index should normally be above 0.9.

Table 13. Investigations of the peripheral circulation in diabetic patients

At the physician's office (regularly)	
Inspection	Dependent rubor pallor with elevation Absence of hair growth Dystrophic toenails Ulcers or gangrenes
Palpation	Decreased pulses Dry and cool skin Impaired sensibility
Pressure measurement	Ankle and arm blood pressure
At the vascular laboratory (if appropriate)	
Distal and/or segmental pressure measurements Oscillography Treadmill testing (with or without distal pressure after exercise) Duplex sonography *For evaluation of the microcirculation* Transcutaneous oxygen pressure Vital capillaroscopy	
At the radiology department (if appropriate)	
Magnetic resonance imaging Angiography	

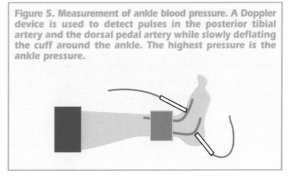

Figure 5. Measurement of ankle blood pressure. A Doppler device is used to detect pulses in the posterior tibial artery and the dorsal pedal artery while slowly deflating the cuff around the ankle. The highest pressure is the ankle pressure.

An ankle-brachial blood pressure index below 0.5 or an ankle pressure below 50 mm Hg indicates severely impaired circulation of the foot.

An ankle-brachial blood pressure index above 1.3 indicates poorly compressible vessels as a result of stiff arterial walls, which usually in diabetic patients are due to atherosclerosis in the media layer of the arterial wall. An arterial angiography should only be performed when this makes it likely that an invasive intervention to restore arterial circulation may be possible.

Treatment

Platelet inhibition with low-dose *aspirin* is indicated in all patients with type 2 diabetes who do not have contra-indication and for patients with severe peripheral vascular disease further inhibition of platelet aggregation by *clopidogrel or dipyridamole* may be indicated.

In patients with non-ischaemic neuropathic ulcers it is of utmost importance to remove any external pressure from the ulcer area sometimes necessitating immobilization of the patient. Amputations have been performed where a careful treatment would have saved the extremity.

The only pharmacological agent so far convincingly shown to have a positive influence on the prognosis of patients with critical limb ischaemia is a synthetic *prostacyclin*. If anatomically possible a *revascularization* procedure, with angioplasty or surgery, should be attempted in all such patients.

Stroke

Recommendation	Class	Level
For stroke prevention, blood pressure lowering is more important than the choice of drug. Inhibition of the renin–angiotensin–aldosterone system may have additional benefits beyond blood pressure lowering *per se*.	IIa	B
Patients with acute stroke and diabetes should be treated according to the same principles as stroke patients without diabetes.	IIa	C

Diabetes is a strong independent risk factor for stroke. The relationship between hyperglycaemia *per se* and stroke is, however, less clear than the relationship between hyperglycaemia and myocardial infarction. Microvascular complications further increase the risk for stroke. In diabetic patients the type of stroke is usually ischaemic.

Prevention of stroke

Measures to prevent stroke should include a multifactorial strategy aimed at treatment of hypertension, hyperlipidaemia, microalbuminuria, hyperglycaemia and the use of antiplatelet medication as outlined elsewhere in these guidelines.

Treatment of acute stroke

The treatment in the acute phase follows similar principles as for the treatment of stroke in the general population. Thrombolysis is an effective treatment for ischaemic stroke if instituted within 3-4 hours. Conservative treatment includes close surveillance in a stroke ward and includes optimisation of circulatory and metabolic conditions, including glycaemic control. Currently it is recommended to acutely reduce high blood pressures, above 220 mm Hg systolic and/or 120 mm Hg diastolic, but with great caution not lowering blood pressure to levels which may enhance ischaemia.

11. Intensive care

Recommendation	Class	Level
Strict blood glucose control with intensive insulin therapy improves mortality and morbidity of adult cardiac surgery patients.	I	B
Strict blood glucose control with intensive insulin therapy improves mortality and morbidity of adult critically ill patients.	I	A

Hyperglycaemia and outcome of critical illness

Stress imposed by critical illness leads to metabolic and endocrine abnormalities. Due to insulin resistance and accelerated glucose production patients usually become hyperglycaemic. In contrast to previous beliefs it is nowadays clearly established that even a modest hyperglycaemia is an important risk factor in terms of mortality and morbidity.

Blood glucose control with intensive insulin therapy in critical illness

Intensive insulin therapy aiming at maintaining blood glucose at a normal level decreases mortality and prevents several critical illness-associated complications as presented in Table 14. Further analyses revealed that it is blood glucose control, and/or other metabolic effects of insulin, that accompany tight blood glucose control, and not the insulin dose *per se* that contributed to improved survival.

Table 14. Published trials on intensive insulin therapy in critical illness

Patient population[a]	Surgical	Medical	Surgical and medical	Surgical	Heart surgery in diabetes
Number of patients	1548	1200/767[b]	1600	61	4864
Randomized study	Yes	Yes	No	Yes	No
Target glucose (mmol/L)	< 6.1	< 6.1	< 7.8	< 6.7	< 8.3
Mortality	↓	↓	↓		↓
Critical illness polyneuropathy	↓				
Bacteraemia/ severe infections	↓	-	-	↓	
Acute renal failure	↓	↓	↓		
Red blood cell transfusions	↓		↓		
Duration of mechanical ventilation	↓	↓			
Length of stay	↓	↓	↓		↓
Deep sternal wound infections					↓

a: See full text document for detailed information

b: Morbidity in all intention-to-treat patients (n = 1200); morbidity and mortality in the patients who required ≥ third day in ICU (n = 767).

12. Health economics and diabetes

Recommendation	Class	Level
Lipid-lowering provides a cost-effective way of preventing complications.	I	A
Tight control of hypertension is cost-effective.	I	A

The total costs for patients with type 2 diabetes have been analysed in eight European countries (Table 15). Due to the strong impact of co-morbidity in type 2 diabetes patients it is not possible to separate which resource use is due to diabetes and which are due to other diseases.

The main cost-driver is not diabetes in itself or its treatment, but the complications. Costs are 1.7,2.0 and 3.5 times higher if the patient has microvascular, macrovascular or both types of complications respectively. The key driver is the cost for hospitalization. Since complications are the most important cost driver the effective prevention of complications is essential and cost-effective.

Table 15. Direct medical costs for patients with type 2 diabetes in eight European countries and percentage of healthcare expenditure in the respective countries (1998)

Country	Total costs (million €)	Cost per patient (€)	Cost of healthcare expenditure (%)
Belgium	1094	3295	6.7
France	3983	3064	3.2
Germany	12438	3576	6.3
Italy	5783	3346	7.4
The Netherlands	444	1889	1.6
Spain	1958	1305	4.4
Sweden	736	2630	4.5
UK	2608	2214	3.4
All countries	29000	2895	5.0

13. Glossary of abbreviations:

ACE-inhibitors	Angiotensin Converting Enzyme-inhibitors
ACS	Acute Coronary Syndrome
ADA	American Diabetes Association
ADP	Adenosine Diphosphate
ARR	Absolute Risk Reduction/1000 person-years
ASA	Acetylsalicyclic Acid
BARI	Bypass Angioplasty Revascularization Investigation
BB(s)	Beta-Blocker(s)
BMI	Body Mass Index
BP	Blood Pressure
CABG	Coronary Artery Bypass Grafting
CAD	Coronary Artery Disease
CHD	Coronary Heart Disease
CHF	Congestive Heart Failure
CPG	Committee for Practice Guidelines
CVD	Cardiovascular Diseases
DES	Drug-Eluting Stents
DM	Diabetes Mellitus
DMF	Diabetes determined by fasting plasma glucose 7.0 mmol/L and 2-h plasma glucose < 11.1 mmol/L
DMP	Diabetes determined by 2-h plasma glucose 11.1 mmol/L and fasting plasma glucose, < 7.0 mmol/L
EASD	European Association for the Study of Diabetes
ECG	Electrocardiogram
ESC	European Society of Cardiology
FPG	Fasting Plasma Glucose
HbA_{1c}	Glycated haemoglobin
HDL	High Density Lipoprotein
IFG	Impaired Fasting Glucose
IGH	Impaired Glucose Homeostasis
IGT	Impaired Glucose Tolerance
LDL	Low Density Lipoprotein
MI	Myocardial Infarction
MODY	Maturity-Onset Diabetes in the Young
NGR	Normal Glucose Regulation
NNT	Numbers Needed to Treat
OGTT	Oral Glucose Tolerance Test
PCI	Percutaneous Coronary Intervention
PG	Plasma Glucose
RRR	Relative Risk Reduction
TG	Triglycerides
UAP	Unstable Angina Pectoris
WHO	World Health Organization

14. Trials and Studies Acronyms

4S	Scandinavian Simvastatin Survival Study
ARTS	Arterial Revascularization Therapy Study
AWESOME	Angina with Extreme Serious Operative Mortality
Evaluation BARI	Bypass Angioplasty Revascularization Investigation
CABRI	Coronary Angioplasty versus Bypass Revascularization Investigation
CARE	Cholesterol and Recurrent Events Trial
EAST	Emory Angioplasty versus Surgery Trial
FINDRISC	FINnish Diabetes Risk SCore
GREACE	Greek Atorvastatin and CHD Evaluation Study
HPS	Heart Protection Study
LIPID	Long-Term Intervention with Pravastatin in Ischaemic Disease Study
LIPS	Lescol Intervention Prevention Study
SoS	The Stent or Surgery Trial

15. References

(1) Conroy RM et al. Estimation of ten-year risk of fatal cardiovascular disease in Europe: the SCORE project. Eur Heart J 2003;24:987-1003.

(2) Swedberg K, Cleland J, Dargie H, Drexler H, Follath F, Komajda M, Tavazzi L, Smiseth OA, Gavazzi A, Haverich A, Hoes A, Jaarsma T, Korewicki J, Levy S, Linde C, Lopez-Sendon JL, Nieminen MS, Pierard L, Remme WJ; Task Force for the Diagnosis and Treatment of Chronic Heart Failure of the European Society of Cardiology. Guidelines for the diagnosis and treatment of chronic heart failure: Executive summary (update 2005). Eur Heart J 2005;26: 1115–1149.

(3) Fuster V, Rydén L, Cannom D S, Crijns H J, Curtis A B, Ellenbogen K A, Halperin J L, Le Heuzey J Y, Kay G N, Lowe J E, Olsson S B, Prystowsky E N, Tamargo J L, Wann S. ACC/AHA/ESC 2006 Guidelines for the management of patients with atrial fibrillation-executive summary: a report of the American College of Cardiology/ American Heart Association Task Force on practice guidelines and the European Society of Cardiology Committee for Practice Guidelines. Eur Heart J 2006; 27;16:1979-2030.

Section IV: Coronary Heart Disease

1. Diagnosis and Treatment of Non-ST-segment Elevation Acute Coronary Syndromes

2. Acute Myocardial Infarction (AMI)

3. Stable Angina Pectoris

4. Percutaneous Coronary Interventions (PCI)

Chapter 1

Diagnosis and Treatment of Non-ST-segment Elevation Acute Coronary Syndromes*
2007

Co-chairperson:
Jean-Pierre Bassand
Department of Cardiology
University Hospital Jean Minjoz
Boulevard Fleming
25000 Besançon
France
Phone: +33 381 668 539
Fax: +33 381 668 582
E-mail: jpbassan@univ-fcomte.fr

Co-chairperson:
Christian W. Hamm
Kerckhoff Heart Center
Benekestr. 2-8
61231 Bad Nauheim
Germany
Phone: +49 6032 996 2202
Fax: +49 6032 996 2298
E-mail: c.hamm@kerckhoff-klinik.de

Task Force Members:
1. Diego Ardissino, Parma, Italy
2. Eric Boersma, Rotterdam, Netherlands
3. Andrzej Budaj, Warsaw, Poland
4. Francisco Fernandez-Avilés, Valladolid, Madrid, Spain
5. Keith A.A. Fox, Edinburgh, United Kingdom
6. David Hasdai, Petah-Tikva, Israel
7. E. Magnus Ohman, Durham, USA
8. Lars Wallentin, Uppsala, Sweden
9. William Wijns, Aalst, Belgium

ESC Staff:
1. Keith McGregor, Sophia-Antipolis, France
2. Veronica Dean, Sophia-Antipolis, France
3. Catherine Desprès, Sophia-Antipolis, France

1. Introduction

These guidelines aim to present management recommendations based on all of the relevant evidence on a particular subject in order to help physicians to select the best possible management strategy for the individual patient. The strength of evidence for or against particular procedures or treatments is weighted, according to predefined scales for grading recommendations and levels of evidence, as outlined below. However, the ultimate judgment regarding the care of an individual patient must be made by the physician in charge of his/her care.

Class I	Evidence and/or general agreement that a given treatment or procedure is beneficial, useful and effective
Class II	Conflicting evidence and/or a divergence of opinion about the usefulness/efficacy of a given treatment or procedure.
Class IIa	Weight of evidence/opinion is in favour of usefulness/efficacy.
Class IIb	Usefulness/efficacy is less well established by evidence/opinion
Class III	Evidence or general agreement that the given treatment or procedure is not useful/effective and in some cases may be harmful

Level of Evidence A	Data derived from multiple randomized clinical trials or meta-analyses
Level of Evidence B	Data derived from a single randomized clinical trial or large non-randomized studies
Level of Evidence C	Consensus of opinion of the experts and/or small studies, retrospective studies, registries

2. Definitions

The different presentations of acute coronary syndromes (ACS) share a common pathophysiological substrate. The leading symptom that initiates the diagnosis and

*Adapted from the ESC Guidelines on the Diagnosis and Treatment of Non-ST Segment Elevation Acute Coronary Syndromes (European Heart Journal 2007; 28 (13) 1598-1660).

therapeutic decision making process is chest pain, but the classification of patients is based on the electrocardiogram (ECG). Two categories of patients may be encountered:

1. **Patients with typical acute chest pain and persistent (> 20 minutes) ST-segment elevation:** This is termed ST-elevation ACS (STE-ACS) and generally reflects an acute total coronary occlusion. Most of these patients will ultimately develop an ST-elevation MI (STEMI). The therapeutic objective is to achieve rapid, complete, and sustained reperfusion by primary angioplasty or fibrinolytic therapy.

2. **Patients with acute chest pain but without persistent ST-segment elevation.** They have rather persistent or transient ST-segment depression or T-wave inversion, flat T-waves, pseudo-normalisation of T-waves, or no ECG changes at presentation.

The initial working diagnosis of non-ST-elevation acute coronary syndrome (NSTE-ACS), based on the measurement of troponins, will subsequently be further qualified as non-ST-elevation MI (NSTEMI) or unstable angina; (Figure 1). In a certain number of patients, coronary artery disease (CAD) will be excluded as the cause of symptoms. The therapeutic management is guided by the final diagnosis.

Figure 1: The spectrum of acute coronary syndromes

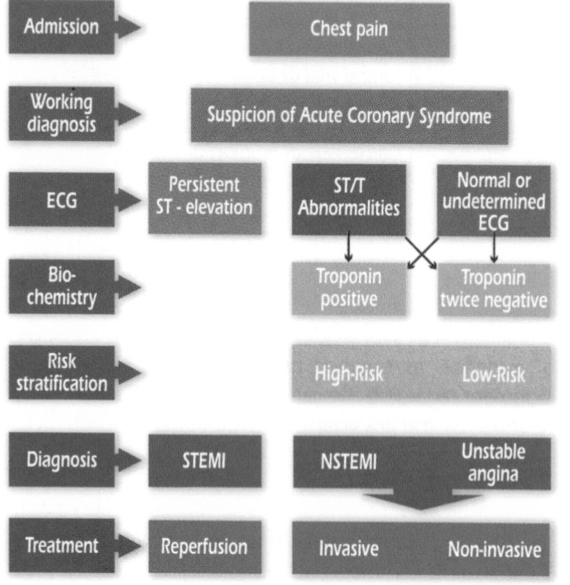

3. Epidemiology and natural history

Data from registries consistently show that NSTE-ACS have become more frequent than ST-elevation ACS. Hospital mortality is higher in patients with STEMI than among those with NSTE-ACS (7% vs 5% respectively), but at 6 months, the mortality rates are very similar in both conditions (12% vs 13% respectively). Long-term follow-up showed that death rates were higher among those with NSTE-ACS than STEMI, with a two fold difference at four years. This difference in mid- and long-term evolution may be due to different patient profiles, since NSTE-ACS patients tend to be older, with more co-morbidities, especially diabetes and renal failure. The difference could also be due to the greater extent of coronary artery and vascular disease, or persistent triggering factors such as inflammation. The implications for therapy are as follows:

- NSTE-ACS is more frequent than STEMI.
- In contrast to STEMI, where most events occur before or shortly after presentation, in NSTE-ACS these events continue over days and weeks.
- Mortality of STEMI and NSTE-ACS after 6 months are comparable.

This implies that treatment strategies for NSTE-ACS need to address the requirements of the acute phase as well as longer-term treatment.

4. Pathophysiology

ACS represent a life-threatening manifestation of atherosclerosis usually precipitated by acute thrombosis, induced by a ruptured or eroded atherosclerotic plaque, with or without concomitant vasoconstriction, causing a sudden and critical reduction in blood flow. In the complex process of plaque disruption, inflammation was revealed as a key pathophysiologic element. In rare cases, ACS may have a non-atherosclerotic aetiology such as arteritis, trauma, dissection, thrombo-embolism, congenital anomalies, cocaine abuse, and complications of cardiac catheterization. Some key pathophysiologic elements are described in more detail in the main document because they are important to understand the therapeutic strategies, particularly the notions of vulnerable plaque, coronary thrombosis, vulnerable patient, endothelial vasodilatory dysfunction, accelerated atherothrombosis, secondary mechanisms of non-ST-elevation ACS and myocardial injury.

5. Diagnosis and risk assessment

The clinical presentation of NSTE-ACS encompasses a wide variety of symptoms. Traditionally, several clinical presentations have been distinguished:

- Prolonged (> 20 minutes) anginal pain at rest,
- New onset (de novo) severe angina Class III of the Classification of the Canadian Cardiovascular Society (CCS),
- Recent destabilisation of previously stable angina with at least CCS III angina characteristics (crescendo angina), or
- Post MI angina.

Prolonged pain is observed in 80% of patients, while de novo or accelerated angina are observed in only 20%. It is important to note that a reliable distinction between ACS with or without ST-elevation cannot be based on symptoms.

Clinical symptoms: Retro-sternal pressure or heaviness ("angina") radiating to the left arm, neck or jaw is the most common symptom. This may be accompanied by other symptoms such as diaphoresis, nausea, abdominal pain, dyspnoea, and syncope. Atypical presentations are not uncommon. These include epigastric pain, recent onset indigestion, stabbing chest pain, chest pain with some pleuritic features, or increasing dyspnea. Atypical complaints are often observed in younger (25-40 years) and older (> 75 years) patients, in women, and in patients with diabetes, chronic renal failure or dementia.

Diagnostic tools: These include:

- physical examination
- electrocardiogram
- biochemical markers
- echocardiography
- imaging of the coronary anatomy.

Clinical history, ECG findings and biomarkers (particularly troponin T or I sampling) are essential for diagnostic (and prognostic) purposes.

Physical examination: Frequently normal. Signs of heart failure or haemodynamic instability must prompt the physician to expedite the diagnosis and treatment of patients. An important goal of the physical examination is to exclude non-cardiac causes.

ECG: ST-segment shifts and T-wave changes are the ECG indicators of unstable coronary artery disease. The number of leads showing ST depression and the magnitude of ST-depression are indicative of extent and severity of ischaemia and correlate with prognosis. ST-segment depression ≥ 0.5 mm (0.05 mV) in two or more contiguous leads, in the appropriate clinical context, is suggestive of NSTE-ACS and linked to prognosis. Minor (0.5 mm) ST-depression may be difficult to measure in clinical practice. More relevant is ST-depression of ≥ 1mm (0.1 mV), which is associated with an 11% rate of death and MI at 1 year. ST-depression of ≥ 2 mm carries about a 6 fold increased mortality risk. ST-depression combined with transient ST-elevation also identifies a high risk subgroup. Deep symmetrical inversion of the T-waves in the anterior chest leads is often related to a significant stenosis of the proximal left anterior descending coronary artery or main stem.

- A normal ECG does not exclude the possibility of NSTE-ACS.

Biomarkers

Troponins: In patients with MI an initial rise in troponins in peripheral blood occurs after 3 to 4 hours. Troponin levels may persist elevated for up to 2 weeks after myocardial infarction. In NSTE-ACS, minor elevation of troponins may be measurable only over 48 to 72 hours. The high sensitivity of troponin tests allows the detection of myocardial damage undetected by CK-MB in up to one third of patients presenting with NSTE-ACS. Minor or moderate elevations of troponins appear to carry the highest early risk in patients with NSTE-ACS.

It should be noted that troponin elevation can be encountered in many conditions that do not constitute acute coronary syndromes (Table 1). Other life threatening conditions presenting with chest pain may also result in elevated troponins and should always be considered as a differential diagnosis.

- The diagnosis of NSTE-ACS should never be made only on the basis of cardiac biomarkers whose elevation should be interpreted in the context of other clinical findings.

Other biomarkers are helpful for differential diagnoses: D-dimer (pulmonary embolism), BNP/NT-proBNP (dyspnoea, heart failure), haemoglobin (anaemia), leucocytes (inflammatory disease), markers of renal function.

Echocardiography: Routine use is recommended to detect wall motion abnormalities and to rule out differential diagnoses.

Differential diagnoses: Other conditions that may mimic NSTE-ACS are summarised in Table 2.

Table 1: Non-coronary conditions with troponin elevations

•	Severe congestive heart failure - acute and chronic
•	Aortic dissection, aortic valve disease or hypertrophic cardiomyopathy
•	Cardiac contusion, ablation, pacing, cardioversion, or endomyocardial biopsy
•	Inflammatory diseases, e.g., myocarditis, or myocardial extension of endo-/pericarditis
•	Hypertensive crisis
•	Tachy- or bradyarrhythmias
•	Pulmonary embolism, severe pulmonary hypertension
•	Hypothyroidism
•	Apical ballooning syndrome
•	Chronic or acute renal dysfunction
•	Acute neurological disease, including stroke, or subarachnoid haemorrhage
•	Infiltrative diseases, e.g., amyloidosis, haemochromatosis, sarcoidosis, scleroderma
•	Drug toxicity, e.g., adriamycin, 5-fluorouracil, herceptin, snake venoms
•	Burns, if affecting > 30% of body surface area
•	Rhabdomyolysis
•	Critically ill patients, especially with respiratory failure, or sepsis

Risk Stratification

Several risk stratification scores have been developed and validated in large patient populations. The GRACE risk score is based on a large unselected population of an international registry with a full spectrum of ACS patients. The risk factors were derived with independent predictive power for in-hospital deaths and post-discharge deaths at 6 months. GRACE risk score makes it possible to assess risk of in-hospital and 6-month death (Table 3) Further details are available at:
http://www.outcomes-umassmed.org/grace/

Table 2: Cardiac and non-cardiac conditions that can mimic NSTE-ACS

Cardiac	Pulmonary	Haematological
Myocarditis Pericarditis Myopericarditis Cardiomyopathy Valvular disease Apical ballooning (Tako-Tsubo syndrome)	Pulmonary embolism Pulmonary infarction Pneunonia Pleuritis Pneumothorax	Sickle cell anaemia
Vascular	**Gastro-intestinal**	**Orthopaedic**
Aortic dissection Aortic aneurysm Aortic coarctation Cerebrovascular disease	Oesophageal spasm Oesophagitis Peptic ulcer Pancreatitis Cholescystitis	Cervical discopathy Rib fracture Muscle injury/ inflammation Costochondritis

Table 3: Mortality in hospital and at 6 months in low, intermediate and high risk categories in registry populations according to the GRACE Risk Score

Risk category (tertiles)	GRACE Risk Score	In-hospital deaths (%)
Low	≤ 108	< 1
Intermediate	109-140	1-3
High	> 140	> 3
Risk category (tertiles)	**GRACE Risk Score**	**Post-discharge to 6 months deaths (%)**
Low	≤ 88	< 3
Intermediate	89-118	3-8
High	> 118	> 8

Recommendations for diagnosis and risk stratification

- Diagnosis and short-term risk stratification of NSTE-ACS should be based on a combination of clinical history, symptoms, ECG, biomarkers and risk score results **(I-B)**.

- The evaluation of the individual risk is a dynamic process that is to be updated as the clinical situation evolves.

    - A 12-lead ECG should be obtained within 10 minutes of first medical contact and immediately read by an experienced physician **(I-C)**. Additional leads (V_3R and V_4R, V_7-V_9) should be recorded. ECG should be repeated in case of recurrence of symptoms, and at 6, 24 hours and before hospital discharge **(I-C)**.

    - Blood must be drawn promptly for troponin (cTnT or cTnI) measurement. The result should be available within 60 minutes **(I-C)**. The test should be repeated after 6-12 hours if the initial test is negative **(I-A)**.

    - Established risk scores (such as GRACE) should be implemented for initial and subsequent risk assessment **(I-B)**.

    - An echocardiogram is recommended to rule in/out differential diagnoses **(I-C)**.

    - In patients without recurrence of pain, normal ECG findings, and negative troponins tests, a non-invasive stress test for inducible ischaemia is recommended before discharge **(I-A)**.

- The following predictors of *long-term* death or MI should be considered in risk stratification **(I-B)**:

    - Clinical indicators: age, heart rate, blood pressure, Killip class, diabetes, previous MI/CAD.

    - ECG markers: ST-segment depression.

    - Laboratory markers: troponins, GFR/CrCl/ Cystatin C, BNP/NT-proBNP, hsCRP.

    - Imaging findings: low ejection fraction, main stem lesion, 3-vessel disease.

    - Risk score result.

6. Treatment

The management of NSTE-ACS includes five therapeutic tools:

- Anti-ischaemic agents

- Anticoagulants

- Antiplatelet agents

- Coronary revascularization

- Long-term management

6.1. Anti-ischaemic agents

These drugs decrease myocardial oxygen consumption (decreasing heart rate, lowering blood pressure or depressing LV contractility) and/or induce vasodilatation.

Recommendations for anti-ischaemic drugs:

- Beta-blockers are recommended in the absence of contraindications, particularly in patients with hypertension or tachycardia **(I-B)**.

- Intravenous or oral nitrates are effective for symptom relief in the acute management of anginal episodes **(I-C)**.

- Calcium channel blockers provide symptom relief in patients already receiving nitrates and beta-blockers; they are useful in patients with contraindications to beta-blockade, and in the subgroup of patients with vasospastic angina **(I-B)**.

- Nifedipine, or other dihydropyridines, should not be used unless combined with beta-blockers **(III-B)**.

6.2. Anticoagulants

Several anticoagulants, which act at different levels of the coagulation cascade, have been investigated in NSTE-ACS:

- Unfractionated heparin (UFH) as intravenous infusion;

- Low molecular weight heparin (LMWH) as subcutaneous injection;

- Fondaparinux as subcutaneous injection;

- Direct thrombin inhibitors (DTIs) as intravenous infusion;

- Vitamin-K antagonists (VKAs) as oral medication.

Most anticoagulants have been shown to be capable of reducing the risk of death and/or MI at the cost of bleeding complications. The recommendations for the use of anticoagulants have mostly been based on the safety - efficacy profile of each drug (balance between risk reduction for ischaemic events, and risk of bleeding).

Recommendations for anticoagulation:

- Anticoagulation is recommended for all patients in addition to antiplatelet therapy **(I-A)**.
- Anticoagulation should be selected according to the risk of ischaemic and bleeding events **(I-B)**.
- Several anticoagulants are available, namely UFH, LMWH, fondaparinux, bivalirudin. The choice depends on the initial strategy (see section 9 Management strategies) urgent invasive, early invasive, or conservative strategies **(I-B)**.
- In an urgent invasive strategy UFH **(I-C)**, or enoxaparin **(IIa-B)** or bivalirudin **(I-B)** should be immediately started. (See section 9 Management strategies).
- In non-urgent situations, when the decision whether to follow early invasive or conservative strategy is pending (see Section 9 Management strategies):
    - Fondaparinux is recommended on the basis of the most favorable efficacy/safety profile **(I-A)**.
    - Enoxaparin with a less favourable efficacy/safety profile than fondaparinux should be used only if the bleeding risk is low **(IIa-B)**.
    - As efficacy/safety profile of LMWH (other than enoxaparin) or UFH relative to fondaparinux is unknown, these anticoagulants cannot be recommended over fondaparinux **(IIa-B)**.
- At PCI procedures the initial anti-coagulant should be maintained also during the procedure regardless whether this treatment is UFH **(I-C)**, enoxaparin **(IIa-B)** or bivalirudin **(I-B)**, while addititional UFH in standard dose (50-100 IU/kg bolus) is necessary in case of fondaparinux **(IIa-C)**.
- Anticoagulation can be stopped within 24 hours of the invasive procedure **(IIa-C)**. In a conservative strategy, fondaparinux, enoxaparin or other LMWH may be maintained up to hospital discharge **(I-B)**.

6.3. Antiplatelet agents

Antiplatelet therapy is necessary for the acute event, and subsequent maintenance therapy. Three related, but complementary strategies provide effective antiplatelet therapy: cyclooxygenase-1 inhibition (aspirin), inhibition of ADP mediated platelet aggregation with thienopyridines (ticlopidine and clopidogrel) and GP IIb/IIIa inhibition (tirofiban, eptifibatide, abciximab).

Premature withdrawal of antiplatelet agents, particularly dual antiplatelet therapy prescribed for the long-term, may lead to recurrence of events, particularly in patients with recent stent implantation. Interruption of dual antiplatelet therapy may become mandatory in certain situations, such as need for urgent surgery or major bleeding that cannot be controlled by local treatment. In this case, different alternative treatments have been proposed, depending on the clinical setting, type of stent and date of implantation, or type of surgery. However, none has formally been proven efficacious. All are based on experts' consensus opinion. LMWH have been advocated without tangible proof of efficacy.

Recommendations for oral antiplatelet drugs

- Aspirin is recommended for all patients presenting with NSTE-ACS without contra-indication at an initial loading dose of 160-325 mg (non-enteric) **(I-A)**, and at a maintenance dose of 75 to 100 mg long-term **(I-A)**.
- For all patients, immediate 300 mg loading dose of clopidogrel is recommended, followed by 75 mg clopidogrel daily **(I-A)**. Clopidogrel should be maintained for 12 months unless there is an excessive risk of bleeding **(I-A)**.
- For all patients with contra-indication to aspirin, clopidogrel should be given instead **(I-B)**.
- In patients considered for an invasive procedure/PCI, a loading dose of 600 mg of clopidogrel may be used to achieve more rapid inhibition of platelet function **(IIa-B)**.
- In patients pre-treated with clopidogrel who need to undergo CABG, surgery should be postponed for 5 days for clopidogrel withdrawal if clinically feasible **(IIa-C)**.

Recommendations for GP IIb/IIIa inhibitors

- In patients at intermediate to high risk, particularly patients with elevated troponins, ST-depression, or diabetes, either eptifibatide or tirofiban for initial early treatment are recommended in addition to oral antiplatelet agents **(IIa-A)**.

Table 4: Summary of antiplatelet and anticoagulant therapies available for the treatment of non-ST-segment elevation ACS

Oral Antiplatelet Therapy
• Aspirin initial dose: 160-325 mg non-enteric formulation, followed by 75-100 mg daily
• Clopidogrel 75 mg/day after a loading dose of 300 mg (600 mg loading dose when rapid onset of action is wanted)
Anticoagulants
• Fondaparinux 2.5 mg subcutaneously daily
• Enoxaparin 1 mg/kg subcutaneously every 12 h
• Dalteparin 120 IU/kg every 12 h
• Nadroparin 86 IU/kg every 12 h
• UFH intravenous bolus 60-70 IU/kg (maximum 5000 IU) followed by infusion of 12-15 IU/kg/h (maximum 1000 IU/h) titrated to aPTT 1.5-2.5 times control
• Bivalirudin intravenous bolus of 0.1 mg/kg and infusion of 0.25 mg/kg/hr. Additional intravenous bolus 0.5 mg/kg and infusion increased to 1.75 mg/kg/hour before PCI
GP IIb/IIIa inhibition
• Abciximab 0.25 mg/kg intravenous bolus followed by infusion of 0.125 μg/kg/min (maximum 10 μg/min) for 12 to 24 h
• Eptifibatide 180 μg/kg intravenous bolus (second bolus after 10 min for PCI) followed by infusion of 2.0 μg/kg/min for 72 to 96 h
• Tirofiban 0.4 μg/kg/min intravenously for 30 minutes followed by infusion of 0.10 μg/kg/min for 48 to 96 h. A high dose regimen (bolus 25 μg/kg + 0.15 μg/kg/min infusion for 18 hours) is tested in clinical trials.

- The choice of combination of antiplatelet agents and anticoagulants should be made in relation to risk of ischaemic and bleeding events **(I-B)**.

- Patients who received initial treatment with eptifibatide or tirofiban prior to angiography, should be maintained on the same drug during and after PCI **(IIa-B)**.

- In high risk patients not pretreated with GP IIb/IIIa inhibitors and proceeding to PCI, abciximab is recommended immediately following angiography **(I-A)**. The use of eptifibatide or tirofiban in this setting is less well established **(IIa-B)**.

- GP IIb/IIIa inhibitors must be combined with an anticoagulant **(I-A)**.

- Bivalirudin may be used as an alternative to GP IIb/IIIa inhibitors plus UFH/LMWH **(IIa-B)**.

- When the anatomy is known and PCI is planned to be performed within 24 hours and using GP IIb/IIIa inhibitors, most secure evidence is for abciximab **(IIa-B)**.

Recommendations for withdrawal of antiplatelet treatment

- Temporary interruption of dual antiplatelet therapy (aspirin and clopidogrel) within the first 12 months after the initial episode is discouraged **(I-C)**.

- Temporary interruption for major or life-threatening bleeding or for surgical procedures where even minor bleeding may result in severe consequences (e.g. brain or spinal surgery) is mandatory **(IIa-C)**.

- Prolonged or permanent withdrawal of aspirin, clopidogrel or both is discouraged unless clinically indicated. Consideration should be given to the risk of recurrence of ischaemic events which depends (among other factors), on initial risk, on presence and type of stent implanted, and on time window between proposed withdrawal and index event and/or revascularization **(I-C)**.

6.4. Coronary revascularization

Revascularization for NSTE-ACS is performed to relieve angina and ongoing myocardial ischaemia, and to prevent progression to MI or death. The indications for myocardial revascularization and the preferred approach (PCI or CABG) depend on the extent and severity of the lesions as identified by coronary angiography, the patient's condition and co-morbidity.

Recommendations for invasive evaluation and revascularization (see also section 9 Management strategies)

- Urgent coronary angiography is recommended in patients with refractory or recurrent angina associated with dynamic ST deviation, heart failure, life threatening arrhythmias or haemodynamic instability **(I-C)**.

- Early (< 72 hours) coronary angiography followed by revascularization (PCI or CABG) in patients with intermediate to high-risk features is recommended **(I-A)**.

- Routine invasive evaluation of patients without intermediate to high risk features is not recommended **(III-C)**, but non-invasive assessment of inducible ischaemia is advised **(I-C)**.

- PCI of non-significant lesions by angiography is not recommended **(III-C)**.

- After critical evaluation of the risk to benefit ratio, and depending on known co-morbidities and potential need for non-cardiac surgery in the short/medium term (e.g. planned intervention or other conditions) requiring temporary withdrawal of dual antiplatelet therapy, consideration should be given to the type of stent to be implanted bare metal stent (BMS) or drug eluting stent (DES) **(I-C)**.

6.5. Long-term management

Long term management implies lifestyle measures and drug treatment in order to keep under control every risk factor impacting on long-term outcome after ACS, but also long-term treatment necessitated by complications of ACS.

Recommendations for lipid lowering therapy

- Statins are recommended for all NSTE-ACS patients (in the absence of contraindications), irrespective of cholesterol levels, initiated early (within 1-4 days) after admission, in the aim of achieving LDLc levels < 100 mg/dL (< 2.6 mmol/L) **(I-B)**.

- Intensive lipid-lowering therapy with target LDLc levels < 70 mg/dL (< 1.81 mmol/L) initiated within 10 days after admission, is advisable **(IIa-B)**.

Recommendations for use of beta-blockers

- Beta-blockers should be given to all patients with reduced LV function **(I-A)**.

Recommendations for use of ACE-Inhibitors

- ACE-inhibitors are indicated long-term in all patients with LVEF ≤ 40% and in patients with diabetes, hypertension or chronic kidney disease, unless contraindicated **(I-A)**.

- ACE-inhibitors should be considered for all other patients to prevent recurrence of ischaemic events **(IIa-B)**. Agents and doses of proven efficacy are recommended **(IIa-C)**.

Recommendations for use of Angiotensin-Receptor Blockers

- Angiotensin-Receptor Blockers should be considered in patients who are intolerant to ACE-inhibitors and/or who have heart failure or MI with LVEF < 40% **(I-B)**.

Recommendations for aldosterone receptor antagonists

- Aldosterone blockade should be considered in patients after MI who are already treated with ACE-inhibitors and beta-blockers, and who have a LVEF < 40% and either diabetes or heart failure, without significant renal dysfunction or hyperkalaemia **(I-B)**.

6.6. Rehabilitation and return to physical activity

Recommendations for rehabilitation and return to physical activity

- After NSTE-ACS, assessment of functional capacity is recommended **(I-C)**.
- Every patient after NSTE-ACS should undergo an ECG-guided exercise test (if technically feasible), or an equivalent non-invasive test for ischaemia, within 4-7 weeks after discharge **(IIa-C)**.
- Based on cardiovascular status and on the results of functional physical capacity assessment, patients should be informed about the timing of resumption and the recommended level of physical activity, including leisure, work and sexual activities **(I-C)**.

7. Complications and their management

Bleeding complications

Bleeding complications have been shown to have a strong impact on the risk of death, myocardial infarction and stroke at 30 days and long-term, with a four- to five-fold increase in the risk of death, myocardial infarction and stroke. Prevention of bleeding has become an important component of the treatment of non-ST-elevation ACS.

The risk factors for the occurrence of bleeding are listed in Table 5. Many of the factors that lead to bleeding complications are also predictive of the risk of ischaemic events (death, myocardial infarction, stroke).

Several reports have recently suggested that transfusion may add to the risk of bleeding, and should be used with a restrictive policy.

Recommendations for bleeding complications

- Assessment of bleeding risk is an important component of the decision-making process. Bleeding risk is increased with higher or excessive doses of anti-thrombotic agents, length of treatment, combinations of several anti-thrombotic drugs, switch between different anticoagulant drugs, as well as with older age, reduced renal function, low body weight, female gender, baseline haemoglobin and invasive procedures **(I-B)**.
- Bleeding risk should be taken into account when deciding on a treatment strategy. Drugs, combination of drugs and non-pharmacological procedures (vascular access) known to carry a reduced risk of bleeding should be preferred in patients at high risk of bleeding **(I-B)**.
- Minor bleeding should preferably be managed without interruption of active treatments **(I-C)**.
- Major bleeding requires interruption and/or neutralisation of both anticoagulant and antiplatelet therapy, unless bleeding can be adequately controlled by specific haemostatic intervention **(I-C)**.
- Blood transfusion may have deleterious effects on outcome, and should therefore be considered individually, but withheld in haemodynamically

Table 5: Multivariate model for major bleeding in patients with non-ST-elevation MI

Variable	Adjusted OR	95% CI	*P*-value
Age (per 10 year increase)	1.22	1.10-1.35	0.0002
Female sex	1.36	1.07-1.73	0.0116
History of renal insufficiency	1.53	1.13-2.08	0.0062
History of bleeding	2.18	1.14-4.08	0.014
Mean arterial pressure (per 20mm Hg decrease)	1.14	1.02-1.27	0.019
Diuretics	1.91	1.46-2.49	< 0.0001
LMWH only	0.68	0.50-0.92	0.012
GP IIb/IIIa inhibitors only	1.86	1.43-2.43	< 0.0001
IV inotropic agents	1.88	1.35-2.62	0.0002
Right-heart catheterization	2.01	1.38-2.91	0.0003

stable patients with haematocrit > 25% or haemoglobin level > 8 g/L **(I-C)**.

Thrombocytopenia

Thrombocytopenia can occur in the course of the treatment of non-ST-elevation ACS. It could be related to drug treatment, particularly use of heparin or GP IIb/IIIa inhibitors. It requires specific measures.

Recommendations for management of thrombocytopenia

- Significant thrombocytopenia (< 100,000/μL^{-1} or > 50% drop in platelet count) occurring during treatment with GP IIb/IIIa inhibitors and/or heparin (LMWH or UFH) requires the immediate interruption of these drugs **(I-C)**.
- Severe thrombocytopenia (< 10,000/μL^{-1}) induced by GP IIb/IIIa inhibitors requires platelet transfusion with or without fibrinogen supplementation with fresh frozen plasma or cryoprecipitate in case of bleeding **(I-C)**.
- Interruption of heparin (UFH or LMWH) is warranted in case of documented or suspected heparin-induced thrombocytopenia (HIT). In case of thrombotic complications, anticoagulation can be achieved with direct thrombin inhibitor (DTI) **(I-C)**.
- Prevention of HIT can be achieved with use of anticoagulants devoid of risk of HIT, such as fondaparinux or bivalirudin, or by brief prescription of heparin (UFH or LMWH) in case these compounds are chosen as anticoagulant **(I-B)**.

8. Special populations and conditions

These include the elderly, female gender, patients with diabetes mellitus, chronic kidney disease or anaemia at baseline, and all may require specific management strategies.

Recommendations for elderly

- Elderly patients (> 75 years) often have atypical symptoms. Active screening for NSTE-ACS should be initiated at lower levels of suspicion than among younger (< 75 years) patients **(I-C)**.
- Treatment decisions in the elderly should be tailored according to estimated life expectancy, patient wishes and co-morbidities to minimize risk and improve morbidity and mortality outcomes in this frail but high-risk population **(I-C)**.
- Elderly patients should be considered for routine early invasive strategy, after careful evaluation of their inherent raised risk of procedure-related complications, especially during CABG **(I-B)**.

Recommendations for women

- Women should be evaluated and treated in the same way as men, with special attention to co-morbidities **(I-B)**.

Recommendations for diabetes

- Tight glycaemic control to achieve normoglycaemia as soon as possible is recommended in all diabetic patients with NSTE-ACS in the acute phase **(I-C)**.
- Insulin infusion may be needed to achieve normoglycaemia in selected NSTE-ACS patients with high blood glucose levels at admission **(IIa-C)**.
- Early invasive strategy is recommended for diabetic patients with NSTE-ACS **(I-A)**.
- Diabetic patients with NSTE-ACS should receive intravenous GP IIb/IIIa inhibitors as part of the initial medical management which should be continued through the completion of PCI **(IIa-B)**.

Recommendations for patients with chronic kidney disease (CKD)

- CrCl and/or GFR should be calculated for every patient hospitalised for NSTE-ACS **(I-B)**. Elderly people, women and low body weight patients merit special attention as near normal serum creatinine levels may be associated with lower than expected CrCl and GFR levels **(I-B)**.
- Patients with CKD should receive the same first-line treatment as any other patient, in the absence of contra-indications **(I-B)**.
- Anticoagulants should be carefully dosed. In patients with CrCl < 30 mL/min or GFR < 30 mL/min/1.73m^2, a careful approach to the use of anticoagulants is recommended, since dose adjustment is necessary with some, while others are contraindicated **(I-C)**.
- UFH infusion adjusted according to aPTT is recommended when CrCl < 30 mL/min or GFR < 30 mL/min/1.73 m^2 **(I-C)**.
- GP IIb/IIIa inhibitors can be used in case of renal failure. Dose adaptation is needed with eptifibatide and tirofiban. Careful evaluation of

Table 6: Recommendations for the use of drugs in case of CKD

Drug	Recommendations in case of CKD
Simvastatin*	Low renal elimination. In patients with severe renal failure (CrCl < 30 mL/min), careful with doses > 10 mg
Ramipril*	Dose adaptation required if CrCl < 30 mL/min (initial dose 1.25 mg daily). Dose must not exceed 5 mg per day.
Losartan*	Recommended for the treatment of hypertension or renal failure in diabetes type 2 with microalbuminuria 50-100 mg per day. Regular monitoring of electrolyte balance and serum creatinine is recommended.
Clopidogrel	No information in patients with renal failure
Enoxaparin*	In case of severe renal failure (CrCl<30mL/min), either contraindicated or dose adjustment required, according to country-specific labelling
Fondaparinux	Contraindicated in severe renal failure (CrCl < 30 mL/min). However, as much lower risk of bleeding complications was observed in Oasis-5 with fondaparinux as compared with enoxaparin, even in patients with severe renal failure, this drug might be the anticoagulant of choice in this situation.
Bivalirudin	If the CrCl < 30 mL/min, reduction of the infusion rate to 1.0 mg/kg/h should be considered. If a patient is on haemodialysis, the infusion should be reduced to 0.25 mg/kg/h. No reduction in the bolus dose is needed.
Tirofiban	Dose adaptation required in patients with renal failure. 50% of the dose only if CrCl < 30 mL/min.
Eptifibatide	As 50% of eptifibatide is cleared through the kidney in patients with renal failure, precautions must be taken in patients with impaired renal function (CrCl < 50 mL/min). The infusion dose should be reduced to 1 μg/kg/min in such patients. The dose of the bolus remains unchanged at 180 μg/kg. Eptifibatide is contra-indicated in patients with creatinine clearance < 30 mL/min.
Abciximab	No specific recommendations for the use of abciximab, or for dose adjustment in case of renal failure. Careful evaluation of haemorrhagic risk is needed before using the drug in case of renal failure.
Atenolol	Half dose recommended for patients with CrCl between 15 and 35 mL/min (50 mg/day). Quarter dose (25 mg/day) recommended if CrCl < 15 mL/min.

*Recommendations are indicated where applicable. It is assumed that the same recommendations are valid for other drugs of the same pharmacological class, but this needs to be assessed on a case by case basis (other LMWH, other statins, ACE-inhibitors, angiotensin receptor inhibitors), since, within the same pharmacological class, the route of elimination may vary. Recommendations for the use of drugs listed in this table may vary depending on the exact labelling of each drug in the country where it is used. Some differences in labelling can appear between countries.

the bleeding risk is recommended for abciximab **(I-B)**.

- Patients with CKD with CrCl < 60 mL/min are at high risk of further ischaemic events and therefore should be submitted to invasive evaluation and revascularization whenever possible **(IIa-B)**.

- Appropriate measures are advised to reduce the risk of contrast induced nephropathy **(I-B)**.

Recommendations for anaemia

- Low baseline haemoglobin is an independent marker of the risk of ischaemic and bleeding events at 30 days. It should be taken into consideration in assessing initial risk **(I-B)**.

- All necessary measures should be taken during the course of initial management to avoid worsening of anaemia by bleeding **(I-B)**.

- Well tolerated anaemia at baseline in patients with NSTE-ACS should not lead to systematic blood transfusion, which should be considered only in case of compromised haemodynamic status **(I-C)**.

9. Management strategies

A stepwise strategy should be applicable to most patients admitted with suspected NSTE-ACS. (Figure 2) It must be appreciated, however, that specific findings in individual patients may result in appropriate deviations from the proposed strategy. For every patient, the physician must make an individual decision taking into account the patient's history (co-morbid illnesses, age etc), his/her clinical condition, findings during the initial assessment on first contact, and the available pharmacological and non-pharmacological treatment options.

First step: initial strategy

Chest pain or discomfort will be the symptom that leads to the patient seeking medical attention or hospitalisation. A patient with suspected NSTE-ACS must be evaluated in a hospital and immediately seen by a qualified physician. Specialised chest pain units provide the best and expeditious care.

The initial step is to assign the patient without delay to a working diagnosis on which the treatment strategy will be based. The criteria are:

- Quality of chest pain and a symptom-oriented physical examination;
- Assessment of the likelihood of CAD (e.g. age, risk factors, previous MI, CABG, PCI;)
- ECG (ST deviation or other ECG abnormalities).

Based on these findings, which should be available within 10 minutes of first medical contact, the patient can be assigned to one of the 3 major working diagnoses:

- STEMI requiring immediate reperfusion;
- NSTE-ACS;
- ACS (highly) unlikely.

Second step: diagnostic validation and risk assessment

After the patient is assigned to the group NSTE-ACS intravenous and oral treatments will be started according to Table 7.

Table 7: Primary therapeutic measures

Oxygen	Insufflation (4 to 8 L/min) if oxygen saturation is < 90%
Nitrates	Sublingually or intravenously (caution if systolic blood pressure < 90 mmHg)
Aspirin	Initial dose of 160-325 mg non-enteric formulation followed by 75-100 mg/d (intravenous administration is acceptable)
Clopidogrel	Loading dose of 300 mg (or 600 mg for rapid onset of action) followed by 75 mg daily
Anticoagulation	Choice between different options depends on strategy: • UFH intravenous bolus 60-70 IU/kg (maximum 5000 IU) followed by infusion of 12-15 IU/kg/h (maximum 1000 IU/h) titrated to aPTT 1.5-2.5 times control • Fondaparinux 2.5 mg/daily subcutaneously • Enoxaparin 1 mg/kg twice/daily subcutaneously • Dalteparin 120 IU/kg twice/daily subcutaneously • Nadroparin 86 IU/kg twice/daily subcutaneously • Bivalirudin 0.1 mg/kg bolus followed by 0.25 mg/kg/h
Morphine	3 to 5 mg intravenous or subcutaneous, depending on pain severity
Oral beta-blocker	Particularly, if tachycardia or hypertension without sign of heart failure
Atropine	0.5-1 mg intravenously, if bradycardia or vagal reaction

The further management will be based on additional information/data:

- Routine clinical chemistry, particularly troponins (on presentation and after 6 to 12 hours) and other markers according to working diagnosis (e.g. D-dimers, BNP, NT-proBNP);
- Repeat, preferably continuous ST segment monitoring (when available);
- Echocardiogram, MRI, CT or nuclear imaging for differential diagnoses (e.g. aortic dissection, pulmonary embolism);
- Responsiveness to antianginal treatment;
- Risk score assessment;
- Bleeding risk assessment.

Risk assessment is an important component of the decision-making process and is subject to constant re-evaluation. It encompasses assessment of both ischaemic and bleeding risk. The risk factors for bleeding and ischaemic events overlap considerably, with the result that patients at high risk of ischaemic events are also at high risk of bleeding complications. Therefore, the choice of the pharmacological environment (dual or triple antiplatelet therapy, anticoagulants) has become critical, as has the dosage of the drugs. In addition, in case invasive strategy is needed, the choice of the vascular approach is very important, since the radial approach has been shown to reduce the risk of bleeding as compared to the femoral approach. In this context, particular attention has to be paid to renal dysfunction, shown to be particularly frequent in elderly patients and among diabetics.

During this step the decision has to be made whether the patient should go on to cardiac catheterization or not.

During this step other diagnoses must be confirmed or excluded, like acute anaemia, pulmonary embolism, aortic aneurysm.

Third step: invasive strategy
Cardiac catheterization is advised to prevent early complications and/or to improve long-term outcome. Accordingly, the need for and timing of invasive strategy has to be tailored according to the acuteness of risk into three categories:

- conservative,
- urgent invasive or
- early invasive.

Conservative strategy: Recommended in patients that fulfil all of the following criteria:

- No recurrence of chest pain;
- No signs of heart failure;
- No abnormalities in the initial ECG or a second ECG (6 to 12 hours);
- No elevation of troponins (arrival and at 6-12 hours).

Low risk, as assessed by a risk score, can support the decision making process for a conservative strategy. The further management in these patients is similar to the evaluation of stable CAD. Before discharge a stress test for inducible ischaemia is useful for further decision making.

Patients who cannot be excluded by the above criteria should go on to cardiac catheterization.

Urgent invasive strategy: Should be undertaken within 2 hours for patients who are early in the process of developing major myocardial necrosis escaping the ECG (e.g. occlusion of the circumflex artery) or are estimated to be at high risk of rapid progression to vessel occlusion. These patients are characterised by:

- Refractory angina (e.g. evolving MI without ST abnormalties);
- Recurrent angina despite intense antianginal treatment associated with ST depression ($\geq$ 2 mm) or deep negative T-waves;
- Clinical symptoms of heart failure or haemodynamic instability ("shock");
- Life threatening arrhythmias (ventricular fibrillation or ventricular tachycardia).

In addition to the medication in Table 7, a GP IIb/IIIa inhibitor (tirofiban, eptifibatide) should be added in symptomatic patients bridging the time to catheterization.

Early invasive strategy: Should be performed within 72 hours in moderate- to high-risk patients.

The following features indicate patients that should undergo routine early angiography:

- Elevated troponin levels;
- Dynamic ST- or T-wave changes (symptomatic or silent) ($\geq$ 0.5 mm);

- Diabetes mellitus;
- Reduced renal function (GFR < 60 mL/min/1.73 m^2);
- Depressed LVEF < 40%;
- Prior MI;
- Early post MI angina;
- PCI within 6 months;
- Prior CABG;
- Intermediate to high risk according to a risk score (Table 3).

A GP IIb/IIIa inhibitor (tirofiban, eptifibatide) should be added to the standard treatment prior to catheterization in case of elevated troponins, dynamic ST/T changes, or diabetes provided there is no overt excessive bleeding risk.

The decision about the timing of catheterization must be re-evaluated continuously and modified according to clinical evolution and occurrence of new clinical findings.

Figure 2: Decision-making algorithm for the management of patients with NSTE-ACS

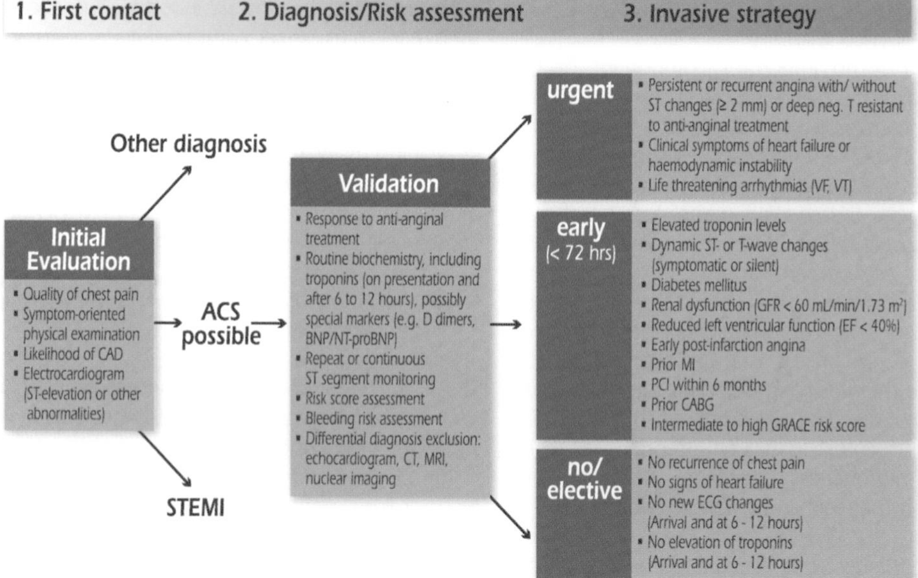

Chapter 2

Acute Myocardial Infarction (AMI)*

2003

Chairperson:
Frans Van de Werf, MD, FESC
Cardiology, Gasthuisberg University Hospital,
Herestraat 49,
B-3000 Leuven
Belgium
E-mail: Frans.VandeWerf@uz.kuleuven.ac.be

Task Force Members:
1. Diego Ardissino, Parma, Italy
2. Amadeo Betriu, Barcelona, Spain
3. Dennis V. Cokkinos, Athens, Greece
4. Erling Falk, Aarhus, Denmark
5. Keith A. A. Fox, Edinburgh, UK
6. Desmond Julian, London, UK
7. Maria Lengyel, Budapest, Hungary
8. Franz-Josef Neumann, München, Germany
9. Witold Ruzyllo, Warsaw, Poland
10. Kristian Thygesen, Aarhus, Denmark
11. Richard Underwood, London, UK
12. Alec Vahanian, Paris, France
13. Freek W.A. Verheugt, Nijmegen, The Netherlands
14. William Wijns, Aalst, Belgium

ESC Staff:
1. Keith McGregor, Sophia-Antipolis, France
2. Veronica Dean, Sophia-Antipolis, France
3. Dominique Poumeyrol-Jumeau, Sophia-Antipolis, France
4. Catherine Despres, Sophia-Antipolis, France

1. Introduction

The management of acute myocardial infarction continues to undergo major changes. Good practice should be based on sound evidence derived from well conducted clinical trials. In view of the great number of trials on new treatments performed in recent years and because of new diagnostic tests, the European Society of Cardiology decided that it was opportune to upgrade the 1996 guidelines and appointed a new Task Force. It must be recognized, that even when excellent clinical trials have been undertaken, their results are open to interpretation and that treatment options may be limited by resources. Indeed, cost-effectiveness is becoming an increasingly important issue when deciding upon therapeutic strategies.

In setting out these new guidelines, the Task Force has attemped to classify the usefulness or efficacy of the recommended routine treatments and the level of evidence on which these recommendations are based. The usefulness or efficacy of a recommended treatment will be presented according to three classes and the strength of evidence will be ranked according to three levels as follows:

Class I	Evidence and/or general agreement that a given treatment is beneficial, useful and effective;
Class II	Conflicting evidence and/or a divergence of opinion about the usefulness/efficacy of the treatment;
Class IIa	Weight of evidence/opinion is in favour of usefulness/efficacy;
Class IIb	Usefulness/efficacy is less well established by evidence/opinion;
Class III	Evidence or general agreement that the treatment is not useful/effective and in some cases may be harmful.

Level of Evidence A	Data derived from multiple randomized clinical trials or meta-analyses
Level of Evidence B	Data derived from a single randomized trial or non-randomized studies
Level of Evidence C	Consensus opinion of the experts

As always with guidelines, they are not prescriptive. Patients vary so much from one another that individual care is paramount and there is still an important place for clinical judgement, experience and common sense.

*Adapted from the Update of the ESC Guidelines on the Management of Acute Myocardial Infarction in Patients Presenting with ST-segment Elevation (European Heart Journal 2003; 24: 28-66)

2. Emergency care

2.1 Initial diagnosis of acute myocardial infarction:

- History of chest pain/discomfort.
- ST-segment elevation or (presumed) new left bundle-branch block on admission ECG. Repeated ECG recordings often needed.
- Elevated markers of myocardial necrosis (CK-MB, troponins). Do not wait for the results to initiate reperfusion treatment !
- 2D echocardiography and perfusion scintigraphy helpful to rule out acute myocardial infarction.

2.2 Relief of pain, breathlessness and anxiety

- Intravenous opioids (e.g. 4 to 8 mg morphine) with additional doses of 2 mg at 5 min intervals.
- O_2 (2–4 l . min^{-1}) if breathlessness or heart failure.
- Consider intravenous beta-blockers or nitrates if opioids fail to relieve pain.
- Tranquillizers may be helpful.

3. Pre-hospital or early in-hospital care

3.1 Recommendations for reperfusion therapy

Reperfusion therapy	CLASS				Level of evidence
	I	IIa	IIb	III	
Reperfusion therapy is indicated in all patients with history of chest pain/discomfort of < 12 hours and associated with ST-segment elevation or (presumed) new bundle-branch block on the ECG	X				A
Primary PCI					
• preferred treatment if performed by experienced team < 90 min after first medical contact	X				A
• indicated for patients in shock and those with contraindications to fibrinolytic therapy	X				C
• GP IIb/IIIa antagonists and primary PCI no stenting with stenting	 X 	 X			 A A
Rescue PCI					
• after failed thrombolysis in patients with large infarcts		X			B

Fibrinolytic treatment	CLASS				Level of evidence
	I	IIa	IIb	III	
In the absence of contraindications (see 3.2) and if primary PCI cannot be performed within 90 min of first medical contact by an experienced team, pharmacological reperfusion should be initiated as soon as possible	X				A
• choice of fibrinolytic agent depends on individual assessment of benefit and risk, availability and cost In patients presenting late (> 4 to 6 hours after symptom onset) a more fibrin-specific agent such as tenecteplase or alteplase is preferred For dosages of fibrinolytic and antithrombin agents, see 3.3 and 3.4		X			B
• prehospital initiation of fibrinolytic therapy if appropriate facilities exist	X				B
• readministration of a non-immunogenic lytic agent if evidence of reocclusion and mechanical reperfusion not available		X			B
• if not already on aspirin 150-325 mg chewable aspirin (no enteric-coated tablets)	X				A
• with alteplase and reteplase a weight-adjusted dose of heparin should be given with early and frequent adjustments according to the aPTT	X				B
• with streptokinase heparin is optional		X			B

3.2 Contraindications to fibrinolytic therapy

Absolute contraindications

- Haemorrhagic stroke or stroke of unknown origin at any time
- Ischaemic stroke in preceding 6 months
- Central nervous system damage or neoplasms
- Recent major trauma/surgery/head injury (within preceding 3 weeks)
- Gastro-intestinal bleeding within the last month
- Known bleeding disorder
- Aortic dissection

Relative contraindications

- Transient ischaemic attack in preceding 6 months
- Oral anticoagulant therapy
- Pregnancy or within 1 week post partum
- Non-compressible punctures
- Traumatic resuscitation
- Refractory hypertension (systolic blood pressure > 180 mm Hg)
- Advanced liver disease
- Infective endocarditis
- Active peptic ulcer

3.3 Fibrinolytic regimens for acute myocardial infarction

	Initial treatment	Antithrombin co-therapy	Specific contraindications
Streptokinase (SK)	1.5 million units in 100 ml of 5% dextrose or 0.9% saline over 30-60 min	None or i.v. heparin for 24 to 48 h	Prior SK or anistreplase
Alteplase (tPA)	15 mg i.v. bolus 0.75 $mg.kg^{-1}$ over 30 min then 0.5 $mg.kg^{-1}$ over 60 min i.v. Total dosage not to exceed 100 mg	i.v. heparin for 24 to 48 h	
Reteplase (r-PA)	10 U + 10 U i.v. bolus given 30 min apart	i.v. heparin for 24 to 48 h	
Tenecteplase (TNK-tPA)	single i.v. bolus 30 mg if <60 kg 35 mg if 60 to <70 kg 40 mg if 70 to <80 kg 45 mg if 80 to <90 kg 50 mg if ≥90 kg	i.v. heparin for 24 to 48 h	

This table describes frequently used fibrinolytic regimens. N.B. Aspirin should be given to all patients without contra-indications.

3.4 Heparin co-therapy

Heparin

i.v. bolus: 60 U . kg^{-1} with a maximum of 4000 U

i.v. infusion: 12 U . kg^{-1} for 24 to 48 h with a maximum of 1000 U . h^{-1}.
Target aPTT: 50-70 ms

aPTT to be monitored at 3, 6, 12, 24 h after starting treatment

3.5 Treatment of pump failure and shock

- **Diagnosis:**
  chest X-ray, echocardiography, right heart catheterisation.

- **Treatment of mild and moderately severe heart failure:**
  O_2
  furosemide:
  20-40 mg intravenously repeated at 1-4 hourly intervals if necessary
  nitrates: if no hypotension
  ACE inhibitors: in the absence of hypotension, hypovolaemia or renal failure.

- **Treatment of severe heart failure:**
  O_2
  furosemide:
  20-40 mg intravenously repeated at 1-4 hourly intervals if necessary
  nitrates: if no hypotension
  inotropic agents: dopamine and/or dobutamine
  haemodynamic assessment with balloon floating catheter
  ventilatory support if inadequate oxygen tension consider early revascularisation.

- Treatment of shock:
  O_2
  haemodynamic assessment with balloon floating catheter
  inotropic agents: dopamine and dobutamine
  ventilatory support if inadequate oxygen tension
  intraaortic balloon pump
  consider ***left ventricular assist devices*** and ***early revascularisation***.

3.6 Recommendations for routine prophylactic therapies in the acute phase

	CLASS				Level of evidence
	I	IIa	IIb	III	
• Aspirin: 150-325 mg (no enteric-coated formulation)	X				A
• Intravenous beta-blocker: for all patients for whom it is not contraindicated Oral beta-blockers: (see table 4.3)			X		A
• ACE inhibitor : oral formulation on first day - to all patients for whom it is not contraindicated - to high-risk patients	 X	X			A A
• Nitrates			X		A
• Calcium antagonists				X	B
• Magnesium				X	A
• Lidocaine				X	B

4. Management of the later in-hospital course

4.1 Risk stratification and indications for revascularisation

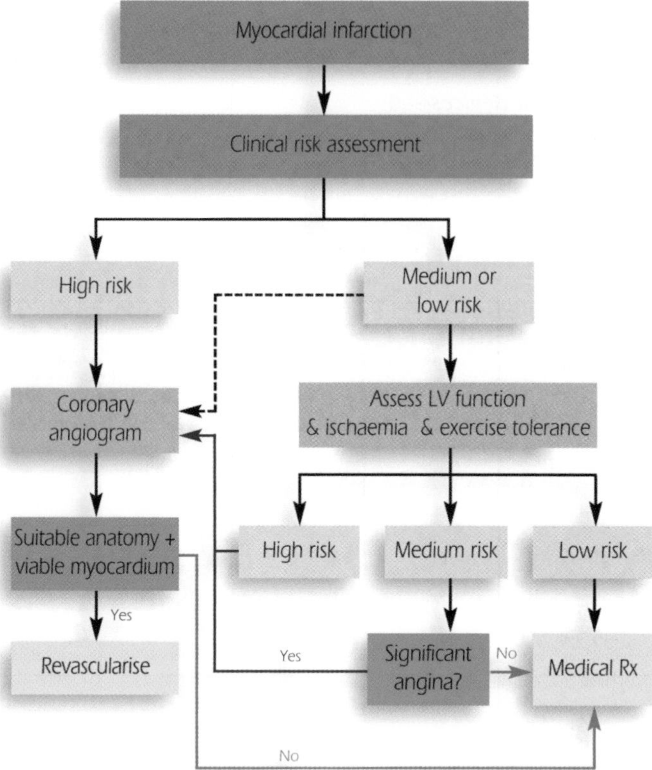

4.2 Rehabilitation

Rehabilitation is aimed at restoring the patient to as full a life as possible, including return to work. It must take into account physical, psychological and socio-economic factors. Rehabilitation is indicated in patients with significant left ventricular dysfunction. The process should start as soon as possible after hospital admission, and be continued in the succeeding weeks and months.

* Limited sales approval in ESC countries.

4.3 Recommendations for secondary prevention

	CLASS				Level of evidence
	I	IIa	IIb	III	
• Stop smoking	X				C
• Optimal glycaemic control in diabetic patients	X				B
• Blood pressure control in hypertensive patients	X				C
• Mediterranean-type diet	X				B
• Supplementation with 1g fish oil n-3 poly-unsaturated fatty acids	X				B
• Aspirin: 75 to 160 mg daily	X				A
If aspirin is not tolerated					
clopidogrel (75 mg daily)			X		C
oral anticoagulant		X			B
• Oral beta-blocker: to all patients if no contraindications	X				A
• Continuation of ACE-inhibition started on the first day (see table 3.6)	X				A
• Statins: if in spite of dietary measures total cholesterol > 190 mg.dL^{-1} (5.06 mmol.L^{-1}) and/or LDL cholesterol > 115 mg.dL^{-1} (2.98 mmol.L^{-1})	X				A
• Calcium antagonists (diltiazem or verapamil) if contraindications to beta-blockers and no heart failure			X		B
• Nitrates in the absence of angina				X	A

Chapter 3

Stable Angina Pectoris*

2006

Chairperson:
Kim Fox
Dept of Cardiology
Royal Brompton Hospital
Sydney Street
London SW3 6NP, UK
Phone: +44 (207) 351 8626
Fax : +44 (207) 351 8629
E-mail: k.fox@rbh.nthames.nhs.uk

Task Force Members:
1. Maria Angeles Alonso Garcia, Madrid, Spain
2. Diego Ardissino, Parma, Italy
3. Pawel Buszman, Katowice, Poland
4. Paolo G. Camici, London, UK
5. Filippo Crea, Roma, Italy
6. Caroline Daly, London, UK
7. Guy De Backer, Ghent, Belgium
8. Paul Hjemdahl, Stockholm, Sweden
9. José Lopez-Sendon, Madrid, Spain
10. Jean Marco, Toulouse, France
11. Joao Morais, Lieiria, Portugal
12. John Pepper, London, UK
13. Udo Sechtem, Stuttgart, Germany
14. Maarten Simoons, Rotterdam, The Netherlands
15. Kristian Thygesen, Aarhus, Denmark

ESC Staff:
1. Keith McGregor, Sophia Antipolis, France
2. Veronica Dean, Sophia Antipolis, France
3. Catherine Després, Sophia Antipolis, France
4. Karine Piellard, Sophia Antipolis, France

1. Introduction

These guidelines aim to present management recommendations based on all of the relevant evidence on a particular subject in order to help physicians to select the best possible management strategy for the individual patient. The strength of evidence for or against particular procedures or treatments is weighed, according to predefined scales for grading recommendations and levels of evidence, as outlined below. However, the ultimate judgement regarding the care of an individual patient must be made by the physician in charge of his/her care.

Class I	Evidence and/or general agreement that a given treatment is beneficial, useful and effective;
Class II	Conflicting evidence and/or a divergence of opinion about the usefulness/efficacy of the treatment or procedure;
Class IIa	Weight of evidence/opinion is in favour of usefulness/efficacy;
Class IIb	Usefulness/efficacy is less well established by evidence/opinion;
Class III*	Evidence or general agreement that the treatment is not useful/effective and in some cases may be harmful.

Level of Evidence A	Data derived from multiple randomized clinical trials or meta-analyses;
Level of Evidence B	Data derived from a single randomized trial or large non-randomized studies;
Level of Evidence C	Consensus opinion of the experts and/or small studies, retrospective studies, registries.

Recommendations for ESC Guidelines Production at www.escardio.org

*Adapted from the ESC Guidelines for the Management of Stable Angina Pectoris Executive Summary (European Heart Journal 2006; 27(11):1341-1381), and Full Text (www.escardio.org)

2. Diagnosis and Assessment

Stable angina is a clinical syndrome characterized by discomfort in the chest, jaw, shoulder, back or arms, typically elicited by exertion or emotional stress and relieved by rest or nitroglycerin. Less typically, discomfort may occur in the epigastric area. It is usual to confine the term to cases in which the syndrome can be attributed to myocardial ischaemia.

Diagnosis and assessment of angina involves clinical assessment, laboratory tests, and specific cardiac investigations. The purpose of investigation can be summarized as follows:

Figure 1. Algorithm for the initial evaluation of patients with clinical symptoms of angina

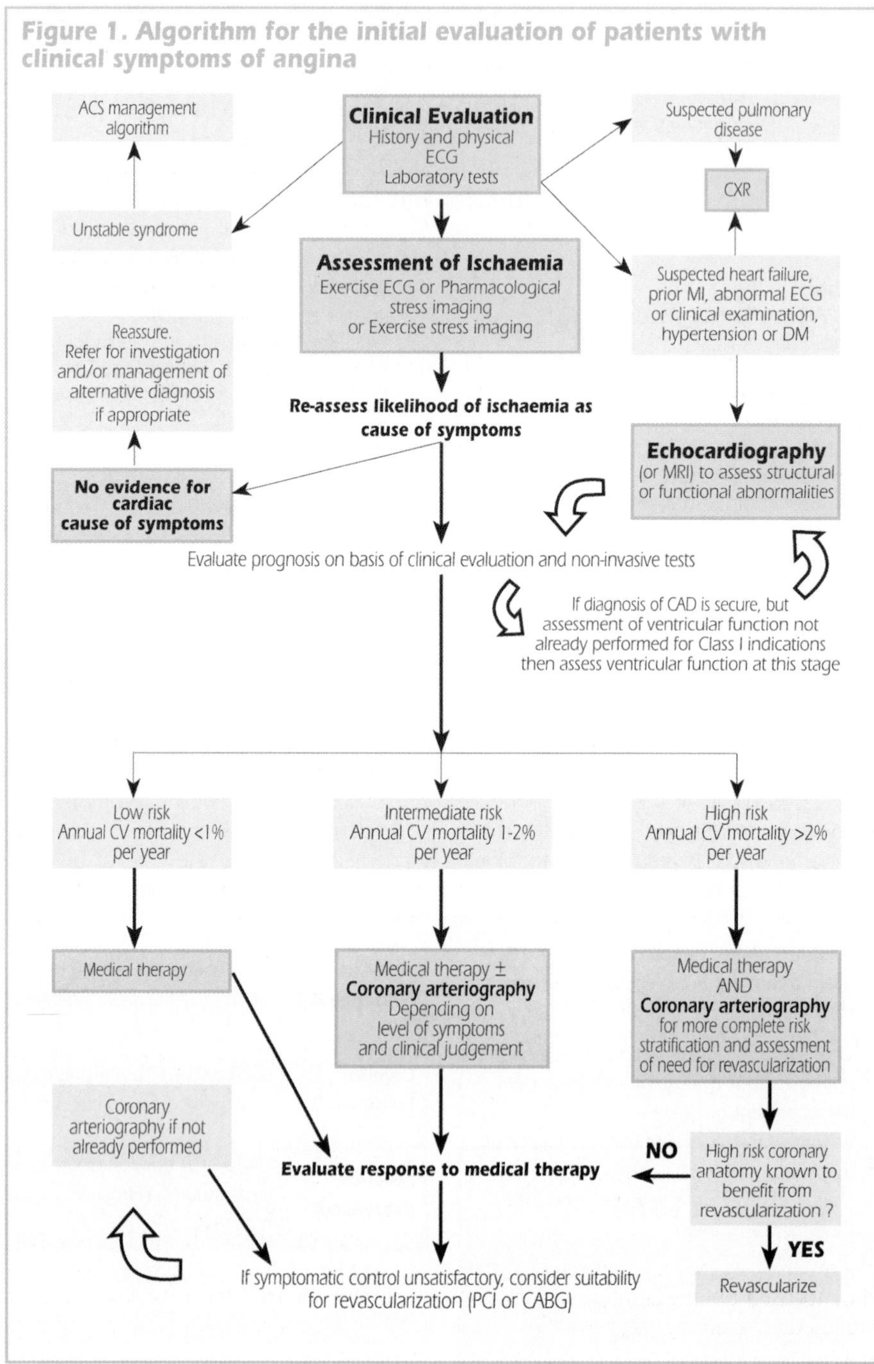

1. Confirmation of the presence of ischaemia in patients with suspected stable angina.

2. Identification or exclusion of associated conditions or precipitating factors.

3. Risk stratification.

4. To plan treatment options.

5. Evaluation of the efficacy of treatment.

An algorithm for the initial evaluation of patients presenting with clinical symptoms suggestive of angina is depicted in Figure 1. Investigations are summarized in Table 2.

2.1 Symptoms and signs

The history is a vital component in the diagnosis of stable angina. The characteristics of discomfort related to myocardial ischaemia (angina pectoris) may be divided into four categories, location, character, duration and relation to exertion and other exacerbating or relieving factors.

It is important to distinguish patients with unstable angina, which may present as:

(i) Rest angina.

(ii) Rapidly increasing or crescendo angina, i.e. previously stable angina, with rapid progressive increase in severity.

(iii) New onset angina, i.e. recent onset of severe angina with marked limitation of ordinary activity within 2 months of initial presentation.

For patients with stable angina it is also useful to classify the severity of symptoms using a grading system such as that of the Canadian Cardiovascular Society Classification (Table 1), Duke Specific Activity Index or Seattle angina questionnaire.

Features of the history important in risk stratification include current smoking, increasing age, prior MI, symptoms of heart failure, and the pattern of occurrence (recent onset or progressive), and severity of angina, particularly if unresponsive to therapy. The pattern of angina occurrence, angina frequency and resting ECG abnormalities are independent predictors of survival and survival free of MI particularly in the first year after assessment.

Physical examination of a patient with (suspected) angina pectoris should be focused on identification or exclusion of causal or associated conditions or precipitating factors and on risk stratification. Key findings to look for are:

Table 1. Classification of angina severity according to the Canadian Cardiovascular Society

Class	Level of symptoms
Class I	"Ordinary activity does not cause angina". Angina with strenuous or rapid or prolonged exertion only.
Class II	"Slight limitation of ordinary activity". Angina on walking or climbing stairs rapidly, walking uphill or exertion after meals, in cold weather, when under emotional stress, or only during the first few hours after awakening.
Class III	"Marked limitation of ordinary physical activity". Angina on walking one or two blocks* on the level or one flight of stairs at a normal pace under normal conditions.
Class IV	"Inability to carry out any physical activity without discomfort" or "angina at rest".

* Equivalent to 100-200 m

- Signs of valvular heart disease or hypertrophic obstructive cardiomyopathy.
- Hypertension.
- Evidence of non-coronary vascular disease.
- Significant comorbid conditions, particularly respiratory pathology.
- Signs of heart failure.
- Assessment of body mass index and waist circumference to assist in identification of metabolic syndrome.

2.2 Laboratory tests

Fasting plasma glucose and fasting lipid profile including total cholesterol (TC), high density lipoprotein (HDL) and low density lipoprotein (LDL) cholesterol, and triglycerides, should be evaluated in all patients with stable angina, to establish the patient's risk profile and ascertain the need for treatment. Elevated TC, LDL and glucose levels are also indicative of prognosis. Lipid profile and glycaemic status should be reassessed periodically to determine efficacy of treatment and to detect new development of diabetes. A full blood count and serum creatinine are also indicated in all patients.

Further laboratory testing, including oral glucose tolerance testing, cholesterol subfractions (ApoA, ApoB), homocysteine, lipoprotein (a) (Lpa), NT-BNP, haemostatic abnormalities and markers of inflammation such as hs CRP, may have a role in selected patients.

Measurement of markers of myocardial damage such as troponins, should be measured if evaluation suggests clinical instability or acute coronary syndrome. Thyroid function should be tested if dysfunction is suspected clinically.

2.3 Chest X-ray

A chest X-ray (CXR) should be requested only in patients with suspected heart failure, valvular disease or pulmonary disease. The presence of cardiomegaly, pulmonary congestion, atrial enlargement and cardiac calcifications have been related to prognosis.

2.4 Resting electrocardiogram (ECG)

All patients with suspected angina pectoris based upon symptoms should have a resting 12-lead electrocardiogram (ECG) recorded, although it should be emphasised that a normal resting ECG is not uncommon even in patients with severe angina and does not exclude the diagnosis of ischaemia. Resting ECG abnormalities, ST depression, Q waves, left anterior hemiblock and left bundle-branch block (LBBB), are associated with an adverse prognosis in stable angina.

2.5 ECG stress testing

In the majority of patients the exercise ECG is the initial test of choice to diagnose coronary disease and risk stratify.

Diagnosis of CAD

ST-segment depression during exercise is used to define a positive test. The reported sensitivity and specificity of the test for the detection of significant coronary disease are 68% and 77% respectively. Exercise ECG testing is not of diagnostic value in presence of LBBB, paced rhythm and Wolff Parkinson White syndrome (WPW). Additionally, results are less reliable in patients with an abnormal resting ECG in the presence of left ventricular hypertrophy, electrolyte imbalance, intraventricular conduction abnormalities and during use of digitalis. For patients with an abnormal resting ECG, an alternative functional test should be employed for diagnostic and prognostic assessment. Exercise ECG testing is also less sensitive and specific in women.

Risk stratification

The exercise ECG has been extensively validated as an important tool in risk stratification in symptomatic patients with known or suspected coronary disease. Prognostic indicators include exercise capacity and exercise-induced ischaemia (clinical and electrocardiographic). Maximum exercise capacity is a consistent prognostic marker and may be measured by maximum exercise duration, maximum MET level achieved, maximum workload achieved in Watts, maximum heart rate and double (rate–pressure) product. The specific variable used to measure exercise capacity is less important than the inclusion of this marker in the assessment.

The clinical value of stress testing is improved considerably by multivariate analysis including several exercise variables in a given patient such as the combination of heart rate at peak exercise, ST-segment depression, the presence or absence of angina during the test, peak workload and ST-segment slope. The combination of exercise and clinical parameters, with or without the use of scores such as the Duke Treadmill Score (DTS), has been shown to be an effective method of discriminating between high and low risk groups.

2.6 Stress testing in combination with imaging

The most well established stress imaging techniques are echocardiography and perfusion scintigraphy. Both may be used in combination with either exercise stress or pharmacological stress, and many studies have been conducted evaluating their use in both prognostic and diagnostic assessment.

Stress imaging techniques are often preferred in patients with previous percutaneous coronary intervention (PCI) or coronary artery bypass graft (CABG) because of its superior ability to localize ischaemia. Novel stress imaging techniques also include stress MRI.

Advantages of stress imaging over conventional exercise ECG testing include:

(i) Superior diagnostic and prognostic performance.

(ii) The ability to quantify and localise areas of ischaemia.

(iii) Ability to provide diagnostic information in the presence of resting ECG abnormalities or inability of the patient to exercise.

Exercise testing with echocardiography

Exercise echocardiography is more sensitive and specific than exercise testing for the detection of coronary disease. Technological advances include the use of contrast agents to enhance endocardial border definition, the use of injectable agents to image myocardial perfusion and advances in detection of ischaemia with tissue Doppler and strain rate imaging.

Stress echocardiography may also be used effectively to risk stratify patients. The risk of future events is influenced by the following:

- number of resting regional wall motion abnormalities;
- number of inducible wall motion abnormalities on stress echocardiography.

Exercise testing with myocardial perfusion scintigraphy

Single photon emission computed tomography (SPECT) may be performed in conjunction with a symptom limited exercise test or pharmacological stress to produce images of regional radionuclide tracer uptake that reflect relative regional myocardial blood flow during stress. These images may then be compared with resting images. Thallium-201 and technetium-99m radiopharmaceuticals are the most commonly used tracers.

SPECT perfusion provides a more sensitive and specific prediction of the presence of coronary artery disease than exercise electrocardiography, and is more sensitive but less specific than stress echocardiography. Stress perfusion imaging has also been extensively validated as a prognostic tool. High risk features include:

- Profound extensive ischaemia.
- Transient ischaemic dilation.
- Pulmonary uptake of tracer.

Pharmacological stress testing with imaging techniques

Exercise imaging is preferable where possible, as it allows for more physiological reproduction of ischaemia and assessment of symptoms. When exercise stress is not possible pharmacological stress may also be employed; either:

(i) Short-acting sympatho-mimetic drugs such as dobutamine.

(ii) Coronary vasodilators (e.g. adenosine and dipyridamole).

On the whole stress echo and stress perfusion scintigraphy, whether using exercise or pharmacological stress, have very similar applications. The choice as to which is employed will depend on local facilities and expertise.

Stress imaging has an important role to play in evaluating patients with a low pre-test probability of disease, particularly women, when exercise testing is inconclusive, in selecting lesions for revascularization, and in assessing ischaemia after revascularization.

Stress Cardiac Magnetic Resonance (CMR)

CMR stress testing in conjunction with a dobutamine infusion can be used to detect wall motion abnormalities induced by ischaemia, or perfusion abmormalities, but is not widely used for this purpose.

2.7 Echocardiography at rest

Resting echocardiography is useful to detect or rule out disorders such as valvular heart disease or hypertrophic cardiomyopathy as a cause of symptoms, and to evaluate ventricular function.

For purely diagnostic purposes echocardiography is useful in patients with clinically detected murmurs, history and ECG changes compatible with hypertrophic cardiomyopathy or previous myocardial infarction, and symptoms or signs of heart failure. However, echocardiography may also contribute useful prognostic information.

In stable angina, the strongest predictor of long-term survival is left ventricular function, with mortality increasing with progressive decreases in function. Left ventricular hypertrophy is also an important prognostic finding. Echocardiography may be used to assess ventricular function in patients who have not had ventricular function assessed by another modality.

Cardiac magnetic resonance may also be used to define structural cardiac abnormalities and evaluate ventricular function, but routine use for such purposes is limited by availability.

Computed Tomography (CT)

Electron beam CT and multi-detector or multi-slice CT have been validated as effective in detection of coronary calcium and quantification of the extent of coronary calcification. CT coronary arteriography can be also be performed by injection of intravenous contrast agents. The negative predictive power of CT angiography used with multi-detector CT is high. Until further data is available to support its wider application CT angiography may be used in patients with a low pre-test probability of disease with an equivocal functional test (exercise ECG or stress imaging).

Magnetic Resonance (MR) Arteriography

Advances in magnetic resonance technology permit non-invasive MR contrast coronary arteriography but remains a research tool rather than part of routine clinical practice.

Non-invasive risk stratification

For the purposes of these guidelines, if an individual with angina is determined, on the basis of a well validated risk prediction model, to have annual cardiovascular mortality of >2%, that individual is deemed high risk, while an annual cardiovascular mortality of <1% is considered low risk, and 1-2% intermediate risk.

Coronary arteriography

Non-invasive testing can establish the likelihood of the presence of obstructive coronary disease with an acceptable degree of certainty, and through appropriate risk stratification may be used to determine the need for coronary arteriography. However, coronary arteriography retains a fundamental position in the investigation of patients with stable angina, providing reliable anatomical information to identify the presence or absence of coronary lumen stenosis, define therapeutic options (suitability of medical treatment or myocardial revascularization) and determine prognosis.

Two vessel and three vessel disease have more severe prognostic implications than single vessel disease. High risk anatomical disease includes left main disease, or multi vessel disease involving the proximal left anterior descending coronary artery (LAD).

When appropriately used, non-invasive tests have an acceptable predictive value for adverse events. When the estimated annual cardiovascular mortality rate is less than or equal to 1%, the use of coronary arteriography to identify patients whose prognosis can be improved is likely to be inappropriate; in contrast it is appropriate for patients whose cardiovascular mortality risk is greater than 2% per annum.

Decisions regarding the need to proceed to arteriography in the intermediate risk group, those with an annual cardiovascular mortality of 1-2% should be guided by a variety of factors including the patient's symptoms, functional status, lifestyle, occupation, comorbidity, and response to initial therapy.

Coronary angiography is also warranted in the following circumstances:

- Serious ventricular arrhythmias or post cardiac arrest (without identifiable non-cardiac cause).
- Early recurrence of moderate or severe symptoms post revascularization.
- High risk of restenosis after PCI if PCI has been performed in a prognostically important site.
- Symptoms require consideration of revascularization.

3. Treatment

3.1 Aims of Treatment

1) To improve prognosis by preventing myocardial infarction and death.

2) To minimize or abolish symptoms.

3.2 General management including non-pharmacological considerations

- Patients and their close associates should be informed of the nature of angina pectoris, and the implications of the diagnosis and the treatments that may be recommended.
- Advice should be given for the management of an acute attack, i.e. to rest, at least briefly, from the activity that provoked the angina and the use of sublingual nitrate for acute relief of symptoms.
- The patient should be informed of potential side-effects of nitrates and appropriate prophylactic use of nitrate.
- Patients should be informed of the need to seek medical advice if angina symptoms persists for >10-20 minutes after rest and/or is not relieved by sublingual nitrate.
- Cigarette smoking should be strongly discouraged.
- Patients should be advised to adopt a "Mediterranean" diet, with vegetables, fruit, fish and poultry being the mainstays. A weight reducing diet should be recommended if the patient is overweight.
- Alcohol in moderation may be beneficial, but excessive consumption is harmful.
- Fish oils rich in omega-3 fatty acids (n-3 polyunsaturated fatty acids) are recommended at least once weekly.
- Physical activity within the patient's limitations should be encouraged.

Table 2. Summary of recommendations for routine non-invasive investigations in evaluation of stable angina

Test	For Diagnosis		For Prognosis	
	Class of Indication	Level of Evidence	Class of Indication	Level of Evidence
Laboratory tests				
Full blood count, creatinine	I	C	I	B
Fasting glucose	I	B	I	B
Fasting lipid profile	I	B	I	B
hs CRP, homocysteine, lp(a), apoA, apoB	IIb	B	IIb	B
ECG				
Initial evaluation	I	C	I	B
During episode of angina	I	B		
Routine periodic ECG on successive visits	IIb	C	IIb	C
Ambulatory ECG monitoring				
Suspected arrhythmia	I	B		
Suspected vasopastic angina	IIa	C		
In suspected angina with normal exercise test	IIa	C		
Chest X-ray				
Suspected heart failure, or abnormal cardiac auscultation	I	B	I	B
Suspected significant pulmonary disease	I	B		
Echocardiogram				
Suspected heart failure, abnormal auscultation, abnormal ECG, Q waves, BBB, marked ST changes	I	B	I	B
Previous MI			I	B
Hypertension or Diabetes Mellitus	I	C	I	B/C
Intermediate or low risk patient not due to have alternative assessment of LV function			IIa	C
Exercise ECG				
First line for initial evaluation, unless unable to exercise/ECG not evaluable	I	B	I	B
Patients with known CAD and significant deterioration in symptoms			I	B
Routine periodic testing once angina controlled	IIb	C	IIb	C
Exercise imaging technique (echo or radionuclide)				
Initial evaluation in patients with uninterpretable ECG	I	B	I	B
Patients with non-conclusive exercise test (but adequate exercise tolerance)	I	B	I	B
For Angina post revascularization	IIa	B	IIa	B
To identify location of ischaemia in planning revascularization	IIa	B		
Assessment of functional severity of intermediate lesions on arteriography	IIa	C		
Pharmacological stress imaging technique				
Patients unable to exercise	I	B	I	B
Patients with non-conclusive exercise test due to poor exercise tolerance	I	B	I	B
To evaluate myocardial viability	IIa	B		
Other indications as for exercise imaging where local facilities favour pharmacological rather than exercise stress	IIa	B	IIa	B
Non-invasive CT arteriography				
Patients with low probability of disease and non-conclusive or positive stress test	IIb	C		

- Concomitant disorders such as diabetes and hypertension should be managed appropriately. Patients with concomitant diabetes and/or renal disease should be treated with a blood pressure goal of <130/80 mmHg. Multifactorial intervention in diabetic patients may reduce both cardiovascular and other diabetic complications markedly.

- Anaemia or hyperthyroidism, if present, should be corrected.

- Sexual intercourse may trigger angina. Nitroglycerin prior to intercourse may be helpful. Phosphodiesterase inhibitors, such as sildenafil, tadafil or vardenafil, can be safely prescribed to men with coronary artery disease but should not be used in those receiving long acting nitrates.

3.3 Pharmacological therapy to improve prognosis

Antithrombotic drugs

Antiplatelet therapy to prevent coronary thrombosis is indicated, due to a favourable ratio between benefit and risk in patients with stable coronary artery disease. Low-dose aspirin (75-150 mg) is the drug of choice in most cases. The thienopyrdine clopidogrel may be considered as an alternative in patients who are aspirin allergic, or in addition to aspirin post-stenting or after an acute coronary syndrome. For patients with a history of gastrointestinal bleeding, aspirin in combination with a proton pump inhibitor may be used rather than clopidogrel.

Anticoagulant drugs (warfarin or thrombin inhibitors), which are combined with aspirin in certain high risk patients, such as post myocardial infarction, are not indicated in the general stable angina population without a separate indication such as atrial fibrillation for example.

Lipid-lowering drugs

Statin treatment reduces the risk of atherosclerotic cardiovascular complications by some 30% in stable angina patients. Subgroup analyses indicate beneficial effects also in diabetic patients with vascular disease and benefits of statin therapy have also been demonstrated in the elderly (>70 years). Similar relative benefits of long-term statin therapy have been observed in patients with different pre-treatment levels of serum cholesterol, even in the "normal" range. Thus, recommendations to treat with statins may be guided as much by the level of cardiovascular risk as by the cholesterol level (within the normal to moderately elevated range).

Statin therapy should always be considered for patients with stable coronary artery disease and stable angina. Therapy should aim at statin dosages documented to reduce morbidity/mortality in clinical trials. The daily statin dosages with solid documentation of mortality benefit are simvastatin 40 mg, pravastatin 40 mg and atorvastatin 10 mg. If this dose is not sufficient to achieve the target total cholesterol and LDL levels mentioned above the dose of statin therapy may be increased as tolerated to achieve the targets.

Recently high-dose atorvastatin treatment (80 mg daily) has been shown to reduce the risk of cardiovascular events compared to 10 mg, but high-dose atorvastatin therapy should be reserved for high risk patients.

Other lipid lowering drugs, e.g. fibrates, prolonged release nicotinic acid and their combinations with statins and other hypolipidaemics may be needed to control the lipid levels in patients with severe dyslipidaemia, particularly those with low levels of HDL-cholesterol and high triglycerides. Adjunctive therapy to statin therapy may be considered on an individualised basis in patients who have severe dyslipidaemia and remain at high risk (estimated cardiovascular mortality >2 % per annum) after conventional measures.

ACE-inhibitors

Angiotensin-converting enzyme (ACE) inhibitors are well established for the treatment of hypertension, heart failure, and LV dysfunction. In addition ramipril and perindopril have been shown to reduce the risk of cardiovascular morbidity and mortality in patients with stable coronary disease without heart failure in two large scale randomized controlled trials. A third trial, using the ACE-inhibitor trandalopril, failed to show a significant reduction in cardiovascular mortality and myocardial infarction.

ACE-inhibitors are indicated for the treatment of patients with stable angina pectoris and co-existing hypertension, diabetes, heart failure, asymptomatic LV dysfunction and post-MI. In angina patients without coexisting indications for ACE-inhibitor treatment the anticipated benefit of treatment (possible absolute risk reduction) should be weighed against costs and risks for side-effects, and the dose and agent used of proven efficacy for this indication in randomized clinical trials.

Beta-blockers

There is evidence of prognostic benefit from the use of beta-blockade in patients with angina who have suffered prior MI or have heart failure, and extrapolated from these data beta-blockers are suggested as a first line anti-anginal therapy in patients without contraindications.

3.4 Pharmacological treatment of symptoms and ischaemia

Symptoms of angina pectoris and signs of ischaemia (also silent ischaemia) may be reduced by drugs that reduce myocardial oxygen demand and/or increase blood flow to the ischaemic area. Commonly used antianginal drugs are beta-blockers, calcium antagonists and organic nitrates (Table 3), potassium channel openers may also be used. Recently sinus node inhibitors have been made available, and metabolic agents may also be used.

General recommendations for pharmacological therapy:

- Anti-anginal drug treatment should be tailored to the needs of the individual patient, and should be monitored individually.
- Short-acting nitrate therapy for all patients for immediate relief of acute symptoms as tolerated.
- Different drug classes may have additive anti-anginal effects in clinical trials.

Table 3: Pharmacological agents to reduce symptoms and ischaemia (recommendations relate to monotherapy, for relief of symptoms, and ischaemia).

Drugs	Action	Comments	Recommendations
Short-acting nitrates	Venodilatation, ↓ diastolic filling - ↓ reduced intracardiac pressure, ↑ subendocardial perfusion.	- Subligual administration. - Situational prophylaxis.	IC
Long-acting nitrates		- Oral or transdermal formulations. - Care to maintain a nitrate free period.	IC
Beta-blockers	↓ oxygen demand by ↓ heart rate ↓ contractility ↓ blood pressure.	- Less side-effects with B1 receptor selective agents. - Titrate dose to symptoms and HR. - Proven to reduce frequency of symptoms and improve exercise tolerance. - May worsen vasospastic angina.	IA
Calcium channel blockers	- Heterogenous class. - Systemic and coronary vasodilation by inhibition of calcium influx via L-type channels. - Verapamil and diltiazem also reduce myocardial contractility, HR and A-V conduction - Dihydropyridine CCB's (e.g. nifedipine, amlodipine and felodipine) are more vaso-selective.	- Proven to reduce frequency of symptoms and improve exercise tolerance. - Efficacy comparable to beta-blockade. - Particularly effective in vasospastic angina.	IA
Potassium channel opener	- Activates potassium channels. - Also has nitrate like vasodilator effects.	- Nicorandil shown to reduce death. - MI and hospitalization for angina in one large RCT in addition to other treatments. - Not available in all countries.	IC
Sinus node inhibitor	- Reduces heart rate via direct inhibition of If channel in sinus node.	- Ivabradine shown to be as effective as beta-blockade in reducing symptoms in a RCT.	IIaB
Metabolic agents	- Increase glucose utilisation relative to fatty acid metabolism.	- Limited haemodynamic effects. - Trimetazidine not available in all countries. - Ranolazine not yet licensed in Europe.	IIbB

- Dosing of one drug should be optimized before adding another one.
- Advisable to switch drug combinations before attempting a three drug regimen.
- Poor compliance should be considered when drug therapy is unsuccessful.
- Patients with symptoms that are poorly controlled on double therapy should be assessed for suitability for revascularization if not already considered.

The following strategy (see algorithm in Figure 2) is recommended for anti-anginal drug treatment in patients who are considered suitable for medical management after initial evaluation and risk stratification.

3.5. Coronary artery bypass surgery (CABG)

There are two main indications for CABG: prognostic and symptomatic. Prognostic benefit of CABG is mainly due to a reduction in cardiac mortality, as there is less evidence for reduction in myocardial infarction. Evidence of prognostic benefit of CABG compared to medical therapy has been demonstrated for patients at moderate to high risk of death. Specific anatomical groups shown to have a better prognosis with surgery than with medical treatment include:

1. Significant stenosis of the left main stem.
2. Significant proximal stenosis of the three major coronary arteries.
3. Significant stenosis of two major coronary arteries, including high grade stenosis of the proximal left anterior descending coronary artery.
4. Three vessel disease with impaired ventricular function.

CABG has also been shown to effectively reduce symptoms of angina and ischaemia in patients with coronary disease.

The overall operative mortality for CABG is between 1-4%, and there are well-developed risk stratification models available for the assessment of risk in individual patients.

Figure 2.
Algorithm for medical management of stable angina.

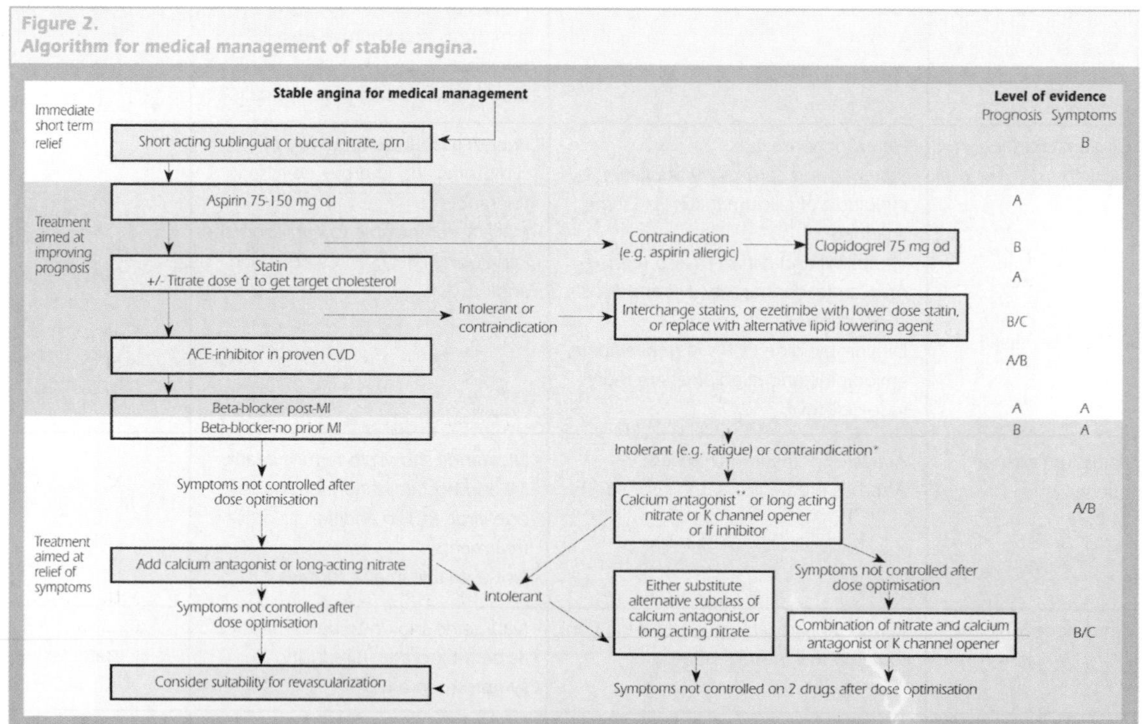

High risk candidates for revascularization on prognostic grounds alone should be identified and referred appropriately.

* Relative contraindications to beta-blockade include asthma, symptomatic peripheral vascular disease and first degree heart block

** Avoid short acting dihydropyridine formulations when not combined with beta-blocker.

Evidence for prognosis refers to evidence of reduction CV death or CV death MI. Evidence for symptoms include reduction in need for revascularization and hospitalization for chest pain.

The risk of surgery should be weighed against quality of life gains, and potential prognostic benefit in the anatomical subgroups above. The use of the internal mammary artery graft to LAD improves survival and reduces the incidence of late myocardial infarction, recurrent angina, and the need for further cardiac interventions. The use of other arterial grafts, also improve long-term patency rates.

3.6 Percutaneous coronary intervention (PCI)

In patients with stable angina and suitable coronary anatomy, the use of stents, the advent of drug eluting stents, and adequate adjuvant therapy allows a competent practitioner to perform either single or multivessel PCI with a high likelihood of initial procedural success and acceptable risk. The risk of death associated with the procedure in routine angioplasty is approximately 0.3% to 1%.

PCI may be considered an alternative to CABG for relief of symptoms in almost all cases. On available evidence, PCI compared to medical therapy does not provide survival benefit in stable angina, but PCI is more often effective than medical treatment in reducing events that impair quality of life (angina pectoris, dyspnoea, and need for re-hospitalization or limitation of exercise capacity). Advances in interventional technology have improved both initial and long term success rates of percutaneous revascularization, and are discussed in detail in the guidelines for PCI.

3.7 PCI versus surgery

Randomized trial evidence suggests that, outside of the population with high risk indicators, which have been proven to benefit prognostically from surgery, either PCI or surgery may be considered as an effective option for the treatment of symptoms.

In non-diabetic patients with 1-2 vessel disease without high-grade stenosis of the proximal LAD in whom angioplasty of one or more lesions has a high likelihood of initial success, PCI is generally the preferred initial approach, influenced by factors such as the less invasive nature and lower risk of the procedure, and the absence of survival advantage of CABG in lower risk subgroups. The individual circumstances and preferences of each patient must be considered carefully when planning the treatment strategy.

3.8 Specific patient and lesion subsets

Patients with severely depressed left ventricular function and/or high surgical risk, patients with left main disease, patients with diabetes and multivessel disease and patients with previous bypass surgery warrant particular consideration when selecting revascularization options:

- Patients in whom surgical risk is prohibitively high may benefit from revascularization by PCI, particularly when residual viability can be demonstrated in the dysfunctioning myocardium perfused by the target vessel(s).

- PCI in left main stem disease is feasible, and good results have been achieved in registries comparing drug-eluting and bare metal stents. However surgery should remain the preferred approach until the outcome of further trials are known.

- Subgroup analyses of randomized trials have shown reduced mortality with bypass surgery compared to PCI in diabetic patients with multivessel disease. Trials are underway to address this important issue, but for the present, PCI should be used with reservation in diabetics with multivessel disease until the results of these trials are available.

- There are no randomized controlled trials comparing treatment options in patients with previous bypass surgery. Re-do surgery may be undertaken on symptomatic grounds where the anatomy is suitable. However, the operative risks are high. In such cases PCI provides a useful alternative to re-do surgery for symptomatic relief.

3.9 Revascularization versus medical therapy

Outside the high risk population known to benefit prognostically from revascularization, an initial pharmacological approach to symptom control may be taken. Revascularization may be recommended for patients with suitable anatomy who do not respond adequately to medical therapy, or for the individual patient who, regardless of age, wishes to remain physically active (performing regular physical exercise).

An adequate response to therapy must be judged in consultation with the patient. Optimal secondary preventative medical therapy, including antiplatelet therapy, statin therapy, +/- beta-blockade, +/- ACE-inhibition should be continued in patients after revascularization irrespective of the need for anti-anginal therapy. Recommendations for revascularization are summarized in Table 4.

Table 4. Summary of recommendations for revascularization in Stable Angina.

Recommendations for revascularization on symptomatic grounds take into account the range of symptomatic grades for which evidence is available and should be construed in this fashion rather than as a directive to perform revascularization across the entire range of symptomatology.

	For Prognosis*		For Symptoms**		
Indication	**Class of Indication**	**Level of Evidence**	**Class of Indication**	**Level of Evidence**	**Studies**
PCI (assuming suitable anatomy for PCI, appropriate risk stratification and discussion with the patient)					
Angina CCS Class I to IV despite medical therapy with single vessel disease			I	A	ACME, MASS
Angina CCS Class I to IV despite medical therapy with multi vessel disease (non diabetic)			I	A	RITA 2, VA-ACME
Stable Angina with minimal (CCS Class I) symptoms on medication and one, two or three vessel disease but objective evidence of large ischaemia	IIb	C			ACIP
CABG (assuming suitable anatomy for surgery, appropriate risk stratification and discussion with the patient)					
Angina and left main stem disease	I	A	I	A	CASS, European Coronary Surgery study, VA Study, Yusef meta-analysis
Angina and three vessel disease with objective large ischaemia	I	A	I	A	
Angina and three vessel disease with poor ventricular function	I	A	I	A	
Angina with two or three vessel disease including severe disease of the proximal LAD	I	A	I	A	
Angina CCS Class I to IV with multi vessel disease (diabetic)	IIa	B	I	B	BARI, GABI, ERACI-I, SoS, ARTs, Yusef et al, Hoffman et al.
Angina CCS Class I to IV with multivessel disease (non diabetic)			I	A	
Angina CCS Class I to IV despite medical therapy and single vessel disease including severe disease of the proximal LAD			I	B	MASS
Angina CCS Class I to IV despite medical therapy and single vessel disease not including severe disease of the proximal LAD			IIb	B	
Angina with minimal (CCS Class I) symptoms on medication and one, two or three vessel disease but objective evidence of large ischaemia	IIb	C			ACIP

* Prognosis = relates to effects on mortality, cardiac or cardiovascular mortality or mortality combined with myocardial infarction.

** Symptoms = relates to changes in angina class, exercise duration, time to angina on treadmill testing, repeat hospitalization for angina or other parameters of functional capacity or quality of life.

CCS = Canadian Cardiovascular Society.

Selection of the method of revascularization should be based on:

1. Risk of periprocedural morbidity and mortality.
2. Likelihood of success, including factors such as technical suitability of lesions for angioplasty or surgical bypass.
3. Risk of restenosis or graft occlusion.
4. Completeness of revascularization.
5. Diabetic status.
6. Local hospital experience in cardiac surgery and interventional cardiology.
7. Patient's preference.

4. Special diagnostic considerations: angina with "normal" coronary arteries

A considerable proportion of patients, especially women, who undergo coronary arteriography because of symptoms of chest pain do not have significant coronary artery disease. In these patients the features of chest pain may suggest one of the following three possibilities:

(i) non-cardiac chest pain;

(ii) atypical angina including vasospastic angina;

(iii) cardiac Syndrome X.

It is important to differentiate Syndrome X and vasospastic angina from non-cardiac chest pain. Intra-vascular ultrasound (IVUS), or assessment of coronary flow reserve or fractional flow reserve may be considered to exclude missed obstructive lesions, if angiographic appearances are suggestive of a non-obstructive lesion rather than completely normal, and stress imaging techniques identify an extensive area of ischaemia. Intracoronary acetylcholine or ergonovine may be administered during coronary arteriography, if the angiogram is visually normal, to assess vasospasm or endothelium dependent coronary flow reserve.

4.1 Syndrome X

The classical description of "Syndrome X" requires the presence of the triad of:

1. Typical exercise induced angina (with or without additional resting angina and dyspnoea).

2. Positive exercise stress ECG or other stress imaging modality.

3. Normal coronary arteries.

A resting echocardiogram should be performed to assess for the presence of LVH and/or diastolic dysfunction. Although the prognosis in terms of survival of patients with Syndrome X appears to be favourable the morbidity is high. Treatment of Syndrome X should focus on symptom relief. Risk factors such as hypertension and hyperlipidaemia that are associated with endothelial dysfunction and may contribute to symptoms should be treated appropriately.

4.2 Vasospastic/Variant Angina

Often referred to as "Prinzmetal angina" it is characterized by typically located pain. It usually occurs at rest, but does not, or only occasionally, occurs with exertion, and is relieved within minutes by nitrates. The pain is classically associated with ST elevation.

Vasospastic angina may coexist with typical exertional angina due to fixed coronary lesions. Vasospasm may occur in response to smoking, electrolyte disturbances (potassium, magnesium), cocaine use, cold stimulation, autoimmune diseases, hyperventilation or insulin resistance. The prognosis of vasospastic angina depends on the extent of underlying coronary artery disease. Ambulatory ST-segment monitoring may be useful. Treatment of vasospastic angina centres on removing the stimulus, and calcium channel blockade or nitrate therapy.

Chapter 4

Percutaneous Coronary Interventions (PCI)*

2005

Chairperson:
Sigmund Silber, MD, FACC, FESC
Professor of Medicine
Cardiology Practice and Hospital, Am Isarkanal 36, 81379 Munich, Germany
Tel: +49 89 742 15130; Fax: +49 89 742 151 31; E-mail: sigmund@silber.com

Task Force Members:
1. Per Albertsson, Göteborg, Sweden
2. Francisco Fernandez-Avilés, Valladolid, Spain
3. Paolo G. Camici, London, UK
4. Antonio Colombo, Milano, Italy
5. Christian Hamm, Bad Nauheim, Germany
6. Erik Jørgensen, Copenhagen, Denmark
7. Jean Marco, Toulouse, France
8. Jan-Erik Nordrehaug, Bergen, Norway
9. Witold Ruzyllo, Warsaw, Poland
10. Philip Urban, Geneva, Switzerland
11. Gregg W. Stone, New York, USA
12. William Wijns, Aalst, Belgium

ESC Staff:
1. Keith McGregor, Sophia-Antipolis, France
2. Veronica Dean, Sophia-Antipolis, France
3. Catherine Després, Sophia-Antipolis, France
4. Xue Li, Sophia-Antipolis, France

1. Introduction and Definitions

Guidelines aim to present all the relevant evidence on a particular issue in order to help physicians to weigh the benefits and risks of a particular diagnostic or therapeutic procedure. They should be helpful in everyday clinical decision-making. To enable clinicians to access the key facts needed to aid in the decision making process at the point of care the ESC has developed pocket guidelines. This succinct PCI Pocket Guidelines aim to assist clinicians making decisions about when to perform PCI.

The ESC *Committee for Practice Guidelines* (CPG) supervises and coordinates the preparation of new *Guidelines and Expert Consensus Documents* produced by Task Forces, expert groups or consensus panels. The chosen experts in these writing panels are asked to provide disclosure statements of all relationships they may have which might be perceived as real or potential conflicts of interest. These disclosure forms are kept on file at the European Heart House, headquarters of the ESC. The CPG is also responsible for the endorsement of these Guidelines and Expert Consensus Documents or statements.

The Task Force has classified and ranked the usefulness or efficacy of the recommended procedures and/or treatments and their levels of evidence as indicated in the tables below:

Table 1-1: Classes of Recommendations.

Class I	Evidence and/or general agreement that a given diagnostic procedure/treatment is beneficial, useful and effective.
Class II	Conflicting evidence and/or a divergence of opinion about the usefulness /efficacy of the treatment.
Class II a	Weight of evidence/opinion is in favour of usefulness/efficacy.
Class II b	Usefulness/efficacy is less well established by evidence/opinion.

Table 1-2: Levels of Evidence.

Level of evidence A	Data derived from multiple randomised clinical trials or meta-analyses.
Level of evidence B	Data derived from a single randomised clinical trial or large non-randomised studies.
Level of evidence C	Consensus of opinion of the experts and/or small studies, retrospective studies, registries.

*Adapted from the Guidelines for Percutaneous Coronary Interventions (PCI) published in the European Heart Journal (2005) and also available at: www.escardio.org.

2. Indications for PCI

a. Indications for PCI in stable Coronary Artery Disease (CAD)

- General Indications for PCI in stable CAD

PCI versus medical therapy or coronary artery bypass graft (CABG) surgery:

PCI gives earlier and more complete relief of angina than medical therapy and is associated with a better exercise tolerance and/or less ischaemia during exercise testing.

In patients with no or mild symptoms, however, the scenario is different and unlikely to be improved by PCI.

Based on trials involving eight year follow-up, there is no significant difference in mortality between PCI and CABG surgery.

The use of stents plays a major role: in early trials without stents, there was a trend favouring CABG surgery over PCI at 3 years that is no longer present in more recent trials with stents. The trend in favour of CABG surgery disappeared despite a reduction in mortality in the CABG surgery arm from 5.2% in trials without stents to 3.5% in the more recent trials with stents. Stenting halved the risk difference for repeat revascularisation.

Both PCI and CABG surgery provided good symptom relief.

- Indications for PCI in special subsets of stable patients

Chronic Total Occlusion (CTO): Still represents the anatomical subset associated with the lowest technical success rates with PCI. When the occlusion can be crossed with a guide wire and the distal lumen has been reached, satisfactory results are obtainable with stent implantation.

PCI as an alternative to CABG surgery in patients with high risk of adverse outcomes: Patients with severely depressed left ventricular function seem to benefit from revascularisation by PCI, in particular when there is evidence for residual viability of the dysfunctional myocardium.

Multi-vessel coronary artery disease and/or diabetes mellitus and many high risk characteristics: CABG surgery was associated with better survival than PCI after adjustment for patient risk profile. The presence of an unprotected left main coronary artery (LM) stenosis identifies an anatomic subset still requiring bypass surgery for revascularisation. Stenting for unprotected LM disease should only be considered in the absence of other revascularisation options.

- Provisional or elective stenting in stable CAD?

There is no doubt that stents are a valuable tool in dissections with threatening vessel closure or insufficient results after balloon angioplasty. In general, stents are superior to balloons for the following reasons:

- Plaque fracture and dissection caused by balloon angioplasty often result in a pseudo-successful procedure and limited luminal enlargement is obtained.
- While abrupt closure within 48 hours following balloon treatment is not uncommon, the treated lesion shows greater acute and subacute stability after stenting.
- The angiographic results that can be obtained after stenting are predictable, irrespective of the stenotic complexity.
- In the medium-long term, stent implantation results in fewer vessel occlusions or reocclusions and lower rates of clinical restenosis.

Table 2-1: Recommendations of PCI indications in stable CAD.

Indication	Classes of Recommendations and Levels of Evidence	Randomised Studies for Levels of Evidence A or B
Objective large ischaemia	I A	ACME* ACIP**
Chronic total occlusion	IIa C	-
High surgical risk, incl. LV-EF < 35%	IIa B	AWESOME
Multi-vessel disease/ diabetics	IIb C	-
Unprotected left main in the absence of other revascularisation options	IIb C	-
Routine stenting of ***de novo*** lesions in native coronary arteries	I A	BENESTENT-I, STRESS
Routine stenting of ***de novo*** lesions in venous bypass grafts	I A	SAVED VENESTENT

Assuming that the lesions considered most significant are technically suited for dilatation and stenting, the classes of recommendation and levels of evidence refer to the use of stainless steel stents. (*the benefit was limited to symptom improvement and exercise capacity; **ACIP is not a pure trial of PCI versus medical treatment as half of the revascularisation patients were treated with bypass graft surgery). For drug-eluting stents, see below.

Thus, PCI can be considered a valuable initial mode of revascularisation in all patients with stable CAD and objective large ischaemia in the presence of almost every lesion subset, with only one exception: chronic total occlusions that cannot be crossed.

In early studies, there was a small survival advantage with CABG surgery compared with PCI without stenting. The addition of stents and newer adjunctive medications improved the outcome for PCI. The decision to recommend PCI or CABG-surgery will be guided by technical improvements in cardiology or surgery, local expertise, and patients' preference. However, until proven otherwise, PCI should be used only with reservation in diabetics with multi-vessel disease and in patients with unprotected left main stenosis. The use of drug-eluting stents might change this situation.

b. Indications for PCI in Acute Coronary Syndromes without ST-Segment Elevation (NSTE-ACS).

- Risk stratification in NSTE-ACS

The importance of stratifying patients with unstable angina (UA) or NSTEMI in high risk versus low risk groups applies to the fact that a clear benefit of early angiography and, when needed, PCI, has been reported only in high risk groups. Patients at high risk for rapid progression to myocardial infarction or death that should undergo coronary angiography within 48 hours are:

Table 2-2: Indications for an invasive strategy in NSTE-ACS

1. Recurrent resting pain
2. Dynamic ST-segment changes (ST-segment depression 0.1 mV or transient [< 30 minutes] ST-segment elevation ≥ 0.1 mV)
3. Elevated Troponin-I, Troponin-T or CK-MB levels
4. Haemodynamic instability within the observation period
5. Major arrhythmias (ventricular tachycardia, ventricular fibrillation)
6. Early post-infarction unstable angina
7. Diabetes mellitus

Characteristics of patients with NSTE-ACS at high acute, thrombotic risk for rapid progression to myocardial infarction or death that should undergo coronary angiography within 48 hours

Furthermore, the following markers of severe underlying disease, i.e. a high long-term risk, might also be helpful for risk assessment in NSTE-ACS:

- Age > 65–70 years.
- History of known CAD, previous MI, prior PCI or CABG.
- Congestive heart failure, pulmonary oedema, new mitral regurgitation murmur.
- Elevated inflammatory markers (i.e., CRP, Fibrinogen, IL 6).
- BNP or NT-proBNP in upper quartiles.
- Renal insufficiency.

Table 2-3: Recommendations for PCI indications in NSTE-ACS (UA or NSTEMI)

Procedure	Indication	Classes of Recommendations and Levels of Evidence	Randomised Studies for Levels of Evidence A or B
Early PCI (< 48 hrs)	High risk NSTE-ACS	I A	FRISC-II TACTICS-TIMI-18 RITA-3
Immediate PCI (< 2.5 hrs)	High risk NSTE-ACS	IIa B	ISAR-COOL
Routine stenting in *de novo* lesions	All NSTE-ACS	I C	-

Figure 1. Coronary angiography and PCI planning in NSTE-ACS

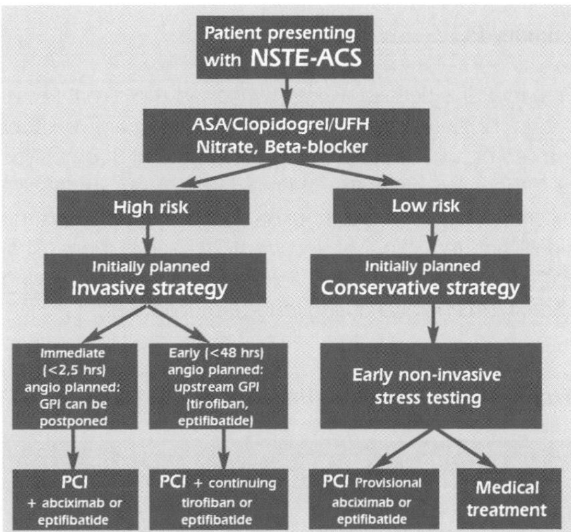

Flow-chart for planning coronary angiography and PCI, if appropriate, according to risk stratification in patients with NSTE-ACS (unstable angina or NSTEMI). GPI = Glycoprotein IIb/IIIa inhibitor. If for some reason the delay between diagnostic catheterisation and planned PCI is up to 24 hours, abciximab can also be administered. Enoxaparin may be considered as a replacement for UFH in high risk NSTE-ACS patients, if invasive strategy is not applicable. For the classes of recommendations and the levels of evidence please see Tables 2-3, 3-1 and 3-2).

A clear benefit from early angiography (< 48 hours) and, when needed, PCI or CABG surgery has been reported only in the high risk groups (Figure 1). Deferral of intervention does not improve outcome. Routine stenting is recommended based on the predictability of the result and its immediate safety (Table 2.3).

c. Indications for PCI in Acute Coronary Syndromes with ST-Segment Elevation (STE-ACS, STEMI)

PCI for STEMI requires an experienced team of interventional cardiologists working together with skilled support staff. This means that only hospitals with an established interventional programme should use PCI for

STEMI instead of intravenous thrombolysis. Most of the trials comparing thrombolysis versus primary PCI were carried out in high volume centres, by experienced operators, with short response times. Therefore, the results do not necessarily apply in other settings. Large variations between individual institutions have been documented. In general, for primary PCI, a higher level of experience and patient volume is required than for PCI in patients with stable coronary artery disease. In patients with multi-vessel disease, primary PCI should be directed only at the infarct-related coronary artery (culprit vessel), with decisions about PCI of non-culprit lesions guided by objective evidence of residual ischaemia at later follow-up.

Fortunately, the implementation of guidelines for patients with acute MI has shown to improve the quality of care. Patients treated during off-hours must have the same outcome as patients treated during routine duty hours.

Primary PCI

Primary PCI is defined as intervention in the culprit vessel within 12 hours after the onset of chest pain or other symptoms, without prior (full or concomitant) thrombolytic or other clot dissolving therapy. The most impressive difference between thrombolysis and primary PCI was the significant reduction of recurrent ischaemia from 21% with thrombolysis to 6%, following primary PCI during short-term and also during long-term follow-up.

Transfer of patients for primary PCI:

There is no doubt that patients presenting within 12 hours after onset of chest pain or other symptoms in hospitals without PCI facilities and having contra-indications to thrombolysis should be immediately transferred to another hospital for coronary angiography and, if applicable, primary PCI, because PCI might be the only chance for quickly opening the coronary artery. Absolute contraindications to thrombolysis are the following conditions:

- Aortic dissection,
- Status post haemorrhagic stroke,
- Recent major trauma/surgery,
- GI bleeding within the last month,
- Known bleeding disorder.

Patients with a contraindication to thrombolysis are known to have a higher morbidity and mortality than those who are eligible. The decision for transferring a patient to a PCI facility will also depend on the individual clinical risk assessment. The choice between PCI and thrombolysis is often dictated by logistical constraints and transport delays (Table 2-4, Figures 2 and 3).

Table 2-4. Recommendations for PCI in NSTE-ACS (STEMI)

Procedure	Indication	Classes of Recommendations and Levels of Evidence	Randomised Studies for Levels of Evidence A or B
Primary PCI	Patients presenting < 12 hours after onset of chest pain/other symptoms and preferably up to 90 min after first qualified medical contact; PCI should be performed by an experienced team	I A	PAMI GUSTO-IIb C-PORT PRAGUE -1 and -2 DANAMI-2
Primary stenting	Routine stenting during primary PCI	I A	Zwolle Stent-PAMI CADILLAC
Primary PCI	When thrombolysis is contraindicated	I C	-
Primary PCI	Preferred more than thrombolysis for patients presenting within > 3 hours and < 12 hours after onset of chest pain/other symptoms	I C	-
Rescue PCI	If thrombolysis failed within 45-60 minutes after starting the administration	I B	REACT
Emergency (multi-vessel) PCI	Cardiogenic shock, in association with IABP even > 12 < 36 hours	I C	-
Routine post-thrombolysis coronary angiography and PCI, if applicable	Up to 24 hours after thrombolysis, independent of angina and/or ischaemia	I A	SIAM III GRACIA-1 CAPITAL-AMI
Ischaemia-guided PCI after successful thrombolysis	Predischarge angina and/or ischaemia after (first) STEMI treated with thrombolysis	I B	DANAMI-1

Within the first 3 hours after onset of chest pain, thrombolysis is a viable alternative (Figure 2). Therefore, within the first 3 hours after onset of chest pain, both reperfusion strategies seem equally effective in reducing infarct size and mortality.

The major reason one could possibly prefer primary PCI over thrombolysis even within the first 3 hours after onset of chest pain is stroke prevention.

In patients presenting 3 to 12 hours after onset of symptoms, myocardial salvage is significantly superior for primary PCI as compared to thrombolysis. It has been demonstrated that with increasing time to presentation, Major Adverse Cardiac Event (MACE) rates increase after thrombolysis but appear to remain relatively stable after PCI. (Figure 2).

Rescue PCI is defined as PCI in a coronary artery that remains occluded despite thrombolytic therapy. Failed thrombolysis is generally suspected when persistent chest pain and non-resolution of ST-segment elevation are evident 45 to 60 min after starting the administration.

Facilitated PCI is defined as planned intervention within 12 hours after onset of chest pain or symptoms, soon after clot dissolving medication to bridge the delay between first medical contact and primary PCI. At the moment, there is no evidence for the recommendation of thrombolysis facilitated primary PCI and no evidence-based recommendation for GP IIb/IIIa inhibitor-facilitated primary PCI to improve patient outcomes.

In cardiogenic shock, emergency PCI may be life saving and should be considered at an early stage. If neither PCI nor surgery is available or can only be provided after a long delay, thrombolytic therapy should be given. In recent years, an increase in revascularisation of patients with AMI complicated for cardiogenic shock was observed, probably due to more frequent admission of eligible patients to hospitals capable of this service (Table 2-4).

Routine angiography early post thrombolysis

Based on the results of randomised clinical trials, routine coronary angiography and - if applicable - PCI early post thrombolysis is recommended (Table 2-4). These trials have contributed to the solution of an old but still pivotal problem: the incidence of re-infarction , the "Achilles' heel" of thrombolysis. Thus, thrombolysis, even if "successful", should not be considered as the final treatment (Table 2-4 and Figure 2).

PCI for patients not having received reperfusion within the first 12 hours

Patients often seek medical attention too late and either do not receive reperfusion therapy or reperfusion therapy fails to successfully recanalise the artery. Late reperfusion therapy is defined as thrombolysis or PCI starting >12 hours after onset of symptoms (for late PCI in cardiogenic shock please see above).

Thrombolytic therapy for the late treatment of patients with STEMI does not reduce infarct size or preserve left ventricular function, probably because it is ineffective in establishing coronary patency. PCI in these patients is supported by the "open artery hypothesis". Although this seems appealing, there is currently no agreement on treatment recommendations for this group of patients.

Figure 2. PCI recommendations in STEMI

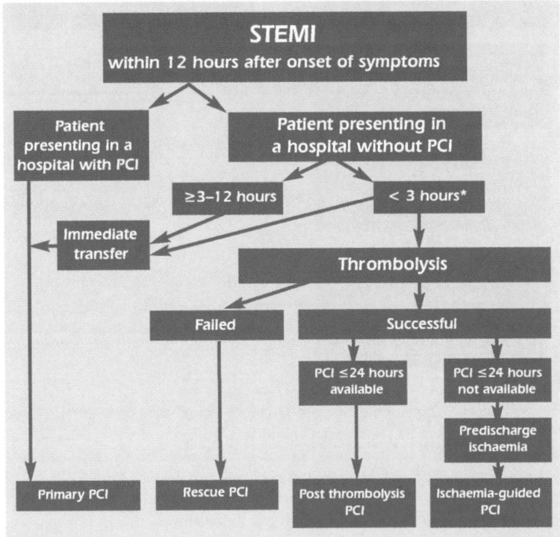

Within the first 3 hours after onset of chest pain or other symptoms, thrombolysis is a viable alternative to primary PCI. *If thrombolysis is contra-indicated or at high risk, immediate transfer for primary PCI is strongly advised. The main rationale for possible preference of primary PCI over thrombolysis within the first 3 hours is stroke prevention. The main rationale for preference of primary PCI over thrombolysis within 3 to 12 hours is to salvage myocardium and to prevent stroke. If thrombolysis is preferred, it should not be considered to be the final treatment. Even after successful thrombolysis, coronary angiography within 24 hours and PCI, if applicable, should be considered. For cardiogenic shock, please see text. For classes of recommendation and levels of evidence please see Table 2-4.

Minimisation of time delays

For all forms of PCI there is unanimous agreement that every effort must be made to minimise any delays between onset of chest pain/other symptoms and the initiation of a safe and effective reperfusion strategy in patients with STEMI. Shortening the total ischaemic time is pivotal, not only for thrombolytic therapy but also for primary PCI (Figure 3). Minimising presentation and treatment delays significantly improves clinical outcome, whereas prolonged symptom-to-treatment times are associated with impaired myocardial perfusion independent of epicardial flow. The effort starts with patient education and includes improvements in organisation of ambulance services as well as optimising procedures within the hospital or private practice (Figure 3).

Figure 3. Solutions to reduce time delays

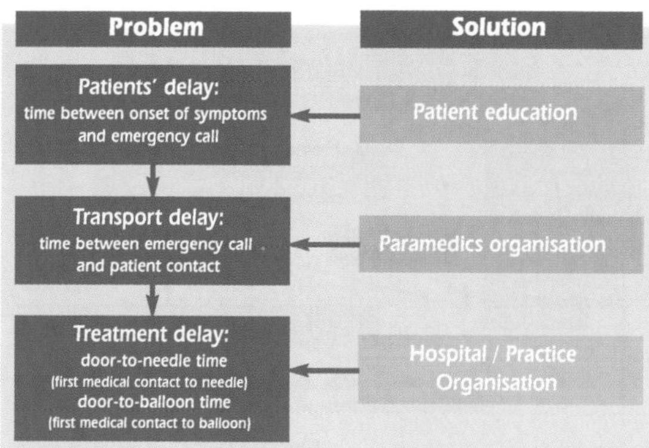

Sources of possible time delays between onset of symptoms and start of reperfusion therapy in patients with STEMI. Solutions to keep the sum of these delays ("total ischaemia time") as low as possible, include improvements in the organisation of ambulance services as well as optimisation of organisation within the hospitals or private practices. Most importantly, patients have to be better educated to minimise the time delay between onset of symptoms and the emergency call.

As far as primary PCI is concerned, all efforts should be made to keep the average time between first medical contact and PCI below 90 minutes, including door to balloon time. Skipping the emergency room and directly transferring STEMI patients to the cath lab additionally reduces door-to-balloon times. However, patients with longer delays should also be treated by primary PCI even when presenting more than 3 hours after onset of symptoms. Only when a substantial delay (e.g. > 2-3 hours) in initiating primary PCI is likely, reperfusion therapy with second or third generation fibrinolytic agents should be considered.

3. Adjunctive Medications for PCI

a. Acetylsalicylic Acid (ASA), Ticlopidine and Clopidogrel

The "double" antiplatelet therapy with ASA and clopidogrel is standard for the pre-treatment of patients with stable CAD undergoing PCI – with or without planned stent implantation (Table 3-1). After implantation of a bare metal stent, clopidogrel must be continued for 3-4 weeks and ASA life-long. In patients presenting with NSTE-ACS, ASA and, if clinically justifiable, immediate administration of clopidogrel, is the basic standard antiplatelet regimen. After the acute phase, the continuation of 100 mg/d ASA + clopidogrel 75mg/d over 9-12 months is beneficial. ASA should be given i.v. to all patients with STEMI as soon as possible after the diagnosis is established - if clinically justifiable. With the concept of primary PCI and primary stenting in STEMI, clopidogrel will be additionally administered in these patients. After brachytherapy, clopidogrel should be administered in addition to ASA for 12 months and after drug-eluting stents for 6 -12 months to avoid late vessel thrombosis.

Table 3-1. Recommendations for Clopidogrel as adjunctive medication for PCI

Indication	Initiation and Duration	Classes of Recommendations and Levels of Evidence	Randomised Studies for Levels of Evidence A or B
Pre-treatment of planned PCI in stable CAD	Loading dose of 300 mg at least 6 hours before PCI, ideally the day before	I C	-
Pre-treatment for primary PCI in STEMI or immediate PCI in NTSE-ACS or ad hoc PCI in stable CAD	Loading dose of 600 mg, immediately after first medical contact, if clinically justifiable	I C	-
After all bare metal stent procedures	3-4 weeks	I A	CLASSICS TOPPS Bad Krozingen
After vascular brachytherapy	12 months	I C	-
After drug-eluting stents	6-12 months	I C	-
After NSTE-ACS	Prolonged for 9-12 months		

b. Unfractionated Heparin (UFH) and Low Molecular Weight Heparins (LMWHs)

UFH is given as an i.v. bolus under activated clotting time (ACT) guidance. Due to their pharmacologic advantages, LMWHs are considered to be more predictable anticoagulants, not requiring laboratory monitoring. However, the data on LMWHs as sole anticoagulant during PCI in stable CAD patients is limited.

UFH is preferred in high risk NSTE-ACS patients with planned invasive strategy and in lower risk patients with planned conservative strategy. If in high risk NSTE-ACS patients an invasive strategy is not applicable for some reason, enoxaparin may be preferred, taking into account an increase in minor bleeding. In patients with STEMI undergoing primary PCI, UFH is the standard therapy.

c. Glycoprotein (GP) IIb/IIIa Inhibitors and Direct Thrombin Inhibitors

Stable CAD

Given the overall low risk of PCI in stable CAD patients, the potential of GP IIb/IIIa inhibitors to increase the risk of bleeding complications and the considerable cost of their use, they are not a part of standard periprocedural medication.

Table 3-2. Recommendations for GP IIb/IIIa inhibitors and Bivalirudin as adjunctive medications for PCI

Medication	Indication	Classes of Recommendations and Levels of Evidence	Randomised Studies for Levels of Evidence A or B
Abciximab, Eptifibatide, Tirofiban in stable CAD	Complex lesions, threatening/ actual vessel closure, visible thrombus, no/slow reflow	IIa C	-
Abciximab, Eptifibatide in NSTE-ACS	Immediately before PCI in high risk patients	I C	-
Tirofiban, Eptifibatide in NSTE-ACS	Pre-treatment before diagnostic angiography and possible PCI within 48 hours in high risk patients ("upstream")	I C	-
Abciximab in NSTE-ACS	In high risk patients with known coronary anatomy in the 24 hours before planned PCI	I C	-
Abciximab in STEMI	All primary PCI (preferably in high risk patients)	IIa A	ADMIRAL, ACE
Bivalirudin	Replacement for UFH or LMWHs (± GP IIb/IIIa inhibitors) to reduce bleeding complications	IIa C	-
Bivalirudin	Replacement for UFH in HIT	I C	-

The use of GP IIb/IIIa inhibitors for PCI in stable angina should be considered on an elective basis. Whenever there is a higher than average risk of acute thrombotic complications (complex interventions, unstable lesions, as bail-out medication in case of threatening/actual vessel closure, visible thrombus or no/slow-reflow phenomenon), GP IIb/IIIa inhibitors are helpful in patients with stable CAD (Table 3-2).

NSTE-ACS

In NSTE-ACS, GP IIb/IIIa inhibitors should be added only in high risk patients, in whom an invasive strategy is planned. For "upstream" management (i.e., initiating therapy when the patient first presents to the hospital and catheterisation is not planned or available within 2.5 hours), tirofiban and eptifibatide show benefit. If cardiac catheterisation is likely to be performed within 2.5 hours, GP IIb/IIIa inhibitors could possibly be postponed and abciximab or eptifibatide initiated in the catheterisation laboratory. If, for some reason, the delay between diagnostic catheterisation and planned PCI is up to 24 hours, abciximab can also be administered.

STEMI

In patients with STEMI, the GP IIb/IIIa inhibitors tirofiban and eptifibatide are less well investigated. In STEMI, stenting plus abciximab seems to be a more evidence-based reperfusion strategy.

Bivalirudin is suggested today as a replacement for UFH (or LMWHs), because of significantly less bleeding compared with UFH alone or UFH + GP IIb/IIIa inhibitors (Table 3-2). Bivalirudin is unanimously recommended for PCI as a replacement for UFH (and LMWHs) in patients with HIT.

4. Adjunctive Devices for PCI

Intracoronary brachytherapy proved to be the only evidence-based non-surgical treatment of in-stent restenosis (Table 4). To avoid late vessel thrombosis, a prolonged intake of clopidogrel for one year after radiation therapy is necessary.

Rotablation is recommended for fibrotic or heavily calcified lesions that can be wired but not crossed by a balloon or adequately dilated before planned stenting. One must know how to manage the complications inherent to rotablation.

PCI of saphenous vein grafts or primary PCI in ACS with a high thrombotic load is at elevated risk for coronary embolisation. Two distal protection devices (GuardWire and FilterWire EX) have proven their safety and efficacy as an adjunctive device for PCI of saphenous vein graft lesions (Table 4).

Whether balloon occlusion and aspiration systems or filter-based catheters will be preferred in other clinical settings such as primary PCI for STEMI, will require more randomised trials with a clinical primary endpoint. At the present time, no definite recommendations can be given regarding the use of embolic protection devices in the setting of STEMI.

Table 4. Recommendations for adjunctive PCI devices

Device	Indication	Classes of Recommendation and Levels of Evidence	Randomised Studies for Levels of Evidence A or B
Brachytherapy	In-stent restenosis in native coronary arteries	I A	SCRIPPS-I GAMMA-1 WRIST LONG-WRIST START INHIBIT
Brachytherapy	In-stent restenosis in saphenous bypass grafts	I B	SVG-WRIST
Cutting Balloon	In-stent restenosis in conjunction with brachy-therapy to avoid geographical miss, slippage of balloons with risk of jeopardising adjacent segments	IIa C	–
Rotablation	Fibrotic or heavily calcified lesions that cannot be crossed by a balloon or adequately dilated before planned stenting	I C	–
DCA	*De novo* ostial or bifurcational lesions in experienced hands	IIb C	–
Distal embolic protection	Saphenous vein grafts	I A	SAFER FIRE
Distal and proximal protection devices	Acute coronary syndromes with high thrombus load in native coronary arteries	IIb C	–
PTFE-covered stents	Emergency tool for coronary perforations	I C	–

DCA, directional coronary arthrectomy; PTFE, polytetrafluoroethylene.

5. Drug-eluting Stents (DES)

Although, a variety of different drugs released from various stent platforms with or without a polymer carrier have been investigated, only two drug-eluting stents have shown significantly positive effects in prospective, randomised studies with clinical primary endpoints at an appropriate time: the Cypher stent (Sirolimus) and the Taxus stent (Paclitaxel).

Evidence-based recommendations for the use of drug-eluting stents must focus on the enrolment criteria of SIRIUS, TAXUS-IV and TAXUS-VI (Table 5). In these patients, target vessel revascularisation rates were single-digit numbers. Subgroup analyses regarding smaller vessels and patients with diabetes are encouraging. Although registry data for in-stent restenosis is promising, randomised trials comparing DES and brachytherapy must be performed in order to give an evidence-based recommendation.

All of the following applications, especially in situations with increased risk of restenosis, must wait for further evidence-based recommendations and are thus presently at IIa C:

- small vessels
- chronic total occlusions
- bifurcational/ostial lesions
- bypass stenoses
- insulin-dependent diabetes mellitus
- multi-vessel disease
- unprotected left main stenoses
- in-stent restenoses

Although randomised trials have yet to be performed, direct stenting (i.e. without pre-dilatation) appears to be safe and effective with the Cypher and the Taxus stents. A convincing reduction of costs in medical care will also be achieved if drug-eluting stents considerably reduce the number of patients undergoing CABG surgery, especially in patients with multi-vessel disease and/or diabetes mellitus.

At the present time, we consider the prolonged (at least 6 months) administration of clopidogrel (in addition to ASA) as mandatory to avoid late stent thrombosis. Therefore, in patients undergoing urgent or scheduled major extracardiac surgery, drug-eluting stents should not be implanted. In these patients, bare stents are probably the safer choice.

Physicians and patients must be made aware that clopidogrel should not be discontinued too early, even for minor procedures like dental care.

Table 5. Recommendations for the use of DES in de novo lesions of native coronary arteries

Drug-eluting stent	Indication	Classes of Recommendations and Levels of Evidence	Randomised Studies for Levels of Evidence A or B
Cypher stent	***De novo*** **lesions in native vessels according to the inclusion criteria**	I B	SIRIUS
Taxus stent	***De novo*** **lesions in native vessels according to the inclusion criteria**	I B	TAXUS-IV
Taxus stent	***De novo*** **long lesions in native vessels according to the inclusion criteria**	I B	TAXUS-VI*

There are only three positive controlled, randomised, adequately powered trials with a primary clinical endpoint at an appropriate time interval.

Main clinical inclusion criteria for SIRIUS, TAXUS-IV and TAXUS-VI were similar: stable or unstable angina or documented ischaemia. The stenoses had to be in native vessels > 50% < 100%. In SIRIUS, reference diameter and lesion length for inclusion were 2.5–3.5 mm and 15–30 mm, respectively. The reference diameter in TAXUS-IV and TAXUS-VI was 2.5–3.75 mm. In TAXUS-IV, the lesion length was 10–28 mm and in TAXUS-VI 18–40 mm. The main common exclusion criteria were acute MI or status post MI with elevated CK/CK-MB, bifurcational or ostial lesions, unprotected left main, visible thrombus, severe tortuosity and/or calcification.

*The moderate release stent used in TAXUS-VI is currently not available.

Section V:
Myocardial Disease

1. Hypertrophic Cardiomyopathy

Chapter 1

Hypertrophic Cardiomyopathy*

2003

Co-chairperson:
Barry J. Maron, MD, FACC, FESC
Minneapolis Heart Institute
Foundation - 920 E 28th Street
Minneapolis, MN 55407 - USA
Phone : +1 (612) 863 3996
Fax: +1 (612) 863 3875
E-mail: hcm.maron@mhif.org

Co-chairperson:
William J. McKenna, MD, FACC, FESC
The Heart Hospital
16-18 Westmoreland Street
London W1G 8PH - UK
Phone: +44 (0)20 7573 8841
Fax: +44 (0)20 7573 8838
E-mail: william.mckenna@uclh.org

Task Force Members:
1. Gordon K. Danielson, Rochester, USA
2. Lukas J. Kappenberger, Lausanne, Switzerland
3. Horst J. Kuhn, Bielefeld, Germany
4. Christine E. Seidman, Boston, USA
5. Pravin M. Shah, Newport Beach, USA
6. William H. Spencer, Charleston, USA
7. Paolo Spirito, Genoa, Italy
8. Folkert J. Ten Cate, Rotterdam, The Netherlands
9. E. Douglas Wigle, Toronto, Canada

ESC Staff:
1. Keith McGregor, Sophia-Antipolis, France
2. Veronica Dean, Sophia-Antipolis, France
3. Dominique Poumeyrol-Jumeau, Sophia-Antipolis, France
4. Catherine Després, Sophia-Antipolis, France

1. Introduction

Hypertrophic Cardiomyopathy (HCM) is a relatively common genetic disorder (1:500) defined by the presence of left ventricular hypertrophy in the absence of a cardiac or systemic cause. It is found in all races and affects men and women equally.

2. Genetics

HCM is inherited as a Mendelian autosomal dominant trait and caused by mutations in any one of 10 genes encoding protein components of the cardiac sarcomere. The most common mutations identified are in the beta-myosin heavy chain, myosin binding protein C and cardiac troponin-T genes. The other genes, which include regulatory and essential myosin light chains, titin, alpha-tropomyosin, alpha-actin, cardiac troponin-I, and alpha-myosin heavy chain, each account for fewer cases. Recently, mutations in the gene encoding the gamma-2-regulatory subunit of the AMP-activated protein kinase have been reported in families with unexplained left ventricular hypertrophy Wolff-Parkinson-White (WPW) syndrome and premature conduction disease. This syndrome is probably more appropriately regarded as a metabolic storage disease distinctive from true HCM.

3. Presentation

HCM can present at any age. Many patients are asymptomatic and are identified incidentally or through screening. When symptoms are present dyspnea, chest pain (which may be anginal or atypical in nature) and impaired consciousness with syncope or presyncope (i.e. dizziness or light-headedness) and palpitation are most common.

4. Diagnosis

4.1 Genetic

Laboratory DNA analysis is the most definitive method for establishing the diagnosis of HCM, however this is not routinely available to most institutions.

4.2 Clinical

ECG: The ECG is abnormal in at least 80% of patients however no specific changes are diagnostic. Left ventricular hypertrophy (LVH) with repolarization abnormalities, pathological Q waves, left and right atrial enlargement are the most common abnormalities detected.

*Adapted from the Clinical Expert Consensus Document on Hypertrophic Cardiomyopathy from the American College of Cardiology and the European Society of Cardiology. (European Heart Journal, 2003, 24 (21): 1965-1991).

Echocardiography: Left ventricular (LV) wall thickening greater than or equal to 15 mm is generally accepted as diagnostic of hypertrophic cardiomyopathy, however, virtually any wall thickness is compatible with the presence of a HCM mutant gene. Hypertrophy is usually associated with a non-dilated and hyperdynamic left ventricle (often with systolic cavity obliteration). Left ventricular outflow tract obstruction, at rest, is seen in approximately one third of patients. Not all patients carrying a HCM causing mutation will express the clinical features (e.g. LVH on echo, abnormal ECG pattern, or disease related symptoms) of the disease. Occasionally mild ECG abnormalities or evidence of diastolic dysfunction assessed by Doppler tissue imaging may precede the development of hypertrophy.

5. Differential diagnosis

Thickening of the LV wall resembling HCM occurs in children (and some adults) with other disease states including Noonan's syndrome, mitochondrial myopathies, Friedreich's ataxia, metabolic disorders, Anderson-Fabry disease, LV non-compaction and cardiac amyloidosis.

6. Pathophysiological features

6.1 Left ventricular outflow tract obstruction (LVOTO)

Obstruction to LV outflow is found in about one third of patients under rest conditions, and may be either subaortic or mid cavity in location. Subaortic obstruction is associated with systolic anterior motion (SAM) of the mitral valve and systolic contact of the anterior or posterior leaflet with the ventricular septum. SAM is usually accompanied by incomplete leaflet apposition with mitral regurgitation (usually mild to moderate in degree). Obstruction in HCM may be fixed (i.e. at rest) or dynamic in which the magnitude of the outflow tract gradient may be labile varying with pharmacological and physiological alterations such as after a heavy meal, ingestion of alcohol or after exercise. Labile gradients are best recorded during and/or immediately following treadmill or bicycle exercise testing.

6.2 Diastolic dysfunction

Diastolic dysfunction with abnormal myocardial relaxation and increased chamber stiffness is common and results in impaired ventricular filling, elevated left atrial and LV end-diastolic pressures (with reduced stroke volume and cardiac output) pulmonary congestion, and impaired exercise performance.

6.3 Myocardial ischaemia

Myocardial ischaemia in HCM is thought to be a consequence of abnormal intramural coronary arterioles with thickened walls (from medial hypertrophy) and narrowed lumen, and/or mismatch between the increased ventricular mass and coronary flow. Ischaemia may lead to myocardial fibrosis and scarring and as a consequence, contribute to systolic and diastolic dysfunction. Ischaemia may also contribute to ventricular arrhythmia and sudden death. The evaluation of ischaemia in HCM however is problematic as non-invasive screening tests such as exercise testing and thallium scintigraphy are difficult to interpret in the presence of ventricular hypertrophy.

Atherosclerotic coronary artery disease is often overlooked and coronary arteriography is indicated in patients with HCM who are over the age of 40 years or who have risk factors for coronary artery disease.

7. Examination

Clinical signs are usually limited to patients with outflow tract obstruction. In these patients there may be a rapid upstroke, arterial pulse, a forceful left ventricular impulse, and a palpable left atrial beat with a prominent "a" wave in the jugular venous pulse. A fourth heart sound is occasionally heard. The murmur of outflow tract obstruction is mid-late systolic and may be increased by physiologic manoeuvres that decrease afterload or venous return (standing or valsalva). The majority of patients with outflow murmurs also have a mitral regurgitation murmur.

8. Treatment

Most patients with HCM have no or only mild symptoms and require no treatment. In patients with symptoms the aim of treatment is to alleviate symptoms and improve exercise capacity.

9. Medical therapy

9.1 Beta-adrenergic blocking agents

Beta-blockers are usually the first line treatment for patients with or without obstruction that have symptoms of exertional dyspnoea or exercise intolerance. The beneficial effects of beta-blockers on symptoms and exercise tolerance appear to be largely due to a decrease in the heart rate with a consequent prolongation of diastole with increased relaxation time and passive ventricular filling. These agents reduce LV contractility, limit latent outflow tract gradient and decrease myocardial oxygen demand and myocardial ischaemia.

9.2 Verapamil

Verapamil in doses up to 480mg per day has favourable effects on symptoms (particularly chest pain) probably by virtue of improving ventricular relaxation and filling as well as reducing myocardial ischaemia and LV contractility. Occasionally adverse haemodynamic side effects can occur as a result of vasodilatation resulting in augmented outflow tract obstruction, pulmonary oedema and cardiogenic shock. Because of these concerns, caution should be exercised in administrating Verapamil to patients with resting left ventricular outflow tract obstruction (LVOTO).

9.3 Disopyramide

Disopyramide has been shown to reduce SAM, outflow tract obstruction and mitral regurgitation and produce symptomatic benefit in patients with resting obstruction. Anticholinergic side effects such as dry mouth and eyes, constipation, indigestion and difficulty in micturition may be reduced by long acting preparations for which cardioactive benefits are more sustained. Because disopyramide may cause accelerated atrioventricular (A-V) nodal conduction and thus increase ventricular rate during atrial fibrillation/flutter supplementary therapy with beta-blockers in low doses is advised. Disopyramide should not be used together with sotalol or amiodarone because of risk of proarrhythmia.

9.4 Diuretics

Diuretics may be used in patients with hypertrophic cardiomyopathy and heart failure symptoms. However, because many patients have diastolic dysfunction and require relatively high filling pressures to achieve adequate ventricular filling diuretics should be administered cautiously and preferably in the absence of marked outflow obstruction.

10. Treatment options for drug-refractory patients

Patients with marked LVOTO at rest or with provocation (peak gradient usually greater than or equal to 50mmHg) and severe limiting symptoms of exertional dyspnoea (New York Heart Association [NYHA] III or IV), chest pain and presyncope or syncope, refractory to maximal medical therapy may be considered for non-medical therapies.

10.1 Surgery

The ventricular septal myectomy operation (Morrow procedure) is the gold standard approach to reduce LVOTO in both adults and children. The myectomy operation should be confined to centres experienced with this procedure.

Myectomy is performed through an aortotomy and involves resection of a carefully defined small amount of muscle from the proximal septum extending from near the base of the aortic valve to beyond the distal margins of mitral leaflets, thereby enlarging the left ventricular outflow tract (LVOT), and reducing left ventricular outflow tract obstruction (LVOTO). Other procedures such as mitral valve replacement or repair are occasionally indicated in selected patients with severe mitral regurgitation due to intrinsic abnormalities of the valve apparatus. Muscular mid-cavity obstruction due to anomalous papilliary muscle requires an extended distal myectomy or alternatively mitral valve replacement. Operative mortality in patients at the most experienced centres is around 1-2% or less but may be higher in elderly patients undergoing additional cardiac surgical procedures. Complications such as complete heart block (requiring permanent pacemaker) and iatrogenic ventricular septal perforation are uncommon.

10.2 Percutaneous Alcohol Septal Ablation (ASA)

This involves the introduction of absolute alcohol into a target septal perforator branch of the left interior descending coronary artery (LAD) guided by myocardial contrast echocardiography. Septal ablation mimics the haemodynamic consequences of myectomy by reducing basal septal thickness and excursion (producing akinetic or hypokinetic septal motion), enlarging the left ventricular outflow tract (LVOT) and thereby lessening mitral valve SAM and mitral regurgitation. After ASA there may be rapid reduction in resting left ventricular outflow tract gradient (LVOTG) but more frequently, a progressive decrease in the gradient occurs during the first 6 to 12 months.

Mortality and morbidity associated with ASA in experienced centres is similar to that of surgical myectomy. Permanent PM implantation due to induced high-grade A-V block has been reduced from 30% to 5% with the use of smaller amounts of alcohol. Myocardial infarction from coronary artery dissection, backward extravasation of alcohol producing LAD occlusion or abrupt coronary no-flow are rare complications. There is also concern that extensive wall thinning could lead to arrhythmogenic susceptibility or even end stage disease and the potential long term risk for arrhythmia related cardiac events is unknown. Proper selection of patients for ASA is crucial.

10.3 Dual chamber pacing

Although initial reports suggested that pacing was associated with a substantial decrease in LVOTO and improvements in symptoms, subsequent randomised studies showed no objective improvements after pacing. Despite this pacing may be an option for severely symptomatic older patients with LVOTO refractory to medical therapy for whom other alternatives are undesirable.

11. Drugs for "end stage"

Up to 5% of patients with HCM may develop systolic dysfunction and heart failure, usually associated with left ventricular wall thinning and chamber enlargement. Drug treatment strategies in such patients involve conversion to after load reducing agents such as ACE inhibitors or angiotensin II receptor blockers or diuretics, digitalis, beta-blockers or spironolactone. Ultimately patients with end stage heart failure may become candidates for heart transplantation.

11.1 Atrial fibrillation (AF)

Paroxysmal or established AF develops in 20-25% of HCM patients and is related to advancing age and left atrial enlargement. AF is associated with heart failure related death, occurrence of fatal and non-fatal stroke as well as long-term disease progression with heart failure symptoms. Electrical or pharmacological cardioversion is indicated in patients presenting within 48 hours of onset of AF assuming the presence of atrial thrombi can be excluded or after a suitable period of anticoagulation therapy. Amiodarone is the most effective antiarrhythmic agent for preventing recurrences of AF. In chronic AF, beta-blockers and verapamil are effective in controlling heart rate, although A-V nodal ablation and permanent pacing is occasionally necessary. Anticoagulant therapy (with warfarin) is indicated in patients with either paroxysmal or chronic AF and the threshold for anticoagulation should be low.

12. Infective endocarditis prophylaxis

In HCM there is a small risk of bacterial endocarditis, which appears largely confined to patients with LVOTO or intrinsic valve disease. Therefore patients with evidence of LVOTO at rest or during exercise should be given antibiotic prophylaxis at the time of dental or selected surgical procedures that create a risk for blood borne bacteraemia.

13. Pregnancy

Patients with HCM generally tolerate pregnancy and delivery well. Absolute maternal mortality is very low and appears to be principally confined to women who are severely symptomatic or have high-risk clinical profiles. Such patients should be afforded specialised joint cardiac and obstetric care during pregnancy and delivery.

13.1 Sudden Cardiac Death

Sudden cardiac death is the most common mode of premature demise in HCM and often occurs in asymptomatic or mildly symptomatic young people. Sudden cardiac death most frequently occurs in adolescents and young adults less than 30 to 35 years although risk extends through mid life and beyond. Sudden cardiac death most commonly occurs during mild exertion or sedentary activities (including sleep).

Available data suggests that ventricular tachyarrhythmias (VT) are the most common mechanism by which sudden cardiac death occurs in HCM. Other triggers/contributing factors include supraventricular arrhythmias, ischaemia, inappropriate vasodilation and conduction disease.

13.2 Risk Stratification

HCM patients (particularly those less than 60 years of age) should undergo clinical assessments on an annual basis, for risk stratification as well as evolution of symptoms. It is possible to identify most high risk patients by non-invasive clinical markers. The highest risk of sudden death has been associated with the following:

- Prior cardiac arrest or spontaneously occurring and sustained VT.
- Family history of premature cardiac death particularly if sudden, in a close relative, or if multiple in occurrence.
- Unexplained syncope, particularly when exertional, recurrent or in young patients.
- Non sustained ventricular tachycardia ≥ 3 beats at rate ≥ 120 beats per minute) on 24 hour ambulatory ECG recordings.
- Abnormal BP response during upright exercise which is attenuated or hypotensive particularly in patients less than 50 years.
- Severe LVH with a Maximal Left Ventricular Wall Thickness (MLVWT) of 30 mm or more.

Some disease causing mutations have been associated with adverse prognosis (e.g. troponin-T and Arg403Gln and Arg719Gln in beta-myosin heavy chain).

However, most of the clinical markers of sudden death risk in HCM are limited by relatively low positive predictive values due in part to relatively low event rates. However, the high negative predictive values of these markers suggest that the absence of these markers can be used to develop a profile of patients with lower likelihood for sudden death.

14. Prevention of sudden cardiac death

Patients with prior cardiac arrest (ventricular fibrillation) or sustained and spontaneously occurring VT are at greatest risk and most deserving of an implantable defibrillator for secondary prevention of sudden death. Otherwise, the highest risk for sudden death has been associated with multiple risk factors. Individual patients with a single major risk factor are also often eligible for primary prevention of sudden death with an implantable defibrillator. Management decisions should be based on individual judgement taking into account the overall clinical profile including age, strength of the risk factor and the level of risk acceptable to the patient and family. Although amiodarone has been associated with improved survival in HCM, and may be suitable in highly selected patients, the implantable cardioverter defibrillator (ICD) is the most effective and reliable prophylactic treatment option available.

15. Exercise recommendations

The consensus is that young patients with HCM should be restricted from intense competitive sports to reduce the risk of sudden cardiac death. Intense physical activity involving burst exertion (e.g. sprinting) or systematic isometric exercise (e.g. heavy lifting) should also be discouraged.

16. Screening

Screening of first-degree relatives and other family members should be encouraged. When DNA based diagnosis is not feasible, the recommended clinical strategies for screening family members involves history and physical examination, 12 lead ECG, and two dimensional echocardiography at annual evaluations during adolescence (12 to 18 years of age). Due to the possibility of delayed onset LVH, it is prudent for adult relatives with normal ECG and echocardiograms beyond age 18 to have subsequent clinical studies performed about every 5 years, particularly if there is a history of late onset disease within the family.

17. HCM in the elderly

HCM, due to sarcomere protein mutations may manifest itself later in life and should be distinguished from non-genetic hypertensive heart disease or age-related changes.

Older patients with HCM generally show relatively mild degrees of LVH and mild symptoms. Some elderly patients, however, have large subaortic gradients caused by systolic apposition of the anterior or posterior mitral valve leaflet with the septum in association with accumulation of calcium within the mitral annulus. Definitive clinical diagnosis of HCM in older patients with LVH and systemic hypertension may be difficult; particularly when the LV wall thickness is less than 20 mm and SAM is absent. In the absence of genotyping, marked LVH disproportionate to the level of blood pressure elevation, unusual patterns of LVH unique to HCM, or obstruction to LV outflow at rest represent presumptive evidence for HCM.

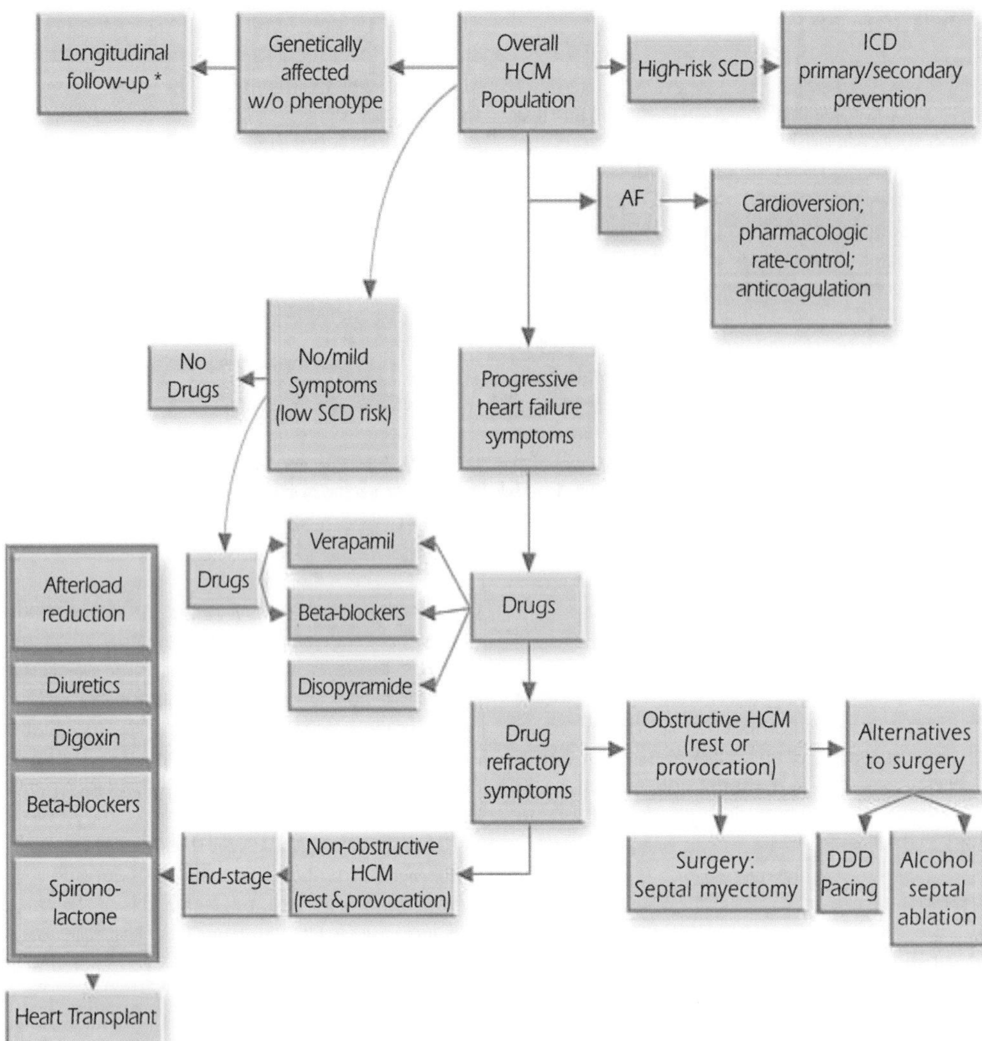

Fig. 1 Clinical presentation and treatment strategies for patient subgroups within the broad clinical spectrum of hypertrophic cardiomyopathy (HCM). See text for details. AF = atrial fibrillation; DDD = dual-chamber; ICD = implantable cardioverter-defibrillator; SCD = sudden cardiac death; and RX = treatment. Table adapted with permission from "Spirito P, Seidman CE, McKenna WJ, Maron BJ. The management of hypertrophic cardiomyopathy. N Engl J Med 1997; 336:775-85". * No specific treatment or intervention indicated, except under exceptional circumstances.

Section VI: Pericardial Disease

1. Management of Pericardial Diseases

Chapter 1

Management of Pericardial Diseases*

2004

Chairperson:
Bernhard Maisch, FESC
Director of the Department of Internal Medicine-Cardiology,
Heart Centre of Philipps-University
Baldingerstrasse 1, D-35043 Marburg, Germany
Phone: + 49 64 21 28 66 462
Fax: + 49 64 21 28 68 954
E-mail: BerMaisch@aol.com

Task Force Members:
1. Petar M. Seferovic, Belgrade, Serbia and Montenegro
2. Arsen D. Ristic, Belgrade, Serbia and Montenegro
3. Raimund Erbel, Essen, Germany
4. Rainer Rienmüller, Graz, Austria
5. Yehuda Adler, Tel Hashomer, Israel
6. Witold Z. Tomkowski, Warsaw, Poland
7. Gaetano Thiene, Padua, Italy
8. Magdi H. Yacoub, Harefield, UK

ESC Staff:
1. Keith McGregor, Sophia Antipolis, France
2. Veronica Dean, Sophia Antipolis, France
3. Catherine Després, Sophia Antipolis, France
4. Xue Li, Sophia Antipolis, France

Introduction

These are the first guidelines on the management of pericardial diseases to be published by the European Society of Cardiology (ESC). These are actually the first official guidelines written on the subject worldwide. The main objective of this document is to present cardiologists with guidelines for the Diagnosis and Management of Pericardial Diseases, focusing on the most clinically relevant abnormalities.

Class I	Evidence and/or general agreement that a given diagnostic procedure/treatment is beneficial, useful and effective;
Class II	Conflicting evidence and/or a divergence of opinion about the usefulness/efficacy of the treatment;
Class IIa	Weight of evidence/opinion is in favour of usefulness/efficacy;
Class IIb	Usefulness/efficacy is less well established by evidence/opinion;
Class III*	Evidence or general agreement that the treatment is not useful/effective and in some cases may be harmful.

* Use of Class III is discouraged by the ESC

Classes of recommendations and levels of evidence

Recommendations for various tests and procedures are ranked in three classes (see opposite)

The level of evidence related to a particular diagnostic or treatment option depends on the available data (see below)

Level of Evidence A	Data derived from multiple randomized clinical trials or meta-analyses
Level of Evidence B	Data derived from a single randomized clinical trial or large non-randomized studies
Level of Evidence C	Consensus opinion of the experts and/or small studies; retrospective studies and registries

*Adapted from the ESC Guidelines on the Diagnosis and Management of Pericardial Diseases (European Heart Jounal 2004; 25: 587-610).

Acute pericarditis

Table 1. Diagnostic pathway and sequence of performance in acute pericarditis (level of evidence B for all procedures)

TECHNIQUE	CHARACTERISTIC FINDINGS
Obligatory (class I):	
Auscultation	Pericardial rub (mono-, bi-, or triphasic)
ECG[a]	*Stage I:* anterior and inferior concave ST-segment elevation. PR segment deviations opposite to P polarity. *Early stage II:* ST junctions return to the baseline, PR deviated. *Late stage II:* T waves progressively flatten and invert *Stage III:* generalised T wave inversions *Stage IV:* ECG returns to prepericarditis state.
Echocardiography	Effusion types B-D (Horowitz) Signs of tamponade (Table 2)
Blood analyses	a) ESR, CRP, LDH, leukocytes (inflammation markers) b) cTnI, CK-MB (markers of myocardial lesion)[b]
Chest X-ray	Ranging from normal to "water bottle" heart shadow. Revealing additional pulmonary/mediastinal pathology.
Mandatory in tamponade (class I), optional in large/recurrent effusions or if previous tests inconclusive (class IIa) in small effusions (class IIb):	
Pericardiocentesis and drainage	Pericardial fluid cytology, and cultures, PCRs and histochemistry for determination of infection or neoplasia.
Optional or if previous tests inconclusive (class IIa):	
CT	Effusions, peri-, and epicardium
MRI	Effusions, peri-, and epicardium
Pericardioscopy, pericardial biopsy	Establishing the specific aetiology

[a] Typical lead involvement: I, II, aVL, aVF, and V3-V6. The ST-segment is always depressed in aVR, frequently inV1, and occasionally in V2. Occasionally, stage IV does not occur and there are permanent T wave inversionsand flattenings. If ECG is first recorded in stage III, pericarditis cannot be differentiated by ECG from diffuse myocardial injury, "biventricular strain," or myocarditis. ECG in EARLY REPOLARISATION is very similar to stageI. Unlike stage I, this ECG does not acutely evolve and J-point elevations are usually accompanied by a slur, oscillation, or notch at the end of the QRS just before and including the J point (best seen with tall R and T waves large in early repolarisation pattern). Pericarditis is likely if in lead V6 the J point is >25% of the height of the T wave apex (using the PR segment as a baseline).

[b] cTnI - cardiac troponin I. It is detectable in 32.2-49%, more frequently in younger, male patients, with ST-segment elevation, and pericardial effusion at presentation. An increase beyond 1.5 ng/ml is rare (7.6-22%), and associated with CK-MB elevation. cTnI increase is not a negative prognostic marker regarding the incidence of recurrences, constrictive pericarditis, cardiac tamponade or residual LV dysfunction.

Management

Figure 1. Diagnosis and management of major pericardial syndromes

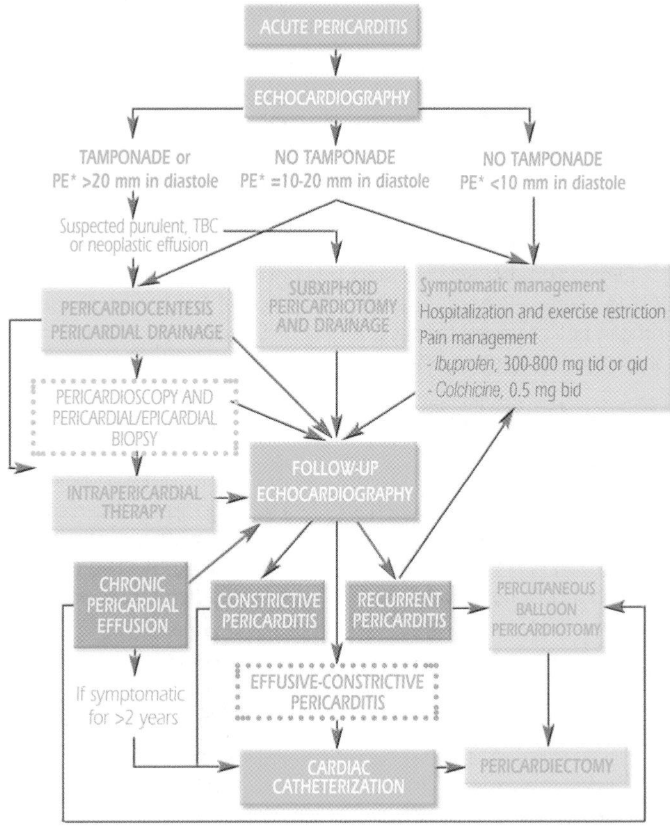

* PE: Pericardial Effusion

Symptomatic management

- Exercise restriction
- Hospitalization is warranted to determine the aetiology and observe for tamponade as well as the effect of treatment.
- Pain management
    - Nonsteroidal anti-inflammatory drugs (NSAID) are the mainstay (class I, level of evidence B).
    - *Ibuprofen* is preferred for its rare side-effects, favourable impact on the coronary flow, and the large dose range. Depending on severity and response, 300-800 mg every 6-8 hours may be initially required and can be continued for days or weeks, best until the effusion has disappeared.
    - *Aspirin* 300-600 mg every 4-6 hours is an alternative regimen.
    - Indomethacin should be avoided in elderly patients due to its flow reduction in the coronary artery.
    - Gastrointestinal protection must be provided.

Treatment and prevention of recurrences

- *Colchicine* (0.5 mg bid) added to a NSAID or as monotherapy also appears to be effective for the initial attack and the prevention of recurrences (class IIa, level of evidence B). It is well tolerated with fewer side-effects than NSAIDs.
- *Percutaneous balloon pericardiotomy* can be considered in cases resistant to medical treatment (class IIb, level of evidence B).
- *Corticosteroids* should be used only in patients with poor general condition or in frequent crises (class IIa, level of evidence C). A common mistake is to use a dose too low to be effective or to taper the dose too rapidly. The recommended regimen is prednisone 1-1.5 mg/kg, for at least one month. If patients do not respond adequately, azathioprine (75-100 mg/day) or cyclophosphamide can be added. Corticoids should be tapered over a three-month period.
- *Pericardiectomy* is indicated only in frequent and highly symptomatic recurrences resistant to medical treatment (class IIa, level of evidence B). Before pericardiectomy, the patient should be on a steroid-free regimen for several weeks.

Pericardial effusion and cardiac tamponade

Table 2. Diagnosis of cardiac tamponade

Clinical presentation:	Elevated systemic venous pressure[a], tachycardia[b], pulsus paradoxus[c], hypotension[d], dyspnoea or tachypnoea with clear lungs.
Precipitating factors:	Drugs (cyclosporine, anticoagulants, thrombolytics, etc.), recent cardiac surgery, indwelling instrumentation, blunt chest trauma, malignancies, connective tissue disease, renal failure, septicaemia[e].
ECG:	Can be normal or non-specifically changed (ST-T wave), electrical alternans (QRS, rarely T), bradycardia (end-stage), Electromechanical dissociation (agonal phase).
Chest X-ray:	Enlarged cardiac silhouette with clear lungs.
M-mode/2D echocardiogram:	Diastolic collapse of the anterior RV free wall[f], RA collapse, LA and very rarely LV collapse, increased LV diastolic wall thickness "pseudohypertrophy", IVC dilatation (no collapse in inspiration), "swinging heart".
Doppler:	1) Tricuspid flow increases and mitral flow decreases during inspiration (reverse in expiration). 2) Systolic and diastolic flows are reduced in systemic veins in expiration and reverse flow with atrial contraction is increased.
M-mode colour Doppler:	Large respiratory fluctuations in mitral/tricuspid flows.
Cardiac catheterization:	1) Confirmation of the diagnosis and quantification of the haemodynamic compromise: • RA pressure is elevated (preserved systolic x descent and absent or diminished diastolic y descent) • Intrapericardial pressure is also elevated and virtually identical to RA pressure (both pressures fall in inspiration) • RV mid-diastolic pressure elevated and equal to the RA and pericardial pressures (no dip-and-plateau configuration) • Pulmonary artery diastolic pressure is slightly elevated and may correspond to the RV pressure. • Pulmonary capillary wedge pressure is also elevated and nearly equal to intrapericardial and right atrial pressure. • LV systolic and aortic pressures may be normal or reduced. 2) Documenting that pericardial aspiration is followed by haemodynamic improvement[g]. 3) Detection of the coexisting haemodynamic abnormalities (LV failure, constriction, pulmonary hypertension). 4) Detection of associated cardiovascular diseases (cardiomyopathy, coronary artery disease).
RV/LV Angiography:	Atrial collapse and small hyperactive ventricular chambers.
Coronary angiography:	Coronary compression in diastole.
Computer tomography:	No visualization of subepicardial fat along both ventricles, which show tube-like configuration and anteriorly drawn atria.

LA = left atrium, LV = left ventricle, RA = right atrium, RV = right ventricle, IVC = inferior vena cava. [a] Jugular venous distension is less notable in hypovolemic patients or in "surgical tamponade". An inspiratory increase or lack of fall of the pressure in the neck veins (Kussmaul sign), when verified with tamponade, or after pericardial drainage, indicates effusive-constrictive disease. [b] Heart rate is usually >100 beats/min, but may be lower in hypothyroidism and in uremic patients. [c] The blood pressure cuff is inflated above the patient's systolic pressure. During slow deflation, the first Korotkoff sound is intermittent. Correlation with the patient's respiratory cycle identifies a point at which the sound is audible during expiration, but disappears when the patient breathes in. As the cuff pressure drops further, another point is reached when the first Korotkoff sound is audible throughout the respiratory cycle. The difference of >10 mmHg in systolic pressure between these two points is accepted as positive pulsus paradoxus. For quick clinical orientation the sign can be also investigated by simply feeling the pulse, which diminishes significantly during inspiration, when the patient is breathing normally. Pulsus paradoxus is absent in tamponade complicating atrial septal defect and in patients with significant aortic regurgitation. Caution: the patient should breathe normally – no deep inspirations. [d] Some patients are hypertensive especially if they have pre-existing hypertension. [e] Febrile tamponade may be misdiagnosed as septic shock. [f] Right ventricular collapse can be absent in elevated right ventricular pressure and right ventricular hypertrophy or in right ventricular infarction. [g] If after drainage of pericardial effusion intrapericardial pressure does not fall below atrial pressure, the effusive-constrictive disease should be considered.

Indications for pericardiocentesis

Class I

- Cardiac tamponade.
- Effusions >20 mm in echocardiography (diastole).
- Suspected purulent or tuberculous pericardial effusion.

Class IIa

- Effusions 10-20 mm in echocardiography in diastole for diagnostic purposes other than purulent pericarditis or tuberculosis (pericardial fluid and tissue analyses, pericardioscopy, and epicardial/pericardial biopsy).
- Suspected neoplastic pericardial effusion.

Class IIb

- Effusions <10 mm in echocardiography in diastole for diagnostic purposes other than purulent; neoplastic or tuberculous pericarditis (pericardial fluid and tissue analyses, pericardioscopy and epicardial/pericardial biopsy). In symptomatic patients diagnostic pericardial puncture should be reserved for dedicated centers.

Contraindications

- Aortic dissection.
- Relative contraindications include uncorrected coagulopathy, anticoagulant therapy, thrombocytopenia <50,000/mm^3, small, posterior and loculated effusions.
- Pericardiocentesis is not necessary when the diagnosis can be made otherwise or the effusions are small and resolving under anti-inflammatory treatment.

How to perform pericardiocentesis

- Obtain recent and reliable echocardiography findings (best immediately before the procedure). The operator performing pericardiocentesis needs to observe the echocardiogram.
- Pericardiocentesis guided by fluoroscopy should be performed in the cardiac catheterization laboratory under local anaesthesia. The subxiphoid approach has been used most commonly, with a 8-17 cm long blunt-tip needle (e.g. Tuohy-17) permitting the passage of the guidewire, directed towards the left shoulder at a 30° angle to the frontal plane.
- Pericardiocentesis guided by echocardiography can be performed in the intensive care unit, or at the bedside. Echocardiography should identify the shortest route to enter the pericardium intercostally (usually in the sixth or seventh rib space in the anterior axillary line). The intercostal arteries should be avoided by puncturing close to the upper margin of the rib.
- It is essential that the needle approaches the pericardium slowly under steady manual aspiration (negative pressure). As soon as the pericardial effusion is aspirated a soft J-tip guidewire should be inserted and after dilatation exchanged for a multi-holed pigtail catheter.
- Strict aseptic conditions, ECG and blood pressure monitoring have to be provided.
- Direct ECG monitoring from the puncturing needle is not an adequate safeguard.
- Right-heart catheterization can be performed simultaneously, allowing the assessment of tamponade, haemodynamic monitoring of pericardiocentesis and exclusion of constriction.
- In large pericardial effusions it is prudent to drain <1 L at the time of initial procedure to avoid the acute right-ventricular dilatation.
- Prolonged pericardial drainage is recommended after pericardiocentesis until the volume of effusion obtained by intermittent pericardial aspiration (every 4-6 h) falls to <25 mL per day.

Analyses of pericardial effusion

Should be carried out according to the clinical presentation.

Class I

- Cytology in suspected **malignant disease**.
- In **suspected tuberculosis** acid-fast bacilli staining, PCR analyses for tuberculosis, mycobacterium culture (preferably with radiometric growth detection e.g., BACTEC-460), adenosine deaminase (ADA), interferon (IFN)-gamma and pericardial lysozyme should be performed.
- In suspected **bacterial infection** cultures of pericardial fluid for aerobes and anaerobes as well as three blood cultures are mandatory. Positive cultures should be followed by sensitivity tests for antibiotics.

Class IIa

- PCR analyses for cardiotropic viruses discriminate viral from auto-reactive pericarditis.
- Tumour markers (carcinoembryonic antigen (CEA), alpha-feto protein (AFP), carbohydrate antigens CA 125, CA 72-4, CA 15-3, CA 19-9, CD-30, CD-25, etc.) should be estimated in suspected neoplastic pericarditis.
- The staining of epithelial membrane antigen, CEA and vimentin can be distinguished between reactive mesothelial and adenocarcinoma cells.

Class IIb

- Analyses of the pericardial fluid specific gravity (>1.015), protein level (>3.0 g/dL; fluid/serum ratio >0.5), LDH (>200mg/dL; serum/fluid >0.6), and glucose (exudates vs. transudates = 77.9±41.9 vs. 96.1±50.7 mg/dL) can separate exudates from transudates but are not directly diagnostic.

Constrictive pericarditis

Table 3. Diagnostic approach in constrictive pericarditis

Clinical presentation:	Severe chronic systemic venous congestion associated with low cardiac output, including jugular venous distension, hypotension with a low pulse pressure, abdominal distension, oedema and muscle wasting.
ECG:	Can be normal, or reveal low QRS voltage, generalized T wave inversion/flattening, LA abnormalities, atrial fibrillation, atrioventricular block, intraventricular conduction defects, or rarely pseudoinfarction pattern.
Chest X-ray:	Pericardial calcifications, pleural effusions.
M-mode/2D echocardiogram:	Pericardial thickening and calcifications[a] as well as the indirect signs of constriction: - RA & LA enlargement with normal appearance of the ventricles, and normal systolic function. - Early pathological outward and inward movement of the interventricular septum ("dip-plateau phenomenon"). - Flattering waves at the LV posterior wall. - LV diameter is not increasing after the early rapid filling phase. - IVC and the hepatic veins are dilated with restricted respiratory fluctuations.[b]
Doppler:	Restricted filling of both ventricles with respiratory variation >25% over the AV-valves.[c]
TEE:	Measurement of the pericardial thickness.
CT/MRI:	Thickened and/or calcified pericardium, tube-like configuration of one or both ventricles, enlargement of one or both atria, narrowing of one or both atrio-ventricular grooves, congestion of the caval veins.
Cardiac catheterization:	"Dip and plateau" or "square route" sign in the pressure curve of the right and/or left ventricle. Equalisation of LV/RV end-diastolic pressures in the range of 5 mmHg or less.[d]
RV/LV angiography:	The reduction of RV & LV size and increase of RA & LA size. During diastole a rapid early filling with stop of further enlargement ("dip-plateau")
Coronary angiography:	In all patients over 35 years and in patients with a history of mediastinal irradiation, regardless of the age.

LA = left atrium, LV = left ventricle, RA = right atrium, RV = right ventricle, IVC = inferior vena cava, TEE = transoesophageal echocardiography. [a] Thickening of the pericardium is not always equal to constrictive physiology. [b] Diagnosis is difficult in atrial fibrillation. Hepatic diastolic vein flow reversal in expiration is observed even when the flow velocity pattern is inconclusive. [c] Patients with increased atrial pressures or mixed constriction and restriction demonstrate <25% respiratory changes. A provocation test with head-up tilting or sitting position with decrease of preload may unmask the constrictive pericarditis. [d] In the early stage or in the occult form, these signs may not be present and the rapid infusion of 1-2 L of normal saline may be necessary to establish the diagnosis. Constrictive haemodynamics may be masked or complicated by valvular- and coronary artery disease.

Table 4. Differential diagnosis: constrictive pericarditis vs. restrictive cardiomyopathy

METHOD	RESTRICTIVE CARDIOMYOPATHY	CONSTRICTIVE PERICARDITIS
Physical findings	Kussmaul's sign ±, apical impulse +++ S_3 (advanced), S_4 (early disease), regurgitant murmurs ++	Kussmaul's sign +, apical impulse – pericardial knock+, regurgitant murmurs –
ECG	Low voltage, pseudoinfarction, left-axis deviation, AF, conduction disturbances.	Low voltage (<50%)
Chest radiography	No calcifications	Calcifications may be present (low diagnostic accuracy)
2D-echocardiography	Small LV cavity with large atria. Increased wall thickness sometimes present (especially thickened interatrial septum in amyloidosis). Thickened valves and granular sparkling (amyloidosis).	Normal wall thickness Pericardial thickening, prominent early diastolic filling with abrupt displacement of IVS.
Doppler studies		
Mitral inflow	No respiration variation of mitral inflow E wave velocity, IVRT. E/A ratio 2, short DT, diastolic regurgitation.	Inspiration: decreased inflow E wave velocity, prolonged IVRT Expiration: opposite changes, short DT, diastolic regurgitation
Pulmonary vein	Blunted S/D ratio (0.5), prominent and prolonged AR. No respiration variation, D wave.	S/D ratio = 1, Inspiration: decreased PV, S and D waves Expiration: opposite changes
Tricuspid inflow	Mild respiration variation of tricuspid inflow E wave velocity, E/A ratio 2, TR peak velocity, no significant respiration change, Short DT with inspiration, diastolic regurgitation.	Inspiration: increased tricuspid inflow E wave velocity, increased TR peak velocity, Expiration: opposite changes, Short DT, diastolic regurgitation
Hepatic veins	Blunted S/D ratio, increased inspiratory reversals. Inspiration: minimally increased HV S and D	Expiration: decreased diastolic flow / increased reversals
Inferior vena cava	Plethoric	Plethoric
Mitral annular motion	Low-velocity early filling (<8 cm/s)	High-velocity early filling (≥8 cm/s)
Colour M-mode	Slow flow propagation	Rapid flow propagation (≥100 cm/s)
Tissue Doppler echocardiography	Peak early velocity of longitudinal expansion (peak Ea) of < 8.0 cm/s or normal	Peak early velocity of longitudinal expansion (peak Ea) of ≥ 8.0 cm/s (89% sensitivity and 100% specificity)
Cardiac catheterization	Dip and plateau LVEDP often >5 mmHg greater than RVEDP, but may be identical, RV systolic pressure >50 mmHg RVEDP < 1/3 RVSP.	Dip and plateau, RVEDP and LVEDP usually equal, Inspiration: Increase in RV systolic pressure. Decrease in LV systolic pressure, with Expiration, opposite
EMB	May reveal specific cause of restrictive cardiomyopathy.	May be normal or show nonspecific hypertrophy or fibrosis.
CT/MRI	Pericardium usually normal.	Pericardium must be thickened or calcified.

Management

- Pericardiectomy is the only treatment for permanent constriction.
- The indications are based upon clinical symptoms, echocardiography findings, CT/MRI, and heart catheterization.
- There are two standard approaches, both aiming at resecting the diseased pericardium as far as possible: 1) The **antero-lateral thoracotomy** (fifth intercostal space) and 2) **median sternotomy** (faster access to the aorta and right atrium for extracorporeal circulation).
- A primary installation of cardiopulmonary bypass is not recommended (diffuse bleeding following systemic heparinization).
- Areas of strong calcification or dense scaring may be left as islands to avoid major bleeding.
- Pericardiectomy for constrictive pericarditis has a mortality rate of 6-12%.
- Major complications include acute perioperative cardiac insufficiency and ventricular wall rupture.
- Cardiac mortality and morbidity at pericardiectomy is mainly caused by the pre-surgically unrecognised presence of **myocardial atrophy or myocardial fibrosis**. Exclusion of patients with extensive myocardial fibrosis and/or atrophy significantly reduces the mortality rate for pericardiectomy.
- Post-operative low cardiac output should be treated by fluid substitution and catecholamines, high doses of digitalis, and intra-aortic balloon pump in most severe cases.
- If indication for surgery was established early, long-term survival after pericardiectomy corresponds to that of the general population.

Viral pericarditis

Diagnosis

- The diagnosis of viral pericarditis is not possible without the evaluation of pericardial effusion and/or pericardial/epicardial tissue, preferably by PCR or in-situ hybridization (class IIa, level of evidence B).
- A four-fold rise in serum antibody levels (two samples within 3-4 weeks) is suggestive but not diagnostic for viral pericarditis (class IIb, level of evidence B).

Management

- In most cases the disease is self-limiting and no specific treatment is necessary.
- Symptomatic treatment for chest pain, eventual rhythm disorders and congestive heart failure is indicated.
- In large effusions and cardiac tamponade pericardiocentesis is necessary.
- In patients with chronic or recurrent symptomatic pericardial effusion and confirmed viral infection, the following specific treatment is under investigation:
  1) CMV pericarditis: hyperimmunoglobulin 4 mL/kg once daily, on days 0, 4 and 8; 2 mL/kg on days 12 and 16;
  2) Coxsackie B pericarditis: Interferon alpha or beta 2.5 million IU/m2 surface area subcutaneously 3 x per week;
  3) Adenovirus and parvovirus B19 perimyocarditis: immunoglobulin treatment 10 g intravenously on day 1 and 3 for 6-8 hours.

Bacterial pericarditis

Diagnosis

- Percutaneous pericardiocentesis must be promptly performed if bacterial pericarditis is suspected.
- Pericardial fluid should undergo Gram, acid-fast and fungal staining, followed by cultures for aerobes, anaerobes and M. tuberculosis (preferably with radiometric growth detection).
- Drug sensitivity testing is essential for treatment selection.
- PCR analyses, increased levels of adenosine deaminase (>40 IU/L), interferon-gamma (200 pg/L), or pericardial lysozyme (6.5 microg/dL) are highly sensitive and specific for diagnosis of tuberculous effusion.

Management (class I, level of evidence B)

- Urgent pericardial drainage, combined with intravenous antibiotic therapy (e.g. vancomycin 1 g bid, ceftriaxone 1-2 g bid, and ciprofloxacin 400 mg/day) is mandatory in purulent pericarditis.
- In selecting antimicrobial therapy the ability of potential agents to kill the causative organism, as well as the minimum inhibitory concentration (MIC - the lowest concentration that inhibits growth) and

minimum bactericidal concentration (MBC – the lowest concentration that decreases a standard inoculum of organisms 99.9% during 24 hours) need to be considered.

- Irrigation with urokinase or streptokinase, using large catheters, may liquify the purulent exudate, but open surgical drainage is preferable.

- The initial treatment of tuberculous pericarditis should include isoniazid 300 mg/day, rifampicin 600 mg/day, pyrazinamide 15-30 mg/kg/day and ethambutol 15-25 mg/kg/day. After two months most patients can be switched to a two-drug regimen (isoniazid and rifampicin) for the total of six months.

- Prednisone (1-2 mg/kg/day) may be given simultaneously with antituberculous therapy for 5-7 days and progressively reduced to discontinuation in 6-8 weeks.

- Patients with tuberculous pericarditis should be put in respiratory isolation if active pulmonary or laryngeal tuberculosis is also suspected. Determination of the absolute lack of infectiousness requires demonstration that cultures become negative. However, in clinical practice, conversion to negative smear results is used as a surrogate for infectiousness. Patients are considered to be non-infectious if they have a clinical response to anti-tuberculous chemotherapy and three consecutive smear-negative sputum samples that were collected on different days.

- Persons with HIV infection and tuberculosis usually can be treated with standard anti-tuberculous regimens with good results, although in some cases, prolonged therapy may be warranted.

- Since treatment of HIV may require protease inhibitors or non-nucleoside reverse transcriptase inhibitors, use of rifampicin may be precluded. The use of corticoid therapy as an adjunct to tuberculostatic treatment is allowed (class I, level of evidence B).

- Pericardiectomy is reserved for recurrent effusions or continued elevation of central venous pressure after 4-6 weeks of antituberculous and corticosteroid therapy.

Pericarditis in renal failure

Diagnosis

- Chest pain, pericardial friction rub and pericardial effusion in a patient with advanced renal failure (acute or chronic). This can occur before dialysis has been instituted or in patients on maintenance chronic haemodialysis or peritoneal dialysis.

- Due to autonomic impairment in uremic patients, heart rate may remain slow (60–80 beats/min) during tamponade, despite fever and hypotension.

- The ECG does not show the typical diffuse ST/T wave elevations observed with other causes of acute pericarditis due to the lack of the myocardial inflammation.

Management

- Frequent haemo- or peritoneal dialysis.

- To avoid haemopericardium, heparin-free haemodialysis should be used.

- Peritoneal dialysis, which does not require heparinization, may be therapeutic in pericarditis resistant to haemodialysis, or if heparin-free haemodialysis cannot be performed.

- NSAIDs and systemic corticosteroids have limited success when intensive dialysis is ineffective.

- Cardiac tamponade and large chronic effusions resistant to dialysis must be treated with pericardiocentesis (class IIa, level of evidence B).

- Large, non-resolving symptomatic effusions should be treated with intrapericardial instillation of corticosteroids after pericardiocentesis or subxiphoid pericardiotomy (triamcinolone hexacetonide 50 mg every 6 hours for 2 to 3 days).

- Pericardiectomy is indicated only in refractory, severely symptomatic patients. Autoreactive pericarditis and pericardial involvement in systemic autoimmune diseases.

Autoreactive pericarditis and pericardial involvement in systemic autoimmune diseases

Diagnosis

- Increased number of lymphocytes and mononuclear cells >5,000/mm^3 (autoreactive lymphocytic), or the presence of antibodies against heart muscle tissue (antisarcolemmal) in the pericardial fluid (autoreactive antibody-mediated).

- Inflammation in epicardial/endomyocardial biopsies by 14 cells/mm^2.

- Exclusion of active viral infection both in pericardial effusion and endomyocardial/epimyocardial biopsies (no virus isolation, no IgM-titer against cardiotropic viruses in pericardial effusion, and negative PCR for major cardiotropic viruses).

- Tuberculosis, Borrelia burgdorferi, Chlamydia pneumoniae, and other bacterial infection excluded by PCR and/or cultures.
- Neoplastic infiltration absent in pericardial effusion and biopsy samples.
- Exclusion of systemic, metabolic disorders and uraemia.

Management

- Intrapericardial treatment with triamcinolone plus colchicine per os 0.5 mg bid for six months is highly efficient with rare side-effects. (class IIa, level of evidence B).
- In systemic autoimmune diseases (rheumatoid arthritis, systemic lupus erythematosus, progressive systemic sclerosis, polymyositis/dermatomyositis, mixed connective tissue disease, seronegative spondyloarthropathies, systemic and hypersensitivity vasculitides, Behçet syndrome, Wegener granulomatosis, and sarcoidosis) intensified treatment of the underlying disease and symptomatic management are indicated (class I, level of evidence B). For tapering of prednisone, ibuprofen or colchicine should be introduced early.

The post-cardiac injury syndrome: postpericardiotomy syndrome

Diagnosis

- Chest pain, pericardial friction rub, ECG changes, pericardial effusion within days to months after cardiac, pericardial injury or both.

Management

- Symptomatic treatment is as in acute pericarditis (NSAIDs or colchicine for several weeks or months, even after disappearance of effusion).
- Long term (3-6 months) oral corticoids or preferably pericardiocentesis and intrapericardial instillation of triamcinolone (300 mg/m^2) are therapeutic options in refractory forms.
- Redo surgery and pericardiectomy are very rarely needed.
- Primary prevention of postperiocardiotomy syndrome using short-term perioperative steroid treatment or colchicine is under investigation.
- Warfarin administration in patients with early post-operative pericardial effusion imposes the greatest risk, particularly in those who did not undergo pericardiocentesis and drainage of the effusion.

Post-infarction pericarditis

(pericarditis epistenocardica and Dressler's syndrome)

Diagnosis

- Pericarditis epistenocardica: detection of pericardial effusion 1-5 days after acute myocardial infarction.
- ECG changes may often be overshadowed by myocardial infarction changes.
- Post-infarction pericardial effusion >10 mm is most frequently associated with haemopericardium, and two thirds of these patients may develop tamponade/free wall cardiac rupture.
- Dressler's syndrome occurs from one week to several months after clinical onset of myocardial infarction with symptoms and manifestations similar to the post-cardiac injury syndrome.

Management

- Hospitalization to observe for tamponade, differential diagnosis and adjustments of treatment.
- Ibuprofen, which increases coronary flow, is the agent of choice.
- Aspirin, up to 650 mg every 4 hours for 2 to 5 days has also been successfully applied (other nonsteroidal agents risk thinning the infarction zone).
- Corticosteroid therapy can be used for refractory symptoms only but could delay myocardial infarction healing (class IIa, level of evidence B).
- In cardiac rupture, urgent surgical treatment is life-saving. However, if immediate surgery is not available or contraindicated pericardiocentesis, an intra-pericardial fibrin-glue instillation could be an alternative in subacute tamponade.

Traumatic pericardial effusion

- Urgent echocardiography, trans-esophageal echo-cardiography (TEE) if available.
- Rescue pericardiocentesis
- Autotransfusion

- Urgent thoracotomy and surgical repair.

Haemopericardium in aortic dissection

Diagnosis

- Urgent echocardiography, in unclear cases TEE
- CT or MRI in complex or unclear cases
- Angiography (only in stable patients).

Management

- Pericardiocentesis is contraindicated due to the risk of intensified bleeding and extension of the dissection.
- Surgery should be performed immediately (class I, level of evidence B).

Neoplastic pericarditis

Diagnosis

- Confirmation of the malignant infiltration within the pericardium (cytology, histology, tumour markers if available) (class I, level of evidence B).
- Of note, in almost 2/3 of the patients with documented malignancy, pericardial effusion is caused by non-malignant diseases, e.g. radiation pericarditis or opportunistic infections.

Management

- Systemic antineoplastic treatment as baseline therapy which can prevent recurrences in up to 67% of cases (class I, level of evidence B).
- Pericardiocentesis to relieve symptoms and establish diagnosis (class IIa, level of evidence B).
- Intrapericardial instillation of cytostatic/sclerosing agent (class IIa, level of evidence B). Cisplatin (single instillation of 30 mg/m^2) is preferred for pericardial metastases of lung cancer and intrapericardial instillation of thiotepa (15 mg on days 1,3 and 5) or cisplatin for breast cancer.
- Pericardial drainage is recommended in all patients with large effusions because of the high recurrence rate (40-70%) (class I, level of evidence B).
- In resistant cases percutaneous balloon pericardiotomy or rarely pericardiectomy may be indicated (patients with very large chronic effusion in whom repeated pericardiocentesis and/or intrapericardial therapy were not successful).
- Radiation therapy is very effective (93%) in controlling malignant pericardial effusion (class IIa, level of evidence B) in patients with radiosensitive tumours such as lymphomas and leukemias. However, radiotherapy of the heart can cause myocarditis and pericarditis by itself.

Pericardial effusion in pregnancy

Diagnosis

- Many pregnant women develop a minimal to moderate clinically silent hydropericardium by the third trimester. Cardiac compression is rare.
- ECG changes of acute pericarditis in pregnancy should be distinguished from the slight ST-segment depressions and T wave changes seen in normal pregnancy.
- Occult constriction becomes manifest in pregnancy due to the increased blood volume.

Management

- Most pericardial disorders are managed as in non-pregnant.
- Caution is necessary while high-dose aspirin may prematurely close the ductus arteriosus.
- Colchicine is contraindicated in pregnancy.
- Pericardiotomy and pericardiectomy can be safely performed if necessary and do not impose a risk for subsequent pregnancies.

Foetal pericardial effusion

- Foetal pericardial fluid can be detected by echocardiography after 20 weeks' gestation and is normally 2 mm or less in depth.
- More fluid should raise questions of hydrops foetalis, Rh disease, hypoalbuminemia, immunopathy or maternally-transmitted mycoplasmal or other infections, and neoplasia.

Drug- and toxin-related pericardial disease

Table 5. Drug- and toxin-related pericardial disease

A. Drug-induced lupus erythematosus		
• Procainamide • Tocainide • Hydralazine	• Methyldopa • Mesalazine • Reserpine	• Isoniazid • Hydantoins
B. Hypersensitivity reaction		
• Penicillins	• Tryptophan	• Cromolyn sodium
C. Idiosyncratic reaction or hypersensitivity		
• Methysergide • Minoxidil • Practolol • Bromocriptine • Psicofuranine • Polymer fume inhalation • Cytarabine	• Phenylbutazone • Amiodarone • Streptokinase • p-Aminosalicylic acid • Thiazides • Streptomycin • Thiouracils	• Sulfa drugs • Cyclophosphamide • Cyclosporine • Mesalazine • 5-Fluorouracil • Vaccines (Smallpox, Yellow fever) • GM-CSF
D. Anthracycline derivatives		
• Doxorubicin	• Daunorubicin	
E. Serum sickness		
• Foreign antisera (e.g., antitetanus)	• Blood products	
F. Venom		
• Scorpion fish sting		
G. Foreign-substance reactions (direct pericardial application)		
• Talc (Mg silicate) • Silicones	• Tetracycline/other sclerosants • Asbestos	• Iron in beta-thalassemia
H. Secondary pericardial bleeding/haemopericardium		
• Anticoagulants	• Thrombolytic agents	
I. Polymer fume fever – Inhalation of burning fumes of polytetrafluoroethylene (Teflon)		

Section VII: Congenital Heart Disease

1. Grown Up Congenital Heart Disease

2. Neonatal Electrocardiogram

Chapter 1

Grown Up Congenital Heart Disease*

2003

Chairperson:
John Deanfield

Address for correspondence:
Professor Andreas Hoffmann
Div. of Cardiology, Univ. Hospital
CH-4031 Basel / Switzerland
Tel: + 41 (0) 61 279 9822
Fax: + 41 (0) 61 279 9823
Email: andreas.hoffmann@unibas.ch

Task Force Members:
1. Margreet Bink-Boelkens, Groningen, The Netherlands
2. Luciano Daliento, Padua, Italy
3. Andreas Hoffmann, Basel, Switzerland
4. Laurence Iserin, Paris, France
5. Harald Kaemmerer, München, Germany
6. Frantisek Kolbel, Praha, Czech Republic
7. Andrew Redington, Toronto, Canada
8. Eric Silove†, Birmingham, UK
9. Keld Sorensen, Braband, Denmark
10. Erik Thaulow, Oslo, Norway
11. Ulf Thilen, Lund, Sweden
12. Pascal Vouhe, Paris, France
13. Carol Warnes, Rochester, USA
14. Gary Webb, Philadelphia, USA

Document writing group:
John Deanfield, Andreas Hoffmann, Harald Kaemmerer, Erwin Oechslin‡

ESC Staff:
1. Keith McGregor, Sophia Antipolis, France
2. Veronica Dean, Sophia Antipolis, France
3. Catherine Després, Sophia Antipolis, France
4. Xue Li, Sophia Antipolis, France

1. Introduction & background

As a result of the success of paediatric cardiology and cardiac surgery over the last 3 decades, there will shortly be more adults than children with congenital heart disease. The need to reintegrate paediatric and adult cardiac services, and in particular to provide smooth "transition" for adolescents is clear.

In this pocket version the special healthcare needs of grown-ups with congenital heart disease and common principles of management are presented in a table format. These represent a consensus view of the panellists, and where possible, are evidence-based.

In this report, we have stratified care recommendations into 3 levels: exclusive follow-up in the specialised unit (level 1), shared care with local informed adult unit (level 2), and predominantly non-specialist care (level 3).

The number of grown-up congenital heart disease patients with individual lesions depends on the incidence at birth, early mortality in childhood as well as the rate of late death. In the absence of hard figures we have developed a simple programme, which enables prediction of late survival rates by entering estimates for each of these outcome determinants. This is available on the ESC Web Site and will be useful for planning of resource requirements and funding.

The establishment of specialised centres to manage the complex grown-up heart disease population is a priority. These centres will provide the basis for research into new areas of cardiology, such as the interaction between congenital and acquired heart problems in older patients. Specialised centres should not 'disenfranchise' local physicians, both in general cardiology and primary care, who have an important role in a hierarchical local, regional and supraregional service.

* Adapted from the ESC Guidelines on the Management of Grown-Up Congenital Heart Disease (European Heart Journal 2003; 24(11): 1035-1084).
†Representative of the Association for European Paediatric Cardiology
‡Chairman of Working Group GUCH 2002-2004

2. Organisation of care

Transition of care	Age 16-18, involving patient, parents, paediatric and adult cardiologist, specialist nurse. Topics should include understanding of disease, future prospects, follow-up visits, medication, prophylaxis of BE, insurance, exercise and sports, career planning, pregnancy and contraception (stepwise approach!).
Levels of care	1) exclusively at specialist centre 2) shared care between adult cardiac unit and specialised centre 3) nonspecialised care
Specialist centre	Serving population of 5-10 million with trained GUCH specialist. The special needs are best covered by a multidisciplinary team in a specialised centre (cath. & EP lab, cong. cardiac surgery, transplantation, MRI, CT, OB/Gyn).

3. Medical issues

Ventricular function	
• Accurate measurement of ventricular performance is the most important part of the preoperative assessment, perioperative management and follow-up.	• Echocardiography (TTE, TOE). Transthoracic windows may be poor; interpretation of results in adults with acquired heart disease may not be transferable to those with CHD! Sequential data are more important than a single measurement.
• Difficult due to the complex anatomy, altered ventricular geometry, effects of previous surgery, extraordinary loading conditions, chronic hypoxia, etc.	• Magnetic resonance imaging. Ventricular end-diastolic/end-systolic volumes, ejection fraction; muscle mass, quantification of regurgitant lesions. Assessment of myocardial performance may add to dimension-based indices.
• Right ventricular (RV) function is very important in CHD patients as the RV may support systemic circulation.	• Radionuclide studies. Wall motion abnormalities, ischaemia.
• Appropriate subspecialty expertise in congenital heart disease is required in the assessment and interpretation of results!	• Invasive studies. Full haemodynamic evaluation.

Arrhythmias and Pacing

General aspects

- Arrhythmias are a frequent cause of morbidity/mortality and the commonest reason for hospital admission.
- Factors predisposing to arrhythmias: underlying cardiac defect, haemodynamic burden, residuae and sequelae of cardiac surgery (scar tissue).
- Electrical and mechanical connection: arrhythmias may result from a haemodynamic burden and lead to severe haemodynamic decline!
- Supraventricular arrhythmias are more frequent than ventricular arrhythmias.

- Supraventricular arrhythmias:
  - Sinus node dysfunction
  - Supraventricular tachycardias (intra-atrial re-entry tachycardia, atrial flutter, atrial fibrillation)

Most frequent after
  - Senning/Mustard procedures
  - Fontan procedures
  - ASD closure (>40 years of age)
  - Repair of Tetralogy of Fallot

- Ventricular arrhythmias:
  - Repair of Tetralogy of Fallot
  - Left ventricular outflow tract obstruction
- Risk stratification for ventricular arrhythmias:
  - Underlying cardiac defect
  - Surgical procedures (time, type)
  - Haemodynamic burden
  - QRS prolongation

- Close integration of the GUCH cardiologist Electrophysiologist with expertise and skills required for patients with CHD, and the GUCH surgeon is mandatory.

Specific recommendations

Pharmacological therapy:
- Limitations: haemodynamic side effects, concomitant sinus node dysfunction, pregnancy.
- Effect of many antiarrhythmics is disappointing.
- Amiodarone is most effective.

Catheter ablation and surgical approaches:
- Lower success rate than in acquired heart disease due to complicated and multiple arrhythmia circuits.
- Combined electrophysiological-surgical revision strategy may be of some success in the most challenging population (Tetralogy of Fallot and 'failing' Fontan patients, Ebstein's anomaly).

Pacemaker (PM):
- Consider limited and abnormal venous access as well as the abnormal cardiac anatomy itself.
- Epicardial systems may be required.
- Fixation of the electrodes may be difficult (consider active fixation).
- Thromboembolic risk in the setting of intracardiac shunts may preclude an endocardial approach.
- Dual chamber pacing and rate response system are desirable.

Implantable Cardioverter Defibrillator (ICD):
- Identification of patients at high risk for malignant arrhythmias and sudden death.

PM and ICD implantation should be performed only by a team with expertise in congenital heart disease.

Cyanosis

- Cyanosis is caused by a right to left shunt at atrial, ventricular or arterial level, may exist with or without pulmonary hypertension.
- It is a multisystem disorder affecting many organ systems.

Haematologic consequences

- Secondary erythrocytosis
- Increased blood viscosity symptoms may include: headache, poor concentration, visual disturbances, fatigue, tinnitus, muscle weakness and pain.
- White blood cell count is normal.
- Platelet count may be normal or reduced.

- Routine phlebotomy is never indicated
- Indication for phlebotomy:
  To relieve moderate to severe hyperviscosity symptoms (no more than 2-3 times per year). To donate autologous blood before surgery if haematocrit > 65%.

- Iron deficiency is frequently caused by unnecessary, repeated phlebotomies and may cause hyperviscosity-like symptoms!

- Do not perform phlebotomy in the setting of iron deficiency! Ec indices insufficient to rule out iron deficiency, add Fe and ferritine measurements.
- Replete iron stores and discontinue administration of ferrous sulfate (325 mg daily) as soon as haemoglobin starts to rise (recheck haemoglobin within 7-10 days). Consider intravenous iron replacement (iron saccharose is safe and well tolerated).

- Dehydration (fever, diarrhoea, etc.) may cause hyperviscosity symptoms.

- Rehydrate and do not perform phlebotomy!

Haemostasis

- Platelet count and function may be reduced
- Intrinsic and extrinsic coagulation pathway may be abnormal:
  - Prolonged aPTT, thrombin time, elevated INR, etc.
- Minor bleeding is common
- Major bleeding is rare

- The use of anticoagulants and antiplatelet agents must be confined to well-defined indications.
- Adjustment of the amount of sodium citrate is mandatory to get accurate coagulation measurements if the haematocrit level is >60%.

Thromboembolic complications

- Dehydration and iron deficiency increase the risk of vascular events!
- Intravenous access does have the potential risk for air embolism into pulmonary and systemic circulations.

- Avoid dehydration and iron deficiency!
- Use an air filter in the setting of an intravenous access.

Renal function

- Glomerular function is decreased
- Proteinuria is common
- Urate clearance is abnormal

- Hyperuricaemia without clinical gout does probably not require treatment.

Miscellaneous

- Acne (potential source of bacteraemia)
- Fragile gingiva
- Infectious disease with high mortality

- Use a soft brush
- Annual flu shot and pneumovax to reduce the risk of infection.

Pulmonary Vascular Disease

• Early diagnosis and improved cardiac surgery have reduced the number of adults with pulmonary vascular disease.	
• Any intervention carries the risk of destabilisation. • Careful management reduces morbidity and mortality. • The quality of life of Eisenmenger patients is good into 3rd decade.	• Policy of 'non-intervention' unless absolutely indicated, is indicated to avoid destabilising the 'balanced physiology. • The decision whether to anticoagulate is controversial.
• The potential for morbidity is high: • haematological and haemostatic abnormalities (see cyanosis) • Pulmonary and cerebral complications are most important.	• There are no data demonstrating improved survival with anticoagulation

• Haemoptysis:
  • Stress/excitement or pulmonary infection may precipitate haemoptysis.
  • Identification of patients at risk is difficult.
	• Do not perform routine bronchoscopy.
	• Consider bedrest.
	• Avoid anticoagulants/antiplatelet agents.
	• Treat pulmonary infection.

• Cerebral complications:
  • TIA/Stroke or abscess
  • No association with higher haematocrit levels
	• Routine phlebotomy does not prevent TIA/stroke.

• Special risk for Eisenmenger patients
  • Dehydration
  • Iron deficiency
  • Cardiac and non-cardiac surgery
  • General anaesthesia
  • Pulmonary infection
  • Anaemia
  • Altitude
  • Intravenous lines
  • Pregnancy (high mortality for both the mother and the foetus)
  • Systemic vasodilatation
	• Avoid dehydration
	• Avoid iron deficiency
	• Careful consideration to any intervention/procedures.
	• Anaesthesia must be performed by cardiac anaesthesist.
	• Annual flu shot / pneumovax
	• No routine phlebotomy (haemoglobin level of 16 g/dl is too low!!).
	• Use an air filter
	• Contraception (methods see below)
	• Systemic vascular resistance may decrease resulting in increase of right to left shunt.

<u>Therapeutic options:</u> • Inhaled prostacyclin/systemic endothelin antagonists/sildenafil • Long-term oxygen therapy • End-stage pulmonary vascular disease	• Symptoms may improve; no clinical trial evidence available yet. • Symptoms may improve, but morbidity and survival will not be modified. • Consider heart-lung transplantation sooner rather than later.

Infective Endocarditis

- Life-long risk of infective endocarditis in most congenital heart defects (exception: secundum ASD, anomalous pulmonary venous connection, VSD after closure, pulmonary valvar stenosis or small patent ductus arteriosus).

- Education of patients and their physicians about risks and importance of early diagnosis.
- Insertion of intrauterine contraceptive devices and delivery should be covered by antibiotics.

- Delay in diagnosis and referral is common.
- Antibiotics are too often prescribed before blood cultures are taken!
- Vegetations may be missed by transthoracic echocardiography.
- Transoesophageal echocardiography increases the detection of vegetations.

- Withdrawal of two blood cultures before administration of antibiotics.
- Prompt referral to specialist unit in the setting of haemodynamic deterioration.
- Management of infective endocarditis should be performed in collaboration with an infectious disease specialist; surgery may be required.
- Treatment of endocarditis: ESC Task Force on Infective Endocarditis, Horstkotte et al; Eur Heart J 2004; 25: 267-276

Imaging

- Non-invasive imaging modalities are the principal methods in the assessment of adults with congenital heart disease.
- Cardiac catheterisation is reserved for specific anatomical and physiological questions (e.g. coronary arteries, pulmonary vascular resistance) or interventions.
- All imaging techniques require staff with expertise in complex congenital heart disease.

- Echocardiography (TTE and TOE)
- Magnetic Resonance Imaging (MRI) is becoming the investigation of choice providing information on anatomy, morphology and physiology:
    - Right ventricular volume and mass
    - Right ventricle to pulmonary artery conduit/valve function
    - Pulmonary arteries
    - Aortic coarctation
    - Systemic/pulmonary venous anomalies
- Ultra fast Computed Tomography (CT) and multislice CT now play a major role in the evaluation of congenital heart disease.

Interventional Catheterisation

• An interventional programme is crucial for a GUCH unit. • Previous experience in children is more relevant than experience in coronary interventions. • Randomised studies against surgical alternatives are almost non-existent.	• The decision to perform interventions should be discussed by a multi-disciplinary team. • Special expertise, training and experience are required.
<u>Balloon dilation</u> • Aortic valvoplasty: residual aortic regurgitation is the most important complication. • Pulmonary valve dilation is usually successful.	• Balloon dilation of previous patch aortoplasty carries a high risk of aortic rupture.
<u>Balloon dilation with stent implantation</u> • Technique of first choice for branch and distal pulmonary arterial stenosis and stenosis in surgical venous pathways (Mustard, Senning, Fontan). • Utility to be proven for aortic coarctation, stenotic aorto-pulmonary collaterals or shunts.	• Questionable in dilation of right ventricular outflow tract obstruction, stenotic right ventricular to pulmonary arterial conduits and systemic arterial stenosis.
<u>Embolisation and occlusion techniques</u> • Method of choice in closure of patent ductus arteriosus/venous and arterial collaterals and fistulous communications. • Standard practice in patent foramen ovale and selected cases of secundum atrial septal defect (suitable atrial and septal anatomy). • Baffle leaks, systemic arterial, coronary and venous fistulous communications may be closed by devices.	• Unanswered questions: little evidence base for PFO closure; degree of acceptable pulmonary hypertension and need for concomitant atrial arrhythmia procedures in secundum ASD.
<u>Percutaneous valve implantation</u> • Implantation of a stent mounted bovine jugular venous valve into the right ventricular outflow tract in patients with severe pulmonary regurgitation after Tetralogy of Fallot repair.	• Advantage: non-surgical management of pulmonary regurgitation. • Disadvantage: lack of long-term results. • Still experimental procedure.

Pregnancy

- Females with (complex) congenital heart disease now reach the childbearing age!
- Most females with congenital heart disease can tolerate pregnancy with proper care.
- Maternal and foetal risks including risk of inherited congenital heart disease have to be assessed.
- Impact of pregnancy on long-term survival is unknown.

- Pre-pregnancy evaluation:
  - Complete history (including family history)
  - Physical examination
  - Doppler-echocardiography (haemodynamic assessment!)
  - Functional capacity (exercise testing)
  - Genetic counselling
  - Review of medications
- Pre-pregnancy counselling, evaluation and risk stratification are mandatory.
  Avoid teratogenic drugs.

High risk patients

- Eisenmenger syndrome
- Severe pulmonary hypertension without shunt
- Severe aortic stenosis (mean gradient >40 mmHg, valve area <0.7 cm^2)
- Severe aortic coarctation
- Significant mitral stenosis (MVA<1.5)
- Reduced systemic ventricular function (EF<35%)
- Mechanical valve prosthesis
- Marfan's syndrome (aortic root >40mm)
- Cyanotic congenital heart disease (O_2 ≤ sat 85%)

- Counselling against pregnancy!
- Management of high risk patients:
  - Referral to a tertiary care centre: the multidisciplinary team (obstetrician, cardiologist expert, anaesthesist, paediatrician) should be involved from early pregnancy, plan monitoring of the pregnancy, mode of delivery and post delivery care.
  - Iron and prenatal vitamins (to prevent anaemia)
  - Foetal cardiac ultrasound
  - Bed rest as pregnancy advances
  - Vaginal delivery is preferable to caesarean section (unless there are obstetric indications).
  - Prophylaxis of venous thromboembolism

Mechanical valves

- Management is challenging
- Heparin therapy carries the risk of thromboembolic complications.
- Warfarin treatment is safer for the mother; the risk of foetal embryopathy appears to be small if warfarin dose is < 5 mg per day.

- Role of low molecular weight heparin is not established.

Cyanotic congenital heart disease

- Foetal risk is porportional to the degree of maternal hypoxia (O_2 sat ≤ 85%).

- Low birth weight for gestational age and prematurity are common.

Contraception

• The risk of pregnancy must be weighed against the risk of contraception. • The patient should choose her own preferred method of contraception.	The physician advises the least hazardous contraceptive method.
Barrier methods	• Safe, high contraceptive efficacy in compliant couples/women>35 years
Oral contraceptive pills Low dose oestrogen combined pills	• Very efficacious, but thrombogenic (e.g. Fontan patients, cyanosis, atrial fibrillation/flutter). • Contraindication if risk of paradoxical embolism, systemic or pulmonary hypertension.
Medroxyprogesterone (Depo-Provera®), levonorgestrel (Norplant®) or progesterone only pills	• Effective, but risk of fluid retention, depression, breakthrough bleeding and higher failure rate than with the combined oral contraceptives.
Intrauterine devices They are not the first choice in patients without previous pregnancy. The risk of pelvic inflammatory disease was overestimated in the past.	• Antibiotic prophylaxis should be given at insertion and at extraction.
Surgical sterilization	• Surgical risk must be considered! • May be the method of choice.

Recurrence Risk/Genetic Counselling

• Data about the recurrence risk in couples where the mother or father has a congenital heart defect are limited. • Genetic counselling should be available in specialised units.	• Recurrence rate of congenital heart disease in offspring ranges from 2-50%. • Single gene disorders and/or chromosome abnormalities have the highest recurrence risks: • Marfan's syndrome, Noonan's syndrome, Holt-Oram syndrome, cong. forms of HCM.
• Foetal echocardiography should be offered at 16-18 weeks gestation. • Chorionic villous sampling or amniocentesis may also be indicated in selected cases. • Teratogenic effect of drugs	• ACE-inhibitors, angiotensin II-receptor antagonists, warfarin, amiodarone.

Co-Morbidity

• Cognitive and intellectual impairment may result from co-existing heritable or chromosomal syndromes in up to 20% of pts.	• Special care and support needed.
• Perinatal and perioperative neurological complications have a serious impact on the adult life and produce an important demand on medical and social institutions.	• Close collaboration among the multi-disciplinary team is the key to solve the broad spectrum of co-morbidities. • Non-cardiac specialists must be involved in the care.
• Acquired heart disease will occur as the population ages.	
• Skeletal abnormalities	
• Cyanotic congenital heart diseases	• See cyanosis
• Psychosocial impact of co-morbidities must be addressed.	

Syndromes associated with cardiac defects and mental deficits

Syndrome	General Features	Cardiac Defect
Foetal Alcohol Syndrome	Facial and growth anomaly, mental retardation	ASD, VSD (30%)
Down (trisomy 21)	Mental retardation, typical facies, lymphedema	AVSD, VSD, aortic valve anomaly in 40%
Noonan	Turner like phenotype, normal chromosomes, mental retardation	Coarctation, HCM, ASD, PS
Turner	Chromosome XO, skeletal and mental deficits	Coarctation in 35%, ± bicuspid aortic valve
Williams Beuren	Facial dysplasia, hypervitaminosis D, hypocalcaemia, mental retardation	Supravalvar aortic stenosis, sometimes with multiple pulmonary artery stenoses.

Emergencies

• The most frequent emergencies are: • Arrhythmias • Heart failure • Infections • Cerebral ischaemia • Aortic root problems	• Patients with more severe complications or more complex congenital heart disease require transfer to the specialist centre. • Appropriate initial treatment in the local hospital must be provided after consultation with the specialist centre.

4. Surgical issues

Cardiac surgery Often staged procedures or late redo's. Risks and benefits often difficult to assess.	Always keep previous operative notes at hand. Careful diagnosis and evaluation. Needs to be discussed with patient.
Preservation of myocardial function.	Avoid or keep aortic cross clamp as short as possible. Consider cold cardioplegia, hypothermia with multidose cardioplegia.
Redo sternotomy (enlarged RV, ant. aorta).	Cardiopulmonary bypass before sternotomy, prosthetic membrane placement when reop. is anticipated.
Pulmonary vascular anomalies (distortion from prev. op, fistulae), aortopulmonary collaterals, pulmonary hypertension.	Careful preop. evaluation, previous cath. intervention in some cases (occlusion of collaterals).
Anaesthesia and perioperative care Individual physiology has to be considered.	Avoid air emboli, optimize volume and flows. Prophylaxis of endocarditis.
Non-cardiac surgery Risk of haemodynamic instability, haemorrhage, endocarditis. Higher risk in emergency procedures. Cyanotic pts are in trouble if systemic resistance falls (increased R-L shunt, hypoxia).	Preop. assessment with GUCH specialist. Anticipate problems. Monitor arterial blood gases and pressure, possibly central venous or PA catheter. Preop. phlebotomy may ameliorate haemostasis if Hct >65%. Avoid any fall in systemic resistance (avoid spinal anaesth).
Transplantation Final palliation to be considered. Outcome less favourable than average Risk stratification necessary.	

5. Psychosocial issues

A specialized service for grown-ups with congenital heart disease must provide support for psychosocial problems related to anxiety about the underlying heart condition, prognosis, social interaction, intellectual development, cognitive function, education, employment, insurance, physical activity. Currently, validated data regarding the relationship between the underlying defect and psychosocial issues are lacking. Intellectual development may be influenced by genotype, the presence of syndromes and the cardiac defect and its treatment. Employment often depends on intellectual and physical capacity, motivation, interaction with peers and discrimination by society. Appropriate employment counselling, based on physical and intellectual capacity and on the underlying defect, is essential. Availability and rates for health and life insurances are not standardized due to a lack of practice guidelines and vary greatly within and between European countries. Problems mostly arise in the private insurance sector. Insurance companies are referring to life tables not based on current outcome data. In the tables of these guidelines insurability is categorized according to contemporary outcome standards. Participation in sports and regular physical exercise have beneficial effects on fitness, psychosocial well-being, confidence, social interaction and on the later risk of acquired cardiac disease. Recommendations on exercise in GUCH need to be based on their ability and on the impact of physical training on cardiac haemodynamics.

It has to be stressed that most GUCH patients say that they are asymptomatic. However, attention should be paid to the fact that the subjective health status is not a good indicator for the objective clinical condition in these cases. Therefore, formal testing, assessing the impact of exercise on the actual haemodynamics and the induction of arrhythmias should be undertaken. Advice to perform social exercise to a level of comfort, but restriction to competitive sports is applicable in most situations. Patient organizations are important as they spread medical information and help with the education of both patients and physicians. In addition they can play a major role in securing and improving patient rights.

Recommendations for sports, physical activity and insurances of grown-ups with congenital heart disease.		
Specific lesion	**Recommendations for sports/physical activity**	**Recommendations for insurance**
Atrial Septal Defect (ASD)	No restrictions unless moderate/severe PVD	Category 1, generally no problem if defect closed early
Ventricular septal defect (VSD), unrepaired	No restrictions if small	Category 1 if small
Ventricular septal defect (VSD), repaired	No restrictions if closed	Category 1
Complete atrioventricular septal defect (cAVSD), postoperative	No restrictions if good repair and no significant arrhythmias	Category 2 if well repaired
Partial atrio-ventricular septal defect (pAVSD), postoperative	No restrictions if good repair and no significant arrhythmias	Category 2
Pulmonary stenosis (PS)	No restrictions unless severe	Category 1 after successful treatment or mild PS
Tetralogy of Fallot (TOF), postoperative	No contraindication unless documented significant arrhythmias, significant ventricular dysfunction or other residua	Category 2
After conduit surgery	Avoid contact sports Otherwise no restrictions if haemodynamically good	Category 2
Aortic valve stenosis (AS), unoperated	No competitive sports if obstruction is moderate or severe	Category 2
Aortic valve stenosis (AS), postoperative	High level activity possible in uncomplicated cases with good LV-function, no impact sports if on anticoagulants	Category 2
Subaortic stenosis (SAS)	No restriction if mild obstruction or after resection	Category 2
Aortic coarctation (CoA), untreated	Restriction prior to repair or interventional treatment	Category 3 for significant untreated CoA
Aortic coarctation (CoA), after repair or interventional treatment (angioplasty ± stenting)	No restrictions if adequate relief of obstruction and no residual arterial hypertension	Category 2
Patent ductus arteriosus (PDA)	No restrictions unless moderate/severe PVD	Category 1 if small PDA or after closure
Ebstein´s anomaly	Recreational sport in asymptomatic pts	Category 2 if asymptomatic without surgery or after successful surgery
After Fontan operation	Recreational sport in asymptomatic pts	Category 3
Marfan syndrome	Avoid contact sports Avoid strenuous exercise Avoid high altitude and diving (cave: spontaneous pneumothorax)	Category 3
After atrial switch operation (Mustard- or Senning-type) operation for transposition of the great arteries	Generally normal activities possible, however, maximal exercise tolerance diminished	Category 3
Congenitally corrected transposition of the great arteries	Recreational sport in asymptomatic pts	Category 3 (in many cases)

6. Specific lesions

This section summarises the current management strategy for the commonest lesions seen in grown-ups with congenital heart disease.

Many recommendations are based on clinical experience rather than on evidence of randomized clinical trials.

We have therefore chosen not to use categories of classes of recommendations and levels of evidence as in other ESC Task Forces.

Levels of care indicated in the tables correspond to those explained earlier, i.e.
1= specialised tertiary care;
2= specialised regional care;
3= care by general practitioner.

Categories for insurance are:
1 = insurable at normal rates;
2 = insurable at elevated rates or with exclusion of specific risks;
3 = cannot usually obtain insurance.

ATRIAL SEPTAL DEFECT	
Introduction & background	• common defect which may be diagnosed first in adult life
Survival → adult life	• small defects - excellent prognosis • large defects - reduced survival, depending on age at treatment
Haemodynamic issues	• PHT • RV dilation/failure • potential for paradoxical embolism • reduced LV compliance
Arrhythmia / pacing	• atrial arrhythmia (atrial fibrillation and flutter) • sick sinus syndrome • pacing rarely required
Investigations	**ECG**: • baseline – if clinically indicated (arrhythmias) **Chest X-ray**: • baseline - otherwise little value **Echo/TOE**: • baseline - location, size, RV size, PA pressure, Qp:Qs, associated lesions • TOE usually performed in older patients and at device closure **Catheter**: • device closure • PVR assessment **MRI**: • rarely helpful **Holter**: • if symptomatic arrhythmia **Exercise test**: • baseline – little value
Indications for intervention	• large defects (>10 mm) unless pulmonary vascular disease (PVR > 8 U/m^2, L-R shunt <1.5, no response to pulmonary vasodilators) • paradoxical embolism
Interventional options	• surgery or device closure (stretched diameter <38mm)
Post treatment outcome	• low risk procedure unless PVD • late intervention less successful
Endocarditis	• very rare • prophylaxis not indicated
Pregnancy/contraception	• no contraindications unless PVD • no restrictions for contraception • consider foetal echocardiography
Recurrence/genetics	• 3% of first degree relatives • familial ASD (with long PR interval) • autosomal dominant
Syndromes	• Holt Oram – upper limb deformity • autosomal dominant
Sport/physical activity	• no restrictions unless moderate/severe PVD
Insurance	• category 1 • generally no problem if defect closed early
Follow-up	• early repair (<30 years) - no problems - discharge • late repair – regular f/u • level 2
Unresolved issues	• surgery vs. device closure • when to close in PHT • concomitant Maze procedure • upper age limit for surgery • PFO closure in patients with suspected paradoxical embolism

VENTRICULAR SEPTAL DEFECT - UNREPAIRED	
Introduction & background	• significant ventricular septal defects usually repaired in childhood • small ventricular septal defect or postoperative septal defect common in adults • Eisenmenger patients becoming less frequent
Survival → adult life	• excellent for small ventricular septal defect • large ventricular septal defect may have pulmonary vascular disease (Eisenmenger) • may develop aortic regurgitation
Haemodynamic issues	• left - right shunt • LV dilatation and impaired function • aortic regurgitation • pulmonary vascular resistance in uncorrected large ventricular septal defect
Arrhythmia / pacing	• rare
Investigations	Chest X-ray: • baseline - cardiomegaly ECG: • routine • rhythm • LVH/RVH Echo: • number, size and location of defects • LV/RV function • aortic regurgitation TOE: • if TTE image inadequate Catheter: • pulmonary vascular resistance • associated lesions MRI: • rarely helpful Holter: • only if symptomatic Exercise test: • only if symptomatic • sports counselling
Indications for intervention	• left – right shunt with left heart volume overload • reversible pulmonary hypertension • aortic regurgitation • associated abnormalities (RV outflow tract, subaortic stenosis) • previous endocarditis
Interventional options	• surgery • catheter closure in muscular VSD(s)
Post treatment outcome	• good surgical results
Endocarditis	• prophylaxis in all
Pregnancy/contraception	• no contraindications in uncomplicated VSD • pregnancy contraindicated in pulmonary vascular disease (Eisenmenger disease)
Recurrence/genetics	• occasionally familial • usual recurrence risk • common cardiac anomaly in syndromes e.g. Down's
Sport/physical activity	• no restriction in small ventricular septal defect
Insurance	• small ventricular septal defects category 1
Follow-up	• infrequent follow-up unless haemodynamic abnormalities (e.g. aortic regurgitation) • small ventricular septal defect level 3, Pulmonary vascular disease (Eisenmenger) level 2, aortic regurgitation/complicated haemodynamics level 1
Unresolved issues	• optimal management of Eisenmenger patients

REPAIRED VENTRICULAR SEPTAL DEFECT	
Introduction & background	• common lesion • most patients now adults
Survival → adult life	• excellent survival • occasional residual shunt • some develop RV or LV outflow tract obstruction • some develop aortic regurgitation
Haemodynamic issues	• residual shunt • ventricular function • aortic regurgitation • new haemodynamic abnormalities (RV outflow obstruction)
Arrhythmia/pacing	• rare AV block, ventricular arrhythmia
Investigations	Chest X-ray: • baseline – cardiomegaly ECG: • rhythm Echo: • residual VSD(s) • LV/RV function • aortic regurgitation TOE if TTE insufficient: • TOE only if TTE inadequate Catheter: • rarely required MRI: • rarely helpful Holter: • only if symptomatic Exercise test: • only if symptomatic • Sports counselling
Indications for intervention	• if residual VSD; see "unrepaired VSD"
Interventional options	• see "unrepaired VSD"
Post treatment outcome	• see "unrepaired VSD"
Endocarditis	• prophylaxis if residual VSD • questionable in closed VSD
Pregnancy / contraception	• no contraindications in uncomplicated closed VSD Pregnancy contraindicated in PVD (Eisenmenger)
Recurrence / genetics	• see: "unrepaired VSD"
Sport / physical activity	• no restriction in closed VSD
Insurance	• category 1
Follow-up	• can discharge if closed VSD without any residual abnormalities • infrequent follow-up for minor residual lesions • Eisenmenger level 2, small VSD level 3, aortic regurgitation/complicated haemodynamics : level 1

<table>
<tr><th colspan="3">COMPLETE ATRIO-VENTRICULAR SEPTAL DEFECT POSTOPERATIVE</th></tr>
<tr><td>Introduction & background</td><td colspan="2">• presentation in infancy</td></tr>
<tr><td>Survival → adult life</td><td colspan="2">• unoperated survivors develop PVD • surgical results markedly improved • status after repair depends mostly on left AV valve function • many patients have Down's syndrome</td></tr>
<tr><td>Haemodynamic issues</td><td colspan="2">• left AV-valve regurgitation (± stenosis) • pulmonary vascular disease
• late sub-aortic stenosis</td></tr>
<tr><td>Arrhythmia / pacing</td><td colspan="2">• risk of complete heart block low (<2%) • atrial arrhythmias especially with left AV-valve dysfunction</td></tr>
<tr><td rowspan="8">Investigations</td><td>Chest X-ray</td><td>• cardiomegaly • pulmonary vascular markings • pulmonary vascular disease</td></tr>
<tr><td>ECG</td><td>• routine (LVH, RVH) • superior QRS-axis
• right bundle branch block
• conduction disturbances</td></tr>
<tr><td>Echo/TOE</td><td>most useful investigation for
• left AV valve morphology and function
• ventricular function • residual lesions (shunt, sub-aortic stenosis)</td></tr>
<tr><td>Catheter</td><td>• rarely required unless re-operation considered</td></tr>
<tr><td>MRI</td><td>• rarely indicated</td></tr>
<tr><td>Holter</td><td>• only in symptomatic patients</td></tr>
<tr><td>Exercise Test</td><td>• rarely indicated</td></tr>
<tr><td>Additional</td><td>• significant left AV valve dysfunction
• significant residual shunt
• subaortic stenosis</td></tr>
<tr><td>Indications for reintervention</td><td colspan="2">• significant left AV-valve dysfunction • significant residual shunt
• sub-aortic stenosis • progressive/symptomatic AV-Block</td></tr>
<tr><td>Interventional options</td><td colspan="2">• re-operation may require valve replacement</td></tr>
<tr><td>Post treatment outcome</td><td colspan="2">• actuarial survival after 20 years > 80% • excellent long-term results unless left AV valve regurgitation (+ stenosis), pulmonary vascular disease, late sub-aortic stenosis</td></tr>
<tr><td>Endocarditis</td><td colspan="2">• prophylaxis in all cases</td></tr>
<tr><td>Pregnancy / contraception</td><td colspan="2">• pregnancy contraindicated in PVD (Eisenmenger) • anticoagulation management in patients with prosthetic valves • avoid oestrogen containing pill in pulmonary hypertension</td></tr>
<tr><td>Recurrence / genetics</td><td colspan="2">• above average recurrence risk Down's syndrome in >50% of complete AVSD • app. 10 - 14% CCD in mothers with AVSD</td></tr>
<tr><td>Sport / physical activity</td><td colspan="2">• no restrictions if good repair and no significant arrhythmias</td></tr>
<tr><td>Insurance</td><td colspan="2">• category 2 if well repaired</td></tr>
<tr><td>Follow-up</td><td colspan="2">• 1-2 yearly intervals with ECG and ECHO in stable cases
• level 2 unless significant haemodynamic problems</td></tr>
<tr><td>Unresolved issues</td><td colspan="2">• only limited data regarding long term prognosis</td></tr>
</table>

<table>
<tr><th colspan="2">PULMONARY STENOSIS</th></tr>
<tr><td>Introduction & background</td><td>Presentation of severe cases mostly in childhood, progression is rare after adolescence</td></tr>
<tr><td>Survival → adult life</td><td>• excellent if relieved effectively • poor if severe valve PS untreated</td></tr>
<tr><td>Haemodynamic issues</td><td>• PS severity • PR severity • Leaflet dysplasia
• right ventricular function</td></tr>
<tr><td>Arrhythmia / pacing</td><td>• atrial arrhythmias in RV failure and tricuspid regurgitation
• pacing not indicated</td></tr>
<tr><td>Investigations</td><td>
<table>
<tr><td>Chest X-ray</td><td>• baseline otherwise little value unless RV failure</td></tr>
<tr><td>ECG</td><td>• rhythm • RV hypertrophy</td></tr>
<tr><td>Echo/TOE</td><td>• investigation of choice for RVOT gradient, pulmonary regurgitation, RV size/function, tricuspid regurgitation</td></tr>
<tr><td>Catheter</td><td>• rarely needed except for balloon dilatation</td></tr>
<tr><td>MRI</td><td>• rarely needed
• assess RV size/function and RA dilation in severe pulmonary regurgitation</td></tr>
<tr><td>Holter</td><td>• not routinely indicated</td></tr>
<tr><td>Exercise test</td><td>• not routinely indicated</td></tr>
</table>
</td></tr>
<tr><td>Indications for intervention</td><td>• valve gradient >30 mmHg at rest or for symptoms</td></tr>
<tr><td>Interventional options</td><td>• balloon valvuloplasty almost always • surgery if valve calcified/dysplastic</td></tr>
<tr><td>Post treatment outcome</td><td>• excellent long-term results unless early failure
• significant pulmonary regurgitation uncommon</td></tr>
<tr><td>Endocarditis</td><td>• low risk. Prophylaxis may not be required in mild cases</td></tr>
<tr><td>Pregnancy / contraception</td><td>• routine pregnancy unless moderate to severe PS or right to left shunt through ASD or PFO</td></tr>
<tr><td>Recurrence / genetics</td><td>• 4% approximately</td></tr>
<tr><td>Syndromes</td><td>• Noonan • congenital rubella • Williams • Alagille</td></tr>
<tr><td>Sport / physical activity</td><td>• unrestricted unless severe</td></tr>
<tr><td>Insurance</td><td>• category 1 after successful treatment or mild PS</td></tr>
<tr><td>Follow-up</td><td>• can discharge if mild with ECHO. Every 1-3 years if more than mild, PR, or desaturation.
• mild PS: level 3, Excellent early result: level 2, Residual gradient or significant PR: level 2</td></tr>
</table>

<table>
<tr><th colspan="3">TETRALOGY OF FALLOT POSTOPERATIVE</th></tr>
<tr><td>Introduction & background</td><td colspan="2">• common lesion • most Fallot patients are now adults</td></tr>
<tr><td>Survival → adult life</td><td colspan="2">• survival rate after surgery excellent (normal in selected groups)
• occasionally unoperated patients survive into adulthood</td></tr>
<tr><td>Haemodynamic issues</td><td colspan="2">• pulmonary regurgitation/PS and RV function • tricuspid regurgitation
• aortic regurgitation • residual lesions • RVOT conduit problems</td></tr>
<tr><td>Arrhythmia / pacing</td><td colspan="2">• late complete heart block rare • ventricular premature beats common in asymptomatic patients • symptomatic VT rare • atrial arrhythmias common and relate to poor haemodynamics • small incidence of late sudden death</td></tr>
<tr><td rowspan="8">Investigations</td><td>Chest X-ray</td><td>• baseline and occasionally follow-up
• cardiomegaly • RV outflow</td></tr>
<tr><td>ECG</td><td>• routine • rhythm • QRS width (usually complete right bundle branch block)</td></tr>
<tr><td>Echo/TOE</td><td>• regularly for PR/RVOTO/RV size and function/tricuspid regurgitation/aortic regurgitation/LV function</td></tr>
<tr><td>Catheter</td><td>• preoperative for residual lesions, coronary anatomy intervention for dilatation/stent of pulmonary arteries
• possibly in future for implantable pulmonary valve</td></tr>
<tr><td>MRI</td><td>• may become investigation of choice for RV size function and pulmonary regurgitation</td></tr>
<tr><td>Holter</td><td>• for symptoms and in poor haemodynamics</td></tr>
<tr><td>Exercise test</td><td>• exercise capacity, arrhythmias</td></tr>
<tr><td>Additional</td><td>• electrophysiological study for syncope, sustained arrhythmia (atrial or ventricular), RFA</td></tr>
<tr><td>Indications for intervention</td><td colspan="2">• significant RVOT or PA branch stenosis • aortic regurgitation
• residual VSD, significant pulmonary regurgitation (with symptoms and RV dilatation)</td></tr>
<tr><td>Interventional options</td><td colspan="2">• surgery, surgery with ablation, balloon dilatation/stenting, RF ablation, catheter intervention for pulmonary valve insertion</td></tr>
<tr><td>Post treatment outcome</td><td colspan="2">• most patients well • RV function may not normalize after pulmonary valve replacement • arrhythmia may persist • risk of sudden death</td></tr>
<tr><td>Endocarditis</td><td colspan="2">• prophylaxis in all</td></tr>
<tr><td>Pregnancy / contraception</td><td colspan="2">• no contraindication to pregnancy in well repaired patient
• monitor ventricular function and arrhythmia
• no additional foetal risk</td></tr>
<tr><td>Recurrence / genetics</td><td colspan="2">• 1.5% for father, 2.5-4% for mother with TOF if deletion of chromosome 22q11- recurrence risk 50%</td></tr>
<tr><td>Syndromes</td><td colspan="2">• 22q11 in 16% of pts</td></tr>
<tr><td>Sport / physical activity</td><td colspan="2">• no contraindication to sport unless documented arrhythmia or significant ventricular dysfunction</td></tr>
<tr><td>Insurance</td><td colspan="2">• Category 2</td></tr>
<tr><td>Follow-up</td><td colspan="2">• one/two yearly with ECG, Echo ± Holter, exercise test
• level 1 if documented residual abnormalities/arrhythmia, level 2 otherwise</td></tr>
<tr><td>Unresolved issues</td><td colspan="2">• risk stratification for sudden death • indication for implantable defibrillator • timing of reoperation for pulmonary regurgitation</td></tr>
</table>

COARCTATION POSTOPERATIVE	
Introduction & background	Most pts present either in early infancy or in adolescence
Survival → adult life	• long-term survival still reduced despite adequate early repair
Haemodynamic issues	• persistent and late developing hypertension at rest and exercise • aortic valve dysfunction • dissection rare
Arrhythmia / pacing	• not an issue
Investigations	**ECG:** • LVH ± repolarization changes **Chest X-ray:** • cardiomegaly • ascending aorta dilation • rib notching **Echo:** • assessment of arch anatomy/ gradient • associated lesions LVH and function **TOE:** • rarely provides additional information **MRI:** • investigation of choice **Holter:** • not indicated unless for ambulatory blood pressure **Exercise test:** • hypertension on exercise • arm/leg gradient • inducible repolarization abnormalities **Catheter:** • if MRI unavailable for arch anatomy • for coronary angiography when indicated for intervention **Additional:** • Screen for intracerebral vascular anomalies advocated by some
Indications for intervention	• significant recoarctation (gradient > 30mm Hg at rest) • aortic aneurysm
Interventional options	• balloon/stenting for anatomically suitable recoarctation • surgery for complex situations ± aneurysms
Post treatment outcome	• excellent but late hypertension and premature atherosclerosis/CVA/MI/heart failure
Endocarditis	• prophylaxis in all cases
Pregnancy / contraception	• relieve residual coarctation prior to pregnancy or during unplanned pregnancy • monitor closely for hypertension • avoid oestrogen containing pill if rest or exercise hypertension
Recurrence / genetics	• recurrence may be familial • 22q11 deletion in complex forms
Syndromes	• Turners (present in approx 30%) • Williams (present in approx 10%) • Shones (associated LV inflow/outflow abnormalities)
Sport / physical activity	• no restrictions if adequate relief of obstruction/no residual hypertension, impact sports to be avoided
Insurance	• category 2
Follow-up	• yearly with same investigations as for unoperated coarctation • level 2
Unresolved issues	• influence of age at repair, type of repair of intervention on late hypertension • late outcome of balloon/stenting • pathophysiology of late hypertension

AORTIC VALVE STENOSIS UNOPERATED	
Introduction & background	• common especially bicuspid aortic valve (1-2% of population) • may occur with other lesions
Survival → adult life	• normal if mild obstruction
Haemodynamic issues	• degree of stenosis may progress • associated aortic regurgitation • LV hypertrophy and function
Arrhythmia / pacing	• VT and VF may occur during exertion with severe obstruction
Investigations	ECG: • LVH and repolarisation changes Chest X-ray: • baseline • calcification Echo: • investigation of choice • LV mass/function • aortic valve/size/morphology/area • LV to aortic gradient • aortic regurgitation TOE: • rarely of value except in endocarditis MRI: • rarely of value Catheter: • for coronary angiography and balloon dilatation Exercise test: • for repolarisation changes and symptoms • surgical decision making
Indications for intervention	• symptoms: severe LV pressure overload • severe aortic stenosis
Interventional options	• balloon valvuloplasty if valve uncalcified - rarely good option in adult • mechanical valve replacement, homograft or Ross procedure depending on patient's age, sex, preferences and local expertise
Post treatment outcome	• recurrence common late after valvotomy • very good in uncomplicated cases of valve replacement
Endocarditis	• prophylaxis indicated in all
Pregnancy / contraception	• low risk in asymptomatic patients even with moderate obstruction • high risk in patients with severe obstruction • transcatheter intervention may be indicated in unplanned pregnancy
Recurrence / genetics	• bicuspid valve may be familial • association with coarctation • recurrence rate may be higher in syndromes
Sport / physical activity	• no competitive sports if obstruction is moderate or severe
Insurance	• category 2
Follow-up	• depends on severity and progression rate ECG/Echo ± exercise test • mild level 3 - moderate/severe level 1
Unresolved issues	• timing of operation in asymptomatic adults with severe AS

VALVAR AORTIC STENOSIS POSTOPERATIVE	
Introduction & background	• common lesion • most interventions in children are balloon dilation or open aortic valvotomy, aortic valve replacement, mechanical or biological prostheses or Ross procedure may have been performed
Survival → adult life	• excellent
Haemodynamic issues	• obstruction • regurgitation • LV function • pulmonary homograft (Ross)
Arrhythmia / pacing	• arrhythmia rare • more common in LV hypertrophy • may cause sudden death
Investigations	**ECG:** • routine • LVH • conduction disturbances • repolarisation changes **Chest X-ray:** • cardiomegaly **Echo:** • see valvar aortic stenosis unoperated • prosthesis function and paravalvular leak **TOE:** • useful in assessment of paravalvular leaks and suspected endocarditis **MRI:** • rarely indicated **Catheter:** • rarely indicated (see valvar aortic stenosis unoperated) **Exercise test:** • surgical decision making for timing of reintervention
Indications for reintervention	• recurrent obstruction (native valve or prosthesis) • regurgitation • occasionally haemolysis
Interventional options	• mechanical valve, homograft or Ross operation • bio-prosthesis may be preferred by elderly • homograft may be preferred in endocarditis
Post treatment outcome	• very good but anticoagulant problems with mechanical valve and late failure
Endocarditis	• prophylaxis in all cases
Pregnancy / contraception	• anticoagulants may cause embryopathy
Recurrence / genetics	• see aortic valve stenosis unoperated
Sport / physical activity	• high level activity possible in uncomplicated cases with good LV function • contact contraindicated in patients on anticoagulants
Insurance	• category 2
Follow-up	• yearly • Ross level 1, otherwise level 2
Unresolved issues	• long-term outcome of Ross procedure • best anticoagulation protocol in pregnancy

CONGENITALLY CORRECTED TRANSPOSITION	
Introduction & background	• rare lesion • usually associated with other abnormalities • may occur with dextrocardia
Survival → adult life	• common to survive to adult life • associated lesions common (VSD, PS, left AV valve regurgitation), determine outcome
Haemodynamic issues	• cyanosis with VSD and PS • PVD if VSD and no PS • systemic ventricular failure with systemic A-V valve regurgitation • referral before systemic ventricular dysfunction • conduit into PA may degenerate
Arrhythmia / pacing	• spontaneous CHB (2% per year) and post surgical heart block • Endocardial pacing in the morphologic LV • Atrial arrhythmias common • Ventricular arrhythmias with systemic ventricular dysfunction • Epicardial pacing if potential for paradoxical embolus
Investigations	Chest X-ray: • baseline • Follow-up for associated lesions • cardiomegaly ECG: • rhythm Echo/TOE: • size and function of systemic ventricle • morphology of left A-V valve • associated lesions Catheter: • pulmonary haemodynamics and anatomy of associated lesions MRI: • rarely required Holter: • for occult arrhythmia detection Exercise test: • helpful for timing of surgery • oximetry • exercise tolerance Additional: • occasionally MUGA for ventricular function
Indications for Intervention	• moderate systemic AV valve regurgitation • significant associated lesions • pacemaker for complete AV block with symptoms, profound bradycardia or chronotropic incompetence
Interventional options	• valve replacement • pulmonary artery banding • "double switch" (controversial in adults)
Post treatment outcome	• good if left A-V valve replacement before systemic ventricular function deteriorates •atrial arrhythmias common
Endocarditis	• prophylaxis in all cases
Pregnancy / contraception	• pregnancy not contraindicated if asymptomatic • monitor ventricular function and rhythm • long-term consequences on systemic ventricular function unknown • avoid oestrogen containing contraceptive pill if cyanosed/pulmonary hypertension
Recurrence / genetics	• 4%
Sport / physical activity	• no restriction on recreational activities
Insurance	• category 3 in most cases
Follow-up	• yearly, with Echo, exercise test ± Holter • level 1 (pre- and postoperative)
Unresolved issues	• classical repair of VSD and PS versus "double switch"

<table>
<tr><th colspan="3">COMPLETE TRANSPOSITION POSTOPERATIVE (Mustard/Senning)</th></tr>
<tr><td>Introduction & background</td><td colspan="2">• common lesion – most Mustard/Sennings patients now adults – operation replaced by arterial switch mid 1980's</td></tr>
<tr><td>Survival → adult life</td><td colspan="2">• low early mortality • significant late morbidity/mortality from arrhythmia/baffle obstruction/RV failure with risk of sudden death</td></tr>
<tr><td>Haemodynamic issues</td><td colspan="2">• intra-atrial baffle obstruction (systemic and pulmonary venous) more common in Mustard than Senning • tricuspid regurgitation/RV failure relatively rare but important to detect early</td></tr>
<tr><td>Arrhythmia / pacing</td><td colspan="2">• progressive loss of sinus rhythm on Holter with follow-up
• slow junctional rhythm may rarely require pacing
• tachyarrhythmias (predominantly atrial flutter) may be related to high incidence of late sudden death
• pacing may be required if antiarrhythmic drugs needed</td></tr>
<tr><td rowspan="7">Investigations</td><td>ECG</td><td>• RVH with basic rhythm (often junctional)</td></tr>
<tr><td>Chest X-ray</td><td>• useful for cardiomegaly
• pulmonary venous obstruction</td></tr>
<tr><td>Echo/TOE</td><td>• TTE for ventricular function/tricuspid regurgitation
• TOE essential if questions remain regarding baffle function</td></tr>
<tr><td>MRI</td><td>• rarely required if TOE available</td></tr>
<tr><td>Holter</td><td>• occult arrhythmia
• not predictive of SD</td></tr>
<tr><td>Exercise test</td><td>• exercise tolerance
• evaluation of arrhythmia</td></tr>
<tr><td>Catheter</td><td>• for intervention and assessment of new symptoms • EP study/RFA for refractory atrial arrhythmias</td></tr>
<tr><td>Indications for intervention</td><td colspan="2">• baffle obstruction • baffle leaks • tricuspid valve dysfunction
• RV failure</td></tr>
<tr><td>Interventional options</td><td colspan="2">• balloon/stenting for pathway obstruction • transcatheter closure for baffle leaks • tricuspid valve replacement • conversion to arterial switch (pulmonary artery banding) • transplantation</td></tr>
<tr><td>Post treatment outcome</td><td colspan="2">• risk of sudden death despite lack of symptoms or overt haemodynamic disturbance</td></tr>
<tr><td>Endocarditis</td><td colspan="2">• prophylaxis in all cases</td></tr>
<tr><td>Pregnancy / contraception</td><td colspan="2">• pregnancy not contraindicated in most cases
• monitor RV function throughout • no contraceptive issues
• long-term consequences on RV function not known</td></tr>
<tr><td>Recurrence / genetics</td><td colspan="2">• familial recurrence of TGA rare</td></tr>
<tr><td>Sport / physical activity</td><td colspan="2">• generally normal activities • maximal exercise tolerance likely to be diminished</td></tr>
<tr><td>Insurance</td><td colspan="2">• category 3</td></tr>
<tr><td>Follow-up</td><td colspan="2">• yearly • level 1</td></tr>
<tr><td>Unresolved issues</td><td colspan="2">• risk stratification for sudden death • fate of systemic RV / tricuspid valve • conversion/transplant strategies</td></tr>
</table>

EBSTEIN'S ANOMALY		
Introduction & background		• wide spectrum of pathologic anatomy which determines onset of severity of symptoms
Survival → adult life		• extremely variable natural history • infant survivors usually reach adulthood
Haemodynamic issues		• cyanosis at rest and/or exercise (right – left shunt at atrial level) • reduced exercise capacity • congestive heart failure (tricuspid stenosis/regurgitation/small RV) • associated lesions • LV abnormalities
Arrhythmia / pacing		• atrial arrhythmias are common • increase with age • related to pre-excitation and atrial dilatation • risk of sudden death
Investigations	Chest X-ray	• marked cardiomegaly • right atrial enlargement
	ECG	• baseline (characteristic pattern) • follow-up for rhythm
	Echo/TOE	• severity of tricuspid valve displacement dysplasia and regurgitation • RV size • associated lesions • LV function
	Catheter	• rarely required unless for coronary angiography in older patients or at EPS
	MRI	• rarely required
	Holter	• useful for arrhythmia monitoring
	Exercise test	• baseline and follow-up • cyanosis • exercise tolerance • arrhythmia
	Additional	• EPS for arrhythmia diagnosis and RFA
	Indications for intervention	• decrease in exercise tolerance • heart failure • increase in cyanosis • arrhythmia
Interventional options		• surgery for tricuspid valve repair or replacement • RFA for arrhythmias/pre-excitation
Post treatment outcome		• symptomatic improvement usual • tricuspid valve replacement – reoperation, thrombotic complications • ongoing arrhythmia problems frequent • risk of sudden death remains • anticoagulants for atrial arrhythmia and prosthetic tricuspid valve
Endocarditis		• prophylaxis in all cases
Pregnancy / contraception		• well tolerated unless cyanosis or heart failure • foetus at risk in cyanosed mother
Recurrence / genetics		• 6% in affected mother. 1% in affected father. Familial occurrence documented.
Sport / physical activity		• recreational sport in asymptomatic patient
Insurance		• unoperated asymptomatic or well post operative category 2
Follow-up		• depends on clinical status • annual follow-up with Echo/Holter + exercise test • level 1 (operated and unoperated)
Unresolved issues		• recurrence of arrhythmias • long-term fate of repairs

FONTAN	
Introduction & background:	• palliative procedure for single ventricle physiology in which all systemic venous return is directed to the lungs - multiple modifications
Survival → adult life	• improved survival with strict selection criteria • late failure even in best cases
Haemodynamic issues	• function of systemic ventricle (preload deprived) • pulmonary vascular resistance • obstruction in Fontan connection • atrial enlargement • pulmonary venous obstruction • AV valve regurgitation • chronic venous hypertension • desaturation/paradoxical embolus in fenestrated Fontan • pulmonary arterio-venous malformations in some
Arrhythmia / pacing	• atrial arrhythmias common • increase with follow-up • sinus node dysfunction • pacing - ventricular pacing requires epicardial system
Investigations	Chest X-ray: • baseline and follow-up • cardiomegaly • pulmonary vascular markings ECG: • rhythm Echo/TOE: most useful investigation for • ventricular function • AV valve regurgitation • residual shunts • obstruction of Fontan connections • thrombus in atrium • routine TOE (2- yearly may be indicated, or if arrhythmia present) Catheter: • for haemodynamic assessment and angiography in clinical deterioration MRI: • obstruction of Fontan connection • occasionally useful for RA size and anastomoses Holter: • routine and for symptomatic arrhythmia Exercise test: • exercise tolerance • evaluation of arrhythmia Additional: • blood/stool for PLE
Indications for intervention	• cyanosis • obstruction to Fontan connection • systemic AV valve regurgitation • ventricular failure • arrhythmia • pulmonary venous obstruction
Interventional options	• consider conversion to TCPC or transplant in failing Fontan • closure of fenestration • AV malformations • RFA • supraventricular arrhythmia • AV sequential pacing
Post treatment outcome	• variable success with catheter ablation of atrial arrhythmias • PLE has < 50% 5 year survival • Fontan conversion results unclear
Endocarditis	• prophylaxis in all
Pregnancy / contraception	• pregnancy possible with perfectly selected patients and proper care • high maternal risk in "failing Fontan" • higher miscarriage rate • foetal risk otf CHD may be higher • avoid oestrogen pill if ejection fraction < 40%, residual shunt, or spontaneous contrast in RA • ACE-inhibitors should be withdrawn • if on anticoagulants – need meticulous management
Sport / physical activity	• recreational sports only
Insurance	• category 3
Follow-up	• at least yearly review with Echo, ECG Holter, exercise testing, blood testing • level 1
Unresolved issues	• indications for and results of Fontan conversion • outcome of TCPC in modern era • role of anticoagulation • medical therapy for failing systemic ventricle • role of ACE-inhibitors

MARFAN's Syndrome

Introduction & background		• abnormal fibrillin gene on chromosome 15q • autosomal dominant inheritance • cardiac defect largely determines outcome
Survival → adult life		• death from cardiac problems • life expectancy reduced but improved by good cardiac follow-up and surgery
Haemodynamic issues		• acute aortic dissection – risk higher if the aortic sinuses >55mm • aortic regurgitation • mitral valve prolapse/regurgitation
Arrhythmia / pacing		• atrial and ventricular arrhythmia in mitral valve prolapse/regurgitation
Investigations	Chest X-ray	• not helpful for follow-up of aorta
	ECG	• rarely useful
	Echo/TOE	• most valuable investigation for serial follow-up of aortic root dimensions, valve function (aortic and mitral)
	Catheter	• rarely indicated
	MRI	• excellent investigation for aortic arch and descending aorta • compliments echocardiography
	Holter	• not routine
	Exercise test	• not routine
	Additional	• non-cardiac assessment (ophthalmic, orthopaedic etc.)
Indications for intervention		• beta-blockers for aortic dilatation • surgery if aortic diameter > 55 mm or rapid increase • significant aortic regurgitation • significant mitral regurgitation
Interventional options		• urgent surgery for dissection • aortic root and valve replacement • valve sparing operation may be indicated
Post treatment outcome		• surgery improves life expectancy but other dissections still possible • beta-blockers delay/prevent progression
Endocarditis		• prophylaxis in valve regurgitation and after aortic surgery
Pregnancy / contraception		• pregnancy contraindicated if aorta is > 45 mm • pregnant women should be on beta-blockers • caesarean section to be discussed if aorta is dilated
Recurrence / genetics		• approximately 50% (autosomal dominant)
Sport / physical activity		• strenuous exercise, high altitude and diving contraindicated (spontaneous pneumothorax)
Insurance		• category 3
Follow-up		• annual follow up for aortic dilatation • more frequent evaluation if aortic diameter increasing • level 1
Unresolved issues		• role of early beta-blockade • long term results of surgery including valve sparing

Chapter 2

Neonatal Electrocardiogram*

2002

Chairperson:
Peter J. Schwartz, MD, FESC, FACC, FAHA
Department of Cardiology
Policlinico S. Matteo IRCCS
Viale Golgi, 19
27100 Pavia
Italy
Phone: +39 (0)382 503567 / 503673
Fax: +39 (0)382 503002
E-mail: PJQT@compuserve.com

Task Force Members:
1. Arthur Garson, Jr., Charlottesville, USA
2. Thomas Paul, Göttingen, Germany
3. Marco Stramba-Badiale, Milan, Italy
4. Victoria L. Vetter, Philadelphia, USA
5. Elisabeth Villain, Paris, France
6. Christopher Wren, Newcastle upon Tyne, UK

ESC Staff:
1. Keith McGregor, Sophia-Antipolis, France
2. Veronica Dean, Sophia-Antipolis, France
3. Dominique Poumeyrol-Jumeau, Sophia-Antipolis, France
4. Catherine Després, Sophia-Antipolis, France
5. Xue Li, Sophia-Antipolis, France

Introduction

Most cardiologists who care for adults have no or minimal experience with electrocardiograms (ECGs) recorded in infants. So far, this has had no practical implications because only seldom are they requested to examine a neonatal ECG. This situation, however, may change as some European countries have begun to consider the possibility of introducing in their National Health Services the performance of an ECG during the first month of life in all newborns, as part of a cardiovascular screening programme.

The main objective of the present report is to present adult cardiologists with a consensus document designed to provide guidelines for the interpretation of the neonatal ECG, focusing on the most clinically relevant abnormalities and on the ensuing management and referral options. This document aims also at providing paediatricians and neonatologists with updated information of clinical relevance that can be detected from a neonatal ECG.

Normal electrocardiogram in the newborn

Changes occur in the normal ECG from birth to adult life, mostly in the first year of life with the majority of normal adult values being abnormal in the newborn. Likewise, many normal newborn values and patterns would be abnormal in the adult. Intervals should be hand measured as computerised systems are often inaccurate in the newborn. Intervals in children increase with increasing age, reaching most of the adult normal values by 7-8 years of age. Values are shown in Table 1.

Heart rate

Normal neonates may have rates of 150-230 beats per minute (bpm), especially if they are crying or agitated.

P Wave

The P wave is generally pointed in lead II and aVF and more rounded in other leads. Lead V1 may be diphasic.

QRS complex

Normal axis is between 55° and 200° at birth, but by 1 month, the normal upper limit has fallen to 160° or less. QRS morphology in the newborn may have more notches than in older children or adults. Normally, there is a Q wave in leads V5-V6. Q wave duration >30 ms is abnormal. A secondary r waves (r′ or R′) in the right chest leads is frequent in normal neonates.

* Adapted from the ESC Guidelines for the Interpretation of the Neonatal Electrocardiogram (European Heart Journal 2002; 23:1329-1344).

Table 1. Normal Neonatal ECG Standards+

Age Group	Heart Rate (bpm)	Frontal Plane QRS Axis # (degrees)	P Wave Amplitude (mm)	P-R Interval # (sec)	QRS Duration # V_5	Q III ^ (mm)	QV_6 ^ (mm)	RV_1 * (mm)	SV_1 * (mm)	R/S V_1 ^	RV_6 * (mm)	SV_6 * (mm)	R/S V_6 ^	SV_1+ RV_6 ^ (mm)	R + S V_4 ^ (mm)
0-1 day	93-154 (123)	+59 to +192 (135)	2.8	0.08-0.16 (0.11)	0.02-0.08 (0.05)	5.2	1.7	5-26	0-22.5	9.8	0-11	0-9.8	10	28	52
1-3 days	91-159 (123)	+64 to +197 (134)	2.8	0.08-0.14 (0.11)	0.02-0.07 (0.05)	5.2	2.1	5-27	0-21	6	0-12	0-9.5	11	29	52
3-7 days	90-166 (129)	+77 to +187 (132)	2.9	0.08-0.14 (0.10)	0.02-0.07 (0.05)	4.8	2.8	3-24	0-17	9.7	0.5-12	0-9.8	10	25	48
7-30 days	107-182 (149)	+65 to +160 (110)	3.0	0.07-0.14 (0.10)	0.02-0.08 (0.05)	5.6	2.8	3-21.5	0-11	7	2.5-16	0-9.8	12	22	47
1-3 months	121-179 (150)	+31 to + 114 (75)	2.6	0.07-0.13 (0.10)	0.02-0.08 (0.05)	5.4	2.7	3-18.5	0-12.5	7.4	5-21	0-7.2	12	29	53

+ From Davignon A, Rautaharju P, Boisselle E, Soumis F, Megelas M, Choquette A. Normal ECG standards for infants and children. Pediatr Cardiol 1979; 1: 123-52.

\# 2nd-98th % tile (mean)

* 2nd-98th % tile (1 mm = 100 μV)

^ 98th % tile (1 mm = 100 μV)

QT Interval

The QT interval is the interval between the beginning of the QRS complex and the end of the T wave and should be measured in leads II, V5 and V6 with the longest value being used. The main difficulty lies in identifying correctly the point where the descending limb of the T wave intersects the isoelectric line. Due to the fast heart rate of infants the P wave may be superimposed on the T wave, particularly when the QT interval is prolonged. In this case, the end of the T wave should be extrapolated by drawing a tangent to the downslope of the T wave and considering its intersection with the isoelectric line. The QT interval duration changes with rate and it is usually corrected (QTc) by using Bazett's formula. Correction of the QT interval requires a stable sinus rhythm without sudden changes in the RR interval. QTc is equal to QT interval in seconds divided by the square root of the preceding RR interval in seconds. To avoid time-consuming calculations, a simple chart where the value of QTc is easily obtained by matching QT and RR interval in millimetres (given the paper speed at 25 mm/sec) has been produced (Appendix 1). When heart rate is particularly slow or fast the Bazett's formula may not be accurate in the correction but it remains the standard for clinical use. The mean QTc on the 4th day of life is 400 ± 20 ms and, at variance with the adult, no gender differences are present. Therefore, the upper normal limit of QTc (2 standard deviations above the mean, corresponding to the 97.5 percentile) is 440 ms. By definition, 2.5% of normal newborns are expected to have a QTc greater than 440 ms. In healthy infants there is a physiological prolongation of QTc by the second month (mean 410 ms) followed by a progressive decline, so that by the sixth month QTc returns to the values recorded in the first week. Despite its apparent simplicity the measurement of the QT interval is fraught with errors. An attempt should be made to measure to the nearest 10 ms (1/4 of a mm) while we recognize that this may be within measurement error.

ST Segment and T Wave

In neonates and infants it is better to consider as the isoelectric line the TP segment instead of the PQ segment. After 1 week, the T wave is negative in lead V1 and positive in V5-V6.

Abnormal electrocardiogram in the newborn

Heart rate

Sinus arrhythmia

Sinus arrhythmia should be differentiated from wandering pacemaker which manifests itself with a gradual change of P wave axis and morphology and that is due to a shift of the pacemaker from the sinus node to the atrium and the atrioventricular (AV) junction. Although wandering pacemaker may accompany other types of bradyarrhythmia, it has no pathological meaning.

Work-up

No work-up should be necessary unless significant bradycardia coexists.

Sinus tachycardia

Sinus tachycardia is a sinus rhythm with a heart rate above the normal limit (166 bpm in the first week and 179 bpm at the age of one month) and it may be caused by fever, infection, anaemia, pain, dehydration (hypovolaemia), hyperthyroidism, myocarditis, beta-adrenergic agonists or theophylline.

Work-up

The evaluation should be performed according to the underlying condition. If myocarditis is suspected an echocardiogram should be performed. Appropriate acute treatment of causes of tachycardia may be considered. Persistence of elevated rates should be further evaluated.

Sinus bradycardia

Sinus bradycardia is a sinus rhythm with a heart rate below the normal limit (91 bpm in the first week and 121 bpm at the age of one month) and it may be caused by central nervous system (CNS) abnormalities, hypothermia, hypopituarism, increased intracranial pressure, meningitis, drugs passed from the mother to infant, obstructive jaundice, typhoid fever. Hypothyroidism is another cause of bradycardia and is often associated with the so-called "mosque sign", a dome-shaped symmetric T wave in the absence of an ST segment.

Transient sinus bradycardia has been observed in newborns from anti-Ro/SSA positive mothers. A lower than normal heart rate has been described in patients affected by the Long QT Syndrome (LQTS) and it may sometimes represent the first sign of the disease during the foetal period.

Work-up

24-hour Holter monitoring may be helpful for further evaluation when a heart rate below 80-90 bpm is present on a surface ECG during infancy. Evaluation for underlying conditions should be performed.

Other bradycardias

Sinus pauses in newborns may last from 800 to 1000 ms. Pauses >2 s are abnormal and may be followed by atrial or junctional escape beats. Even a healthy neonate may show periods of junctional rhythm, i.e. a sequence of narrow QRS complexes in the absence of preceding P waves. Infants with augmented vagal tone may have sinus bradycardia, or significant sinus pauses of several seconds, during feeding, sleep, defecation. Apparent life-threatening events (ALTE), described as loss of consciousness, pallor and hypotonia, have been related to vagal overactivity, which may manifest as sinus pauses or abrupt bradycardia. ALTE may be associated with apnoeic episodes, or gastro-oesophageal reflux, that may precede severe bradycardia. Infants with LQTS may also have sinus pauses.

Work-up

24-hour Holter monitoring may be useful for the assessment of significant bradycardia. Long pauses, secondary to excessive vagal tone may be eliminated by the use of atropine, and rarely require pacemakers. Treatment of other underlying diseases should be undertaken.

P Wave

Abnormal P waves may be seen in infants with atrial enlargement or non-sinus origin of the P wave. Right atrial enlargement or/and hypertrophy produces increased P wave amplitude with normal duration, best seen in lead II. Left atrial enlargement and/or hypertrophy produces an increased (>0.1 mV) and prolonged (>40 ms) negative terminal deflection of the P wave in lead V1. Left atrial enlargement also causes exaggerated notching of the P wave in lead II, although this is not a specific sign.

Work up

An echocardiogram should be performed when clinically indicated.

Atrioventricular conduction

Complete (3rd degree) atrioventricular block

Approximately 1 out of every 15 000 to 20 000 live births results in a baby with isolated AV block. Most of them are ascribed to the presence of anti Ro/SSA and La-SSB antibodies in the mothers. 2% to 5% of women with known antibodies will have a first child with AV block. Mortality rate in patients with neonatal AV block is still high, especially during the first 3 months. Acquired complete AV block is rare in neonates. It is mainly caused by infections (viral myocarditis, HIV) or may be related to tumours.

1st and 2nd degree atrioventricular block

Neonates may present with 1st or 2nd degree AV block which may rarely progress to complete AV block. Neonates with LQTS may show 2:1 AV block because they have a fast atrial rate and the P wave falls within the very prolonged T wave. In spite of high doses of beta-blockers and pacing, there is still significant mortality. Heart block associated with prolonged QT interval may be caused by cisapride, diphemanil or doxapram.

Work up

Clinical history of autoimmune disease and plasma titres of maternal antibodies (anti Ro/SSA and antiLa/SSB) should be assessed. In the absence of maternal antibodies, ECG should also be performed on the parents and siblings (see intraventricular abnormalities). Neonates with 1st degree AV block should be followed with additional ECGs in the following months. Neonates and infants with 2nd or 3rd degree AV block need a complete paediatric cardiology work-up, including an echocardiogram. The only effective treatment of congenital complete AV block in neonates with symptoms or a low ventricular escape rhythm is permanent artificial pacing.

Intraventricular conduction

Bundle Branch Block

Congenital isolated complete right bundle branch block (RBBB) and left bundle branch block (LBBB) are very rare in neonates. The classical ECG in Ebstein's anomaly of the tricuspid valve displays a prolonged PR interval and a wide RBBB pattern. Left anterior fascicular block is found in association with atrioventricular canal defects and tricuspid atresia. In severe cardiomyopathy, interruption of the left bundle carries a poor prognosis. Hereditary bundle branch block is an autosomal dominant genetic disease, which induces RBBB, left or right QRS axis deviation or AV block.

Non-specific intraventricular conduction abnormalities

They are very rare in neonates and infants with normal hearts and may be caused by myocarditis or endocarditis.

Work up

Neonates and infants with intraventricular conduction abnormalities need a complete paediatric cardiology work-up. Evaluation of possible underlying causes should be performed. ECG should also be performed on the parents and siblings.

Wolff-Parkinson-White (WPW) syndrome

In newborns and infants preexcitation may be subtle and only be detected in the mid-precordial leads and it is often intermittent. The prevalence of WPW syndrome is high in the presence of 2 of the 4 following characteristics:

- PR interval =100 ms,
- QRS duration =80 ms,
- lack of a Q wave in V6,
- left axis deviation.

Short PR intervals are also observed in mannosideosis, Fabry's disease, and Pompe's disease. A short PR interval in a normal heart may be caused by a low right atrial pacemaker with a negative P wave in lead aVF and positive or isoelectric in lead I. The prevalence of WPW syndrome in the paediatric population is 0.15-0.3%, with an incidence of 4 per 100 000 persons per year. In children with structural heart disease (Ebstein´s anomaly of the tricuspid valve, l-transposition of the great arteries, hypertrophic cardiomyopathy and cardiac tumours) the prevalence is 0.330.5%. The incidence of sudden death in preexcitation syndrome during childhood is 0.5% and cardiac arrest may be the initial presentation.

Work up

Congenital heart disease is more common in infants and young children with preexcitation, with a prevalence as high as 45% for infants with an ECG pattern consistent with a right-sided accessory pathway. Thus, a complete 2-dimensional echocardiography work-up is recommended. Assessment of the conduction properties of the accessory pathway, i.e. the antegrade effective refractory period and the shortest RR-interval with preexcitation, by trans-oesophageal programmed stimulation may be useful in selected patients for risk stratification and mode of therapy.

QRS axis and amplitude

A relative right axis deviation is seen in normal neonates. Left axis deviation is seen in atrioventricular or ventricular septal defect, tricuspid atresia, and WPW syndrome, but occasionally also in normal infants.

Right ventricular hypertrophy

It may be suspected from a QR complex in V1, an upright T wave in V1 (normal in the first week of life), increased R wave amplitude in V1, and increased S wave amplitude in V6 (according to the Davignon criteria). Sensitivity and specificity have not been tested in the neonate. QR patterns are commonly seen with pressure overload congenital lesions, rSR′ patterns in volume overload lesions.

Left ventricular hypertrophy

ECG signs in children (not specifically tested in neonates) are T wave abnormalities in leads V5 and V6, increased R wave amplitude in V6, increased S wave amplitude in V1 (according to the Davignon criteria), and a combination of these last two variables. Left to right shunt lesions may result in left ventricular hypertrophy, but this may be in association with right ventricular hypertrophy and manifested as biventricular hypertrophy.

Low QRS voltage

In the limb leads the total amplitude of R+S in each lead ≤0.5 mV may be indicative of myocarditis or cardiomyopathy.

Work-up

Evaluation of the underlying causes should be performed. An echocardiogram should be performed when clinically indicated.

Ventricular repolarisation

QT interval prolongation

Measurements of the QT interval should be performed by hand. QT duration may change over time and it is recommended to repeat the ECG in those infants found to have a prolonged QTc on the first ECG. While exceptions do exist, the more prolonged the QTc interval, the greater the likelihood of its clinical significance. A QTc close to 500 ms implies a clear abnormality even taking into account potential measurement errors.

QT prolongation may be caused by hypocalcemia with a distinctive lengthening of the ST segment, hypokalemia and hypomagnesemia, with a decrease of T wave amplitude and increase of U wave amplitude, CNS abnormalities, with T wave inversion, macrolide antibiotics (spyramycin, erythromycin, clarithromycin), trimethoprim, cisapride. Neonates born from mothers positive for the anti-Ro/SSA antibodies may show transient QT interval prolongation in the first 6 months of life.

Finally, some of the neonates with QT interval prolongation may be affected by the congenital Long QT Syndrome (LQTS), whose prevalence appears to be close to 1/3000-1/5000, and is characterised by the occurrence of syncopal episodes due to torsades de pointes ventricular tachycardia (VT) and by a high risk of sudden cardiac death among untreated patients. Importantly, in 12% of patients with LQTS sudden death is the first manifestation of the disease and in 4% this happens in the first year of life. This point alone mandates the treatment of all those diagnosed as affected, even if there are no symptoms. LQTS is a genetic disease due to mutations of several genes all encoding ionic (potassium or sodium) currents involved in the control of ventricular repolarisation. In most cases, several members of the same family are gene-carriers. Low penetrance exists in LQTS, which means that gene-carriers may not show the clinical phenotype and may have a normal QT interval. Therefore, a normal QT in the parents does not rule out familial LQTS. In addition, approximately 30% of cases are due to "de novo" mutations which imply unaffected parents and no family history. "De novo" LQTS mutations have been demonstrated in infant victims of cardiac arrest and sudden death diagnosed as Sudden Infant Death Syndrome. Beta-blockers are the first choice therapy in LQTS and if beta-blockers are unable to prevent new cardiac events, additional drug therapy, left cardiac sympathetic denervation, pacemakers or the implantable cardioverter defibrillator should be considered based on evidence, with due consideration for body size.

Work-up

The likelihood of having LQTS increases with increasing QTc; however, since a small percentage of LQTS patients has a QTc < 440 ms, the correlation between QT prolongation and presence of the syndrome is not absolute. Therefore, the following discussion is presented as guidelines based upon experience and current knowledge, and is likely to be updated frequently. Given the life-threatening potential of the disease, once the diagnosis of LQTS becomes probable, it is recommended that these infants are referred to a specialist as soon as possible.

- First ECG: QTc above 440 ms, the upper limit of normal.

Exclude other causes of acquired QT interval prolongation and obtain a detailed family history for the possibility of familial LQTS. In the family, episodes of early sudden death, fainting spells, and seizures-epilepsy should alert to this possibility. The ECG should be repeated after a few days to confirm the abnormal finding. Subsequent management depends on: 1) presence or absence of family history suggestive for LQTS, and 2) the degree of QT interval prolongation. The presence of complex ventricular arrhythmias would have additional importance. The following stepwise approach involves infants with and without family history for LQTS. If family history is positive, then a) as LQTS is an autosomal dominant disease b) the infant has a 50% probability of being affected and complete diagnostic procedures should be performed, as always with LQTS families (Figure 1).

- The 2nd ECG is normal.

If the first QTc was <470 ms, dismiss the case. If the first QTc was ≥470 ms, then plan a 3rd ECG after 1-2 months to remain on the safe side.

- The 2nd ECG shows a QTc between 440 and 470 ms.

In these cases with persistent borderline QT prolongation, electrolytes, including calcium and magnesium, should be checked. Clinical history of autoimmune disease and plasma titres of maternal antibodies (anti Ro/SSA and antiLa/SSB) should be assessed. T wave morphology may be helpful; for example, the presence of notches on the T

Figure 1. QT prolongation management flow-chart

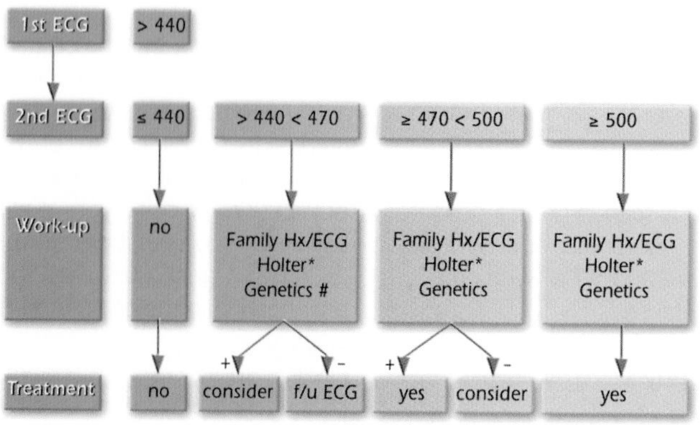

Electrolytes, echocardiogram, intracranial ultrasound are recommended in the appropriate clinical situation. In cases of positive genetics and QTc > 440 ms, therapy is indicated. # In cases of a positive family history (Hx) for LQTS ;* See text on this page.

wave in the precordial leads further suggests the presence of LQTS. Additionally, mild bradycardia can also be found in LQTS. ECGs should be obtained from the parents and siblings of the neonate. In the absence of family history of LQTS, symptoms or arrhythmias, a 24-hour Holter monitoring should be obtained to look for T wave alternans, complex ventricular arrhythmias or marked QTc prolongation, and the ECG should be periodically checked during the first year. No treatment is currently recommended. With a positive family history, the probability of LQTS becomes high. Additional diagnostic procedures (24-hour Holter monitoring, echocardiogram and genetic screening) should be performed and initiation of therapy could be considered.

- The 2nd ECG shows a QTc ≥470 and <500 ms.

All diagnostic procedures listed above should be performed and a 3rd ECG should be planned within a month. In case of a positive family history, therapy should be initiated. Even without family history, therapy should be considered. Even in infants with very prolonged QTc in the first month of life, the ECG may normalised. If subsequent ECGs and diagnostic procedures do not confirm the presence of LQTS, it is logical to progressively withdraw therapy and to return to periodic observations.

- The 2nd ECG shows a QTc ≥500 ms

Infants with a QTc ≥500 ms are very likely to be affected by LQTS and to become symptomatic. All diagnostic procedures listed above should be performed and these infants should be treated.

Highest risk

The presence of QTc close to 600 ms, or of T wave alternans, or of 2:1 AV block secondary to major QT prolongation, or of hearing loss identify infants at extremely high risk.

ST segment elevation

ST segment elevation may be caused by pericarditis (most frequent), hyperkalemia, intracranial haemorrhage, pneumothorax and pneumopericardium, subepicardial injury due to anomalous left coronary artery or to Kawasaki disease with cardiac involvement. ST segment elevation with a RBBB pattern in the right precordial leads (V1 and V2) is the typical finding of the Brugada syndrome, a genetic disorder associated with a high incidence of sudden cardiac death secondary to ventricular fibrillation, in the absence of cardiac structural abnormalities. The ST segment elevation is typically downsloping or "coved" and it is followed by a negative T wave, at variance with the early repolarisation syndrome where ST segment elevation has an upward concavity, it is confined to mid-precordial leads and it is associated with a positive T wave. The diagnosis of the Brugada syndrome is made difficult by the intermittent nature of the ECG abnormalities, as 40% of cases may be normal transiently. Rare cases of Brugada syndrome have been reported during infancy.

Work-up

Whenever the underlying cause has been identified, it should be treated. If the Brugada syndrome is suspected, careful family history should be collected, a 24-hour Holter monitoring should be obtained, and the patient should be referred to a specialist.

Atrial and ventricular arrhythmias

Atrial/junctional

Premature atrial beats

Premature atrial beats (PABs) usually have a different morphology and mean vector from sinus P waves. It is relatively common in the same strip to see PABs conducted normally, aberrantly and blocked.

Work-up

In patients with frequent PABs, a follow-up ECG at one month may be performed. Relatively long periods of blocked atrial bigeminy may simulate sinus bradycardia. The distinction is important since blocked atrial bigeminy is most often benign while severe sinus bradycardia may accompany systemic illness.

Supraventricular tachycardia

Supraventricular tachycardia (SVT) has an extremely regular R-R interval after the first 10–20 beats most often at rates 260–300 bpm. Persistent aberration of SVT in infants is exceedingly rare, implying the diagnosis of VT with a QRS complex different from sinus (table 2).

Work-up

It is important to document SVT with a 12-lead ECG before attempting conversion of the rhythm unless the infant is critically ill. After sinus rhythm is achieved, the WPW pattern should be sought on a 12-lead ECG. Treatment to prevent further episodes of SVT in infancy is generally recommended. An echocardiogram is indicated to determine ventricular function or the presence of congenital heart disease.

Table 2. Distinguishing Tachyarrhythmias in Infants

	Sinus Tachycardia	SVT	Atrial Flutter	VT
History	Sepsis, fever, hypovolaemia, etc.	Usually normal	Most have a normal heart	Many with abnormal heart
Rate	Almost always <230 bpm	Most often 260 - 300 bpm	Atrial 300 - 500 bpm. Vent. 1:1 to 4:1 conduction	200 - 500 bpm
R-R interval variation	Over several seconds may get faster and slower	After first 10 - 20 beats, extremely regular	May have variable block (1:1, 2:1, 3:1) giving different ventricular rates	Slight variation over several beats
P Wave Axis	Same as sinus almost always visible P waves	60% visible P waves, P waves do not look like sinus P waves	Flutter waves (best seen in LII, LIII, aVF, V1)	May have sinus P waves continuing unrelated to VT (AV dissociation), retrograde P waves, or no visible P waves
QRS	Almost always same as slower sinus rhythm	After first 10 - 20 beats, almost always same as sinus	Usually same as sinus, may have occasional beats different from sinus	Different from sinus (not necessarily "wide")

SVT = Supraventricular tachycardia; VT = Ventricular tachycardia

Atrial flutter

In general, there is variable AV conduction from 1:1 to 4:1 yielding an irregular ventricular rate and the QRS complex is usually the same as in sinus rhythm. Due to the occasional association with WPW, this pattern should be specifically sought. Other types of supraventricular arrhythmias such as atrial fibrillation or multifocal tachycardia are extremely rare in the neonate.

Work-up

Conversion to sinus rhythm should be attempted. An echocardiogram is worthwhile to determine ventricular function and the possible presence of congenital heart disease.

Ventricular arrhythmias

Premature ventricular beats

In infants, the QRS duration of premature ventricular beats (PVBs) may be normal or slightly prolonged, but if the complex has a different morphology from the sinus and it is not preceded by premature P wave, the diagnosis is PVB. It is not possible to distinguish PVBs from PABs with aberrancy on the basis of QRS morphology.

Work-up

The QT interval should be measured (see section on ventricular repolarisation). In complex ventricular arrhythmias, a 24-hour Holter monitoring may be worthwhile. An echocardiogram may be performed to determine ventricular function or structural abnormalities. Occasionally maternal drugs that cause ventricular arrhythmias may be transferred in utero or post-natally in breast milk.

Ventricular tachycardia

SVT in infants with a different QRS beyond the first 10–20 beats is rare and a diagnosis of VT should be strongly considered. The rate of VT may be 200–500 bpm. There may be sinus P waves unrelated to VT (AV dissociation), retrograde P waves or no visible P waves. The diagnosis of VT should be strongly considered if the patient has PVBs during times of sinus rhythm with a similar morphology to the tachyarrhythmia.

Work-up

An underlying cardiac or CNS abnormality may be found in infants with VT. The QT interval should be measured (see section on ventricular repolarisation), a 24-hour Holter monitoring and echocardiogram should be obtained. Treatment is generally indicated.

Accelerated ventricular rhythm

It is also known as "slow VT", the rate is approximately the same as the infant's sinus rate (<200 bpm), and the rhythms tend to alternate.

Work-up

While these infants most often have a normal heart, a work-up similar to VT is indicated.

Appendix 1, Part 1. QTc

R-R Interval

QT Interval

mm		8,50	8,75	9,00	9,25	9,50	9,75	10,00	10,25	10,50	10,75	11,00	11,25	11,50	11,75	12,00	12,25	12,50	12,75	13,00	13,25		mm
	msec	340	350	360	370	380	390	400	410	420	430	440	450	460	470	480	490	500	510	520	530	msec	
6,00	240	412	406	400	395	389	384	379	375	370	366	362	358	354	350	346	343	339	336	333	330	240	6,00
6,25	250	429	423	417	411	406	400	395	390	386	381	377	373	369	365	361	357	354	350	347	343	250	6,25
6,50	260	446	439	433	427	422	416	411	406	401	396	392	388	383	379	375	371	368	364	361	357	260	6,50
6,75	270	463	456	450	444	438	432	427	422	417	412	407	402	398	394	390	386	382	378	374	371	270	6,75
7,00	280	480	473	467	460	454	448	443	437	432	427	422	417	413	408	404	400	396	392	388	385	280	7,00
7,25	290	497	490	483	477	470	464	459	453	447	442	437	432	428	423	419	414	410	406	402	398	290	7,25
7,50	300	514	507	500	493	487	480	474	469	463	457	452	447	442	438	433	429	424	420	416	412	300	7,50
7,75	310	532	524	517	510	503	496	490	484	478	473	467	462	457	452	447	443	438	434	430	426	310	7,75
8,00	320	549	541	533	526	519	512	506	500	494	488	482	477	472	467	462	457	453	448	444	440	320	8,00
8,25	330	566	558	550	543	535	528	522	515	509	503	497	492	487	481	476	471	467	462	458	453	330	8,25
8,50	340		575	567	559	552	544	538	531	525	518	513	507	501	496	491	486	481	476	471	467	340	8,50
8,75	350			583	575	568	560	553	547	540	534	528	522	516	511	505	500	495	490	485	481	350	8,75
9,00	360				592	584	576	569	562	555	549	543	537	531	525	520	514	509	504	499	494	360	9,00
9,25	370					600	592	585	578	571	564	558	552	546	540	534	529	523	518	513	508	370	9,25
9,50	380						608	601	593	586	579	573	566	560	554	548	543	537	532	527	522	380	9,50
9,75	390							617	609	602	595	588	581	575	569	563	557	552	546	541	536	390	9,75
10,00	400								625	617	610	603	596	590	583	577	571	566	560	555	549	400	10,00
10,25	410									633	625	618	611	605	598	592	586	580	574	569	563	410	10,25
10,50	420										640	633	626	619	613	606	600	594	588	582	577	420	10,50
10,75	430											648	641	634	627	621	614	608	602	596	591	430	10,75
11,00	440												656	649	642	635	629	622	616	610	604	440	11,00
11,25	450													663	656	650	643	636	630	624	618	450	11,25
11,50	460														671	664	657	651	644	638	632	460	11,50
11,75	470															678	671	665	658	652	646	470	11,75
12,00	480																686	679	672	666	659	480	12,00
12,25	490																	693	686	680	673	490	12,25
12,50	500																		700	693	687	500	12,50
12,75	510																			707	701	510	12,75
13,00	520																				714	520	13,00
	msec	340	350	360	370	380	390	400	410	420	430	440	450	460	470	480	490	500	510	520	530	msec	
mm		8,50	8,75	9,00	9,25	9,50	9,75	10,00	10,25	10,50	10,75	11,00	11,25	11,50	11,75	12,00	12,25	12,50	12,75	13,00	13,25		mm

Chart for calculation of QTc (for heart rates between 81 and 176 bpm)*. QTc, according to the Bazett's formula, is obtained by matching QT and RR interval inmillimetres, given the paper speed at 25 mm/sec. Corresponding values of RR interval and uncorrected QT interval are also indicated.

Appendix 1, Part 2. QTc

R-R Interval

QT Interval

mm		13,50	13,75	14,00	14,25	14,50	14,75	15,00	15,25	15,50	15,75	16,00	16,25	16,50	16,75	17,00	17,25	17,50	17,75	18,00	18,25	18,50		mm
	msec	540	550	560	570	580	590	600	610	620	630	640	650	660	670	680	690	700	710	720	730	740	msec	
6,00	240	327	324	321	318	315																	240	6,00
6,25	250	340	337	334	331	328	325	323	320	318	315												250	6,25
6,50	260	354	351	347	344	341	338	336	333	330	328	325	322	320	318	315							260	6,50
6,75	270	367	364	361	358	355	352	349	346	343	340	338	335	332	330	327	325	323	320	318	316		270	6,75
7,00	280	381	378	374	371	368	365	361	359	356	353	350	347	345	342	340	337	335	332	330	328	325	280	7,00
7,25	290	395	391	388	384	381	378	374	371	368	365	363	360	357	354	352	349	347	344	342	339	337	290	7,25
7,50	300	408	405	401	397	394	391	387	384	381	378	375	372	369	367	364	361	359	356	354	351	349	300	7,50
7,75	310	422	418	414	411	407	404	400	397	394	391	388	385	382	379	376	373	371	368	365	363	360	310	7,75
8,00	320	435	431	428	424	420	417	413	410	406	403	400	397	394	391	388	385	382	380	377	375	372	320	8,00
8,25	330	449	445	441	437	433	430	426	423	419	416	413	409	406	403	400	397	394	392	389	386	384	330	8,25
8,50	340	463	458	454	450	446	443	439	435	432	428	425	422	419	415	412	409	406	404	401	398	395	340	8,50
8,75	350	476	472	468	464	460	456	452	448	445	441	438	434	431	428	424	421	418	415	412	410	407	350	8,75
9,00	360	490	485	481	477	473	469	465	461	457	454	450	447	443	440	437	433	430	427	424	421	418	360	9,00
9,25	370	504	499	494	490	486	482	478	474	470	466	463	459	455	452	449	445	442	439	436	433	430	370	9,25
9,50	380	517	512	508	503	499	495	491	487	483	479	475	471	468	464	461	457	454	451	448	445	442	380	9,50
9,75	390	531	526	521	517	512	508	503	499	495	491	488	484	480	476	473	470	466	463	460	456	453	390	9,75
10,00	400	544	539	535	530	525	521	516	512	508	504	500	496	492	489	485	482	478	475	471	468	465	400	10,00
10,25	410	558	553	548	543	538	534	529	525	521	517	513	509	505	501	497	494	490	487	483	480	477	410	10,25
10,50	420	572	566	561	556	551	547	542	538	533	529	525	521	517	513	509	506	502	498	495	492	488	420	10,50
10,75	430	585	580	575	570	565	560	555	551	546	542	538	533	529	525	521	518	514	510	507	503	500	430	10,75
11,00	440	599	593	588	583	578	573	568	563	559	554	550	546	542	538	534	530	526	522	519	515	511	440	11,00
11,25	450	612	607	601	596	591	586	581	576	572	567	563	558	554	550	546	542	538	534	530	527	523	450	11,25
11,50	460	626	620	615	609	604	599	594	589	584	580	575	571	566	562	558	554	550	546	542	538	535	460	11,50
11,75	470	640	634	628	623	617	612	607	602	597	592	588	583	579	574	570	566	562	558	554	550	546	470	11,75
12,00	480	653	647	641	636	630	625	620	615	610	605	600	595	591	586	582	578	574	570	566	562	558	480	12,00
12,25	490	667	661	655	649	643	638	633	627	622	617	613	608	603	599	594	590	586	582	577	574	570	490	12,25
12,50	500	680	674	668	662	657	651	645	640	635	630	625	620	615	611	606	602	598	593	589	585	581	500	12,50
12,75	510	694	688	682	676	670	664	658	653	648	643	638	633	628	623	618	614	610	605	601	597	593	510	12,75
13,00	520	708	701	695	689	683	677	671	666	660	655	650	645	640	635	631	626	622	617	613	609	604	520	13,00
	msec	540	550	560	570	580	590	600	610	620	630	640	650	660	670	680	690	700	710	720	730	740	msec	
mm		13,50	13,75	14,00	14,25	14,50	14,75	15,00	15,25	15,50	15,75	16,00	16,25	16,50	16,75	17,00	17,25	17,50	17,75	18,00	18,25	18,50		mm

Chart for calculation of QTc (for heart rates between 81 and 176 bpm)*. QTc, according to the Bazett's formula, is obtained by matching QT and RR interval inmillimetres, given the paper speed at 25 mm/sec. Corresponding values of RR interval and uncorrected QT interval are also indicated.

Section VIII:
Pregnancy and Heart Disease

1. Cardiovascular Disease during Pregnancy

Chapter 1

Cardiovascular Disease during Pregnancy*

2003

Chairperson:
Celia Oakley, MD, FRCP, FESC, FACC
Professor (Emeritus) of Clinical Cardiology
Imperial College School of Medicine
Hammersmith Hospital
London W12 0NN
UK
Phone: +44 (0) 1844 208246
or +44 (0) 20 8383 3141
Fax: +44 (0) 1844 202968
or +44 (0) 20 8740 8373
Email: oakleypridie@aol.com

Task Force Members:
1. Anne Child, London, UK (Genetics)
2. Bernard Iung, Paris, France (Cardiology)
3. Patrizia Presbitero, Milan, Italy (Cardiology)
4. Pilar Tornos, Barcelona, Spain (Cardiology)

ESC Staff:
1. Keith McGregor, Sophia-Antipolis, France
2. Veronica Dean, Sophia-Antipolis, France
3. Dominique Poumeyrol-Jumeau, Sophia-Antipolis, France
4. Catherine Després, Sophia-Antipolis, France

1. Introduction

Cardiovascular diseases during pregnancy represent a very heterogeneous group as regards the diseases involved and the risks related to pregnancy. Management is based on haemodynamic principles: full diagnosis of the maternal heart condition plus knowledge of the physiological changes in pregnancy. Likely outcome is determined by these. Good management depends on team work between local physicians and general practitioners, involved cardiologists, obstetricians and anaesthetists and where appropriate, geneticists and neonatologists. Pregnant women do not like to travel and shared care between local doctors and the specialist centre should be practised whenever possible. Most women with heart disease do well but some conditions are dangerous.

2. Physiological changes during pregnancy

An increase in blood volume follows an increase in capacity of the vascular bed caused by hormonal changes which relax smooth muscle. The changes begin as early as the 5th week.

- Both blood volume and cardiac output rise by 30 to 50% (more in multiple pregnancy).
- Stroke volume increases more than heart rate. A resting tachycardia gives warning of inability to raise stroke output and is dangerous when left ventricular filling is slow or coronary flow reserve reduced.
- Diastolic BP falls, is lowest in mid-trimester and rises towards the end with little change in systolic pressure.
- Coagulation factors rise and fibrinolytic activity diminishes. The risk of thromboembolism increases.
- The post-partum period is also not risk-free since haemodynamic conditions do not return to normal for up to one month after the delivery.

*Adapted from the ESC Expert Consensus Document on the Management of Cardiovascular Diseases during Pregnancy. (European Heart Journal 2003; 24(8): 761-781)

3. In general

3.1 Pre-existing conditions which may confer high maternal risk

- Pulmonary hypertension of any cause
- Left ventricular inflow or outflow obstruction – mitral or aortic stenosis and some cases of hypertrophic cardiomyopathy
- The fragile aorta e.g. in Marfan syndrome or coarctation
- Valvular prostheses requiring anticoagulant treatment
- Any patients reaching NYHA* class III or IV during pregnancy
- Severe cyanotic congenital heart disease

3.2 Low maternal risk

- Any patient in NYHA* class I to II before pregnancy except for those at high maternal risk (see above)
- Left to right shunts
- Valvular regurgitation
- Modest left ventricular outflow obstruction
- Right ventricular outflow obstruction (unless severe)

3.3 Maternal conditions causing high foetal risk

- Any maternal condition reaching NYHA* class III or IV in pregnancy
- Haemodynamic instability
- Need for warfarin dosage above 5 mg/day
- Pre-eclampsia and eclampsia
- Severe cyanotic congenital heart disease

The presence of functional NYHA* class III and IV during pregnancy requires immediate hospitalization and prompt treatment. Unless haemodynamic improvement is obtained termination of pregnancy or delivery should be considered.

* NYHA = New York Heart Association

3.4 Heart conditions which may develop in pregnancy or parturition

- Hypertension and pre-eclampsia
- Peripartum cardiomyopathy
- Myocardial infarction (usually due to dissection)
- Aortic dissection
- Pulmonary embolism
- Tachyarrhythmias (all types)

4. Congenital Heart Disease

4.1 High risk patients

- *Eisenmenger syndrome or severe pulmonary hypertension without septal defects*
  These patients face a high mortality and should be strongly advised against pregnancy. If pregnant and if termination is refused they should be admitted to hospital in the second trimester for bed rest, oxygen, oximetry, prophylactic heparin and foetal monitoring. Vasodilators need to be avoided during delivery and good hydration maintained. Most deaths occur suddenly during the post-partum period.
- *Severe left ventricular outflow obstruction*
  Failure of the left ventricular outflow velocity to rise, tachycardia, angina or dyspnoea indicate need for rest, beta-blockers and percutaneous aortic valvotomy or surgery if appropriate. If surgery is needed, the foetus should be delivered by C-section before the intervention.
- *Severe maternal cyanosis*
  Oxygen saturation falls during pregnancy but is maximised by rest and oxygen. Foetal growth is impaired. The risk depends on the severity of cyanosis. The risk is high if O_2 saturation is $< 85\%$. Prophylactic heparin should be given.

4.2 Patients at low or moderate risk

- *Pulmonary stenosis*
  Generally, pulmonary stenosis is better tolerated than aortic stenosis but in the presence of severe stenosis, pregnancy may precipitate right ventricular failure, arrhythmia or tricuspid regurgitation. It only rarely needs intervention by balloon valvotomy during pregnancy.

- *Coarctation of the aorta*
  Uncorrected coarctation is only rarely seen. Management of hypertension is never fully successful because of surges on effort despite rest and a beta-blocker. It brings risk of stroke and dissection. Repair reduces but does not remove these risks.

- *Previous surgery with residual defects but good ventricular function*
  After correction of the Tetralogy of Fallot, the risk is low in patients with good repairs. Patients with systemic right ventricle after intra-atrial correction of transposition or univentricular circulations after a Fontan repair can do well provided ventricular function is still sound. Patients with complex congenital defects need careful individual assessment for ventricular function, conduction defects, pulmonary vascular disease, arrhythmic and thromboembolic risk. The risk of foetal defect is low including the 22q11 deletion syndrome.

5. Marfan syndrome and other inherited conditions affecting the aorta

Women with aortic root diameter < 4 cm and no substantial mitral or aortic regurgitation face a 1% risk of aortic dissection or rupture.

Mitral regurgitation is not usually a problem but, if severe, should be repaired before pregnancy.

Patients with aortic root dilatation ≥ 4 cm face about a 10% risk but this risk is reduced after elective aortic root replacement.

Beta-blockers should be continued throughout pregnancy including operated patients.

6. Acquired valvular heart disease

- Rheumatic heart valve disease is still common in developing countries.

- Mitral regurgitation is well tolerated unless atrial fibrillation develops with a fast ventricular rate.

- In aortic regurgitation tachycardia reduces the time for diastolic regurgitation and it is well tolerated even when severe.

6.1 Mitral stenosis

- Left atrial pressure rises due to increased stroke and blood volume and shortened diastole. Tachycardia warns of this. Close follow-up with serial Doppler echocardiography is needed, in particular during the 2nd and 3rd trimesters.

- A mitral valve area < 1.5 cm^2 carries risk. A selective beta-blocker should be started in patients with dyspnoea in a dose sufficient to control sinus rate and a diuretic may be needed.

- Prophylactic balloon valvotomy is not recommended but should be performed in an experienced centre if pulmonary congestion persists or if systolic pulmonary pressure remains > 50 mmHg despite medical therapy.

6.2 Aortic stenosis

Most cases are congenital or are associated with mitral stenosis. The risk is generally low if mean aortic gradient remains ≤ 50 mmHg during pregnancy.

6.3 Heart valve prostheses

Haemodynamic tolerance is generally good. The problem is the absolute need for anticoagulant treatment in patients with mechanical prostheses.

In managing these patients it needs to be remembered that:

- Pregnancy is a hypercoagulable state.

- Vitamin K antagonists cross the placenta and may cause embryopathy.

- The risk of embryopathy is dose related. It is negligible if the dose is 5 mg or less.

- Heparin is less effective.

- Maternal risk of thromboembolism is minimised if warfarin is continued throughout.

- Elective caesarean section at 36 weeks avoids the transfer to heparin which is necessary to avoid neonatal cerebral haemorrhage during vaginal delivery.

- The choice should be made after the patient and her partner have been fully informed.

- The safety and efficacy of low molecular weight heparin has not been established for patients with mechanical heart valves so should not be recommended at the present time.

7. Cardiomyopathies

7.1 Peripartum cardiomyopathy (PPCM)

- This is unexplained left ventricular dysfunction which develops during the last month of pregnancy or within five months of delivery confirmed by echocardiography.
- It presents with heart failure, less often embolism or arrhythmia.
- The worst cases present early post-partum and may need inotropic agents and a ventricular assisting device. As ventricular function usually improves even in the most fulminating cases, every effort should be made to avoid transplantation.
- Early biopsy usually shows myocarditis and immuno suppressives may be helpful.
- Anticoagulants are important. ACE-inhibitors are contra-indicated before delivery.
- The risk of recurrence should lead to discouragement of further pregnancies even after an apparent recovery of left ventricular function.

7.2 Dilated cardiomyopathy (DCM)

Patients with dilated cardiomyopathy should be advised against pregnancy because of a high chance of deterioration.

Termination should be advised if the ejection fraction is < 45% and/or the left ventricular dimensions are definitely above normal.

- Echocardiography should be performed before conception if possible in all patients with a family history of DCM or PPCM.
- Pregnancy is inadvisable if left ventricular function is reduced.
- Patients with a family history of DCM may have a higher risk of PPCM.
- Pregnant patients with DCM are at high risk.

7.3 Hypertrophic cardiomyopathy (HCM)

- Women with HCM usually tolerate pregnancy well but fatalities have been reported. There is no evidence for an increased risk in pregnancy.
- After a diagnosis is first made in pregnancy, an asymptomatic patient can usually be reassured.
- Pulmonary oedema may occur in patients with severe diastolic dysfunction who are very tachycardia sensitive. They are at risk and need rest and a beta-blocker and cautious use of a diuretic.
- If atrial fibrillation develops low molecular weight heparin provides suitable anticoagulation.
- Cardioversion will be needed if atrial fibrillation (AF) persits.
- Normal delivery is advised on a selected date with continued beta-blocker, avoidance of vasodilatation and careful replacement of blood loss.
- The genetic risk needs to be discussed.

8. Arrhythmias

- Both ectopic beats and sustained arrhythmias become more frequent or develop for the first time.
- Treatment is the same as outside pregnancy but as conservative as possible.
- Blood levels of antiarrhythmic drugs need to be checked because of altered pharmacokinetics.
- Cardioversion should be used if tachyarrhythmia is sustained and causing haemodynamic instability. Cardioversion is safe for the foetus.
- Selective beta-1 blocking drugs are preferred for prophylaxis of supraventricular arrhythmias.
- Vagal stimulation and, failing that, intravenous adenosine are first choice for treatment of supraventricular tachycardia.
- Radiofrequency ablation can, if necessary, be performed.
- Ventricular tachycardia is much less common and should be terminated by cardioversion if not well haemodynamically tolerated.

n.b. The reader should consult the ESC Guidelines for the Management of Patients with Supraventricular Arrhythmias for more details.

9. Hypertensive disorders

9.1 Pre-existing hypertension

- Control of pre-existing hypertension should begin before conception and reduces the risk of exacerbation of high BP but has not been shown to reduce super-imposed pre-eclampsia or perinatal mortality.
- Foetal growth should be monitored.
- Methyl dopa remains the first choice and beta-blockers have had extensive and safe use (Atenolol has been reported to reduce foetal growth).
- **ACE-inhibitors and angiotensin receptor inhibitors** are contra-indicated during the second and third trimesters.

9.2 Pre-eclampsia

- There is no specific treatment.
- Pre-eclampsia is completely reversible and usually abates after delivery.
- The aim is to safeguard the mother while securing maturation of the foetus.
- Antihypertensive treatment has not been shown to improve foetal outcome.

9.3 Treatment of acute hypertension

Nifedipine, labetalol and hydralazine are used. Magnesium sulphate is indicated for severe pre-eclampsia and eclampsia but delivery is the only definitive treatment.

Close maternal and foetal surveillance are essential and prompt delivery is indicated if the condition of either worsens.

Section IX: Valvular Heart Disease

1. Valvular Heart Disease

Chapter 1

Valvular Heart Disease*

2007

Chairperson:
Alec Vahanian
Cardiology Department
Hôpital Bichat
46 rue Henri Huchard
75018, Paris, France
Phone: +33 1 40 25 67 60
Fax: +33 1 40 25 67 32
E-mail: alec.vahanian@bch.aphp.fr

Task Force Members:
1. Helmut Baumgartner, Vienna, Austria
2. Jeroen Bax, Leiden, The Netherlands
3. Eric Butchart, Cardiff, UK
4. Robert Dion, Leiden, The Netherlands
5. Gerasimos Filippatos, Athens, Greece
6. Frank Flaschkampf, Erlangen, Germany
7. Roger Hall, Norwich, UK
8. Bernard Iung, Paris, France
9. Jaroslaw Kasprzak, Lodz, Poland
10. Patrick Nataf, Paris, France
11. Pilar Tornos, Barcelona, Spain
12. Lucia Torracca, Milan, Italy
13. Arnold Wenink, Leiden, The Netherlands

ESC Staff:
1. Keith McGregor, Sophia Antipolis, France
2. Veronica Dean, Sophia Antipolis, France
3. Catherine Després, Sophia Antipolis, France

1. Introduction

Valvular heart disease (VHD) is common and often requires intervention. Due to the predominance of degenerative valve disease, the two most frequent valve diseases are now calcific aortic stenosis (AS) and mitral regurgitation (MR), while aortic regurgitation (AR) and mitral stenosis (MS) have become less common. The increase in age of patients with valvular heart disease is associated with a higher frequency of comorbidity, which contributes to increased operative risk and renders decision-making for intervention more complex. Another important aspect of contemporary heart valve disease is the growing proportion of previously operated patients who present with further problems.

Class I	Evidence and/or general agreement that a given treatment is beneficial, useful and effective;
Class II	Conflicting evidence and/or a divergence of opinion about the usefulness/efficacy of a given treatment or procedure;
Class IIa	Weight of evidence/opinion is in favour of usefulness/efficacy;
Class IIb	Usefulness/efficacy is less well established by evidence/opinion;

The guidelines focus on VHD in adults and adolescents, are oriented towards management, and will not deal with endocarditis and congenital valve diseases in adults and adolescents.

The committee emphasises the fact that many factors ultimately determine the most appropriate treatment in individual patients within a given community. Furthermore, due to the lack of evidence-based data in the field of VHD most recommendations are largely the result of expert consensus opinion. Therefore, deviations from these guidelines may be appropriate in certain clinical circumstances.

Level of Evidence A	Data derived from multiple randomized clinical trials or meta-analyses
Level of Evidence B	Data derived from a single randomized trial or non-randomized studies
Level of Evidence C	Consensus of opinion of the experts and/or small studies, retrospective studies, registries

*Adapted from the ESC Guidelines on the Management of Valvular Heart Disease (European Heart Journal 2007;28: 230-268).

2. Patient evaluation

Clinical evaluation is the first step in the diagnosis of VHD and the assessment of its severity.

Echocardiography is the key technique to confirm the diagnosis of VHD as well as to assess its severity and prognosis.

When assessing the severity of VHD it is necessary to check consistency between the different echocardiographic measurements as well as with the anatomy and mechanisms of VHD. It is also necessary to check their consistency with clinical assessment.

The evaluation of the severity of stenotic VHD should combine the assessment of valve area and flow-dependent indices. AS with a valve area <1.0 cm^2 or <0.6cm^2/m^2 body surface area (BSA) is considered severe. Severe AS is unlikely if cardiac output is normal, and there is a mean pressure gradient <50 mmHg.

In MS, planimetry, when it is feasible, is the method of choice to evaluate valve area. MS usually does not have clinical consequences at rest when valve area is >1.5 cm^2, unless in patients with particularly large body size. No generally accepted grading of tricuspid stenosis severity exists. A mean gradient >5 mmHg is considered indicative of clinically significant tricuspid stenosis. The quantification of severe regurgitation should not rely entirely on one single figure, but requires an integrative approach (Table 2).

Table 2: Criteria for the definition of severe valve regurgitation: An integrative approach

	AR	MR	TR
Specific signs of severe regurgitation	• Central jet width ≥65% of LVOT* • Vena contracta >0.6 cm*	• Vena contracta width 30.7 cm with large central MR jet (area >40% of LA) or with a wall impinging jet of any size, swirling in LA* • Large flow convergence*** • Systolic reversal in pulmonary veins • Prominent flail MV or ruptured papillary muscle	• Vena contracta width >0.7 cm in echo • Large flow convergence*** • Systolic reversal in the hepatic veins
Supportive signs	• Pressure half-time <200 ms • Holodiastolic aortic flow reversal in descending aorta • Moderate or greater LV enlargement**	• Dense, triangular CW Doppler MR jet • E-wave dominant mitral inflow (E >1.2 m/s)**** • Enlarged LV and LA size***** (particularly when normal LV function is present)	• Dense, triangular CW TR signal with early peak • Inferior cava dilatation and respiratory diameter variation <<50% • Prominent transtricuspid E-wave, especially if >1 m/s • RA, RV dilatation
Quantitative parameters			
R Vol (ml/beat)	≥60	≥60	
RF (%)	≥50	≥50	
ERO (cm^2)	≥0.30	≥0.40	

AR = aortic regurgitation, CW = continuous wave, ERO = effective regurgitant orifice area, LA = left atrium, LV = left ventricle, LVOT = left ventricular outflow tract, MR = mitral regurgitation, MV = mitral valve, R Vol = regurgitant volume, RA = right atrium, RF = regurgitant fraction, RV = right ventricle, TR = tricuspid regurgitation

* At a Nyquist limit of 50-60 cm/s.

** In the absence of other aetiologies of LV dilatation.

*** Large flow convergence defined as flow convergence radius 30.9 cm for central jets, respectively, with a baseline shift at a Nyquist of 40 cm/s; cut-offs for eccentric jets are higher and should be angled correctly.

**** Usually above 50 years of age or in conditions of impaired relaxation, in the absence of mitral stenosis or other causes of elevated LA pressure.

***** In the absence of other aetiologies of LV and LA dilatation and acute MR.

Adapted from Zoghbi WA, Enriquez-Sarano M, Foster E, et al. Recommendations for evaluation of the severity of native valvular regurgitation with two-dimensional and Doppler echocardiography. J Am Soc Echocardiogr 2003;16:777-802.

In MR and MS, transthoracic echocardiography (TTE) provides precise assessment of valve morphology, which is important for the selection of candidates for surgical valve repair and percutaneous mitral commissurotomy (PMC). Echocardiography should include a comprehensive evaluation of all valves, the ascending aorta, and indices of left ventricular (LV) enlargement and function, LV dimensions being indexed to BSA. Transoesophageal echocardiography (TEE) should be considered when TTE is of suboptimal quality or to exclude left atrial thrombosis before PMC or if prosthetic dysfunction or endocarditis is suspected. It should be performed intraoperatively to monitor the results of valve repair or complex procedures. TTE also plays an important role in monitoring the results of PMC during the procedure.

Exercise testing is useful to unmask the objective occurrence of symptoms in patients who claim to be asymptomatic. Exercise testing is recommended in truly asymptomatic patients with AS provided it is performed under close monitoring.

Low-dose dobutamine stress echocardiography is useful in AS with impaired LV function to distinguish the rare cases of pseudo-severe AS from truly severe AS. In addition this test may detect the presence of contractile reserve (increase > 20% of stroke volume). The use of stress tests to detect coronary artery disease associated with severe VHD is discouraged because of their low diagnostic value.

In expert centres **multislice computed tomography** can be useful to exclude coronary artery disease in patients who are at low risk of atherosclerosis.

At present, **magnetic resonance imaging** is not indicated in VHD in routine clinical practice; however, it can be used as an alternative technique when echocardiography is not feasible.

Coronary angiography is widely indicated to detect associated coronary artery disease when surgery is planned (Table 3). It can be omitted in patients with acute aortic dissection, large aortic vegetation, or occlusive prosthetic thrombosis leading to an unstable haemodynamic condition.

The performance of **cardiac catheterization** should be restricted to situations where non-invasive evaluation is inconclusive or discordant with clinical findings.

The **assessment of comorbidity** is directed by the clinical evaluation.

Endocarditis prophylaxis should be considered in any patient with VHD, and adapted to the individual patient risk.

The decision to intervene in a patient with VHD relies on an **individual risk-benefit analysis**. Multivariate scores, such as the Euroscore (http://www.euroscore.org/calc.html), are useful in this setting. Decision-making should also take into account the patient's life expectancy, quality of life, as well as local resources and very importantly, the decision of the informed patient. In the elderly, age, *per se*, should not be considered a contra-indication for surgery.

3. Indications for treatment in native valve diseases

3.1 Aortic regurgitation

Indications for surgery

In chronic AR, the goals of the operation are to avoid left ventricular systolic dysfunction and/or aortic complications (Table 4).

Table 3: Indications for coronary angiography in patients with valvular heart disease

	Class
Before valve surgery in patients with severe valvular heart disease and any of the following: • history of coronary artery disease • suspected myocardial ischaemia* • left ventricular systolic dysfunction • in men aged over 40 and post-menopausal women • ≥1 cardiovascular risk factor	IC
When coronary artery disease is suspected to be the cause of severe mitral regurgitation (ischaemic mitral regurgitation)	IC

* Chest pain, abnormal non-invasive testing.

Table 4: Indications for surgery in aortic regurgitation

	Class
Severe AR	
Symptomatic patients (dyspnoea NYHA class II, III, IV or angina)	IB
Asymptomatic patients with resting LVEF ≤50%	IB
Patients undergoing CABG or surgery of ascending aorta, or on another valve	IC
Asymptomatic patients with resting LVEF >50% with severe LV dilatation: End diastolic dimension >70 mm or End systolic dimension >50 mm (or >25 mm/m² BSA)*	 IIaC IIaC
Whatever the severity of AR	
Patients who have aortic root disease with maximal aortic diameter**: ≥45 mm for patients with Marfan's syndrome ≥50 mm for patients with bicuspid valves ≥55 mm for other patients	 IC IIaC IIaC

Severity is defined from clinical and echocardiographic assessment.

In asymptomatic patients repeated and high quality measures are necessary before surgery.

* Patient's stature should also be considered. Indexing is helpful. Changes in sequential measurements should be taken into account. ** Decision should take into account the shape and thickness of ascending aorta as well as the shape of the other parts of aorta. For patients who have an indication for surgery on the aortic valve, lower thresholds can be used for combining surgery on the ascending aorta.

AR = aortic regurgitation, BSA = body surface area, CABG = coronary artery bypass grafting, LV = left ventricular, EF = ejection fraction

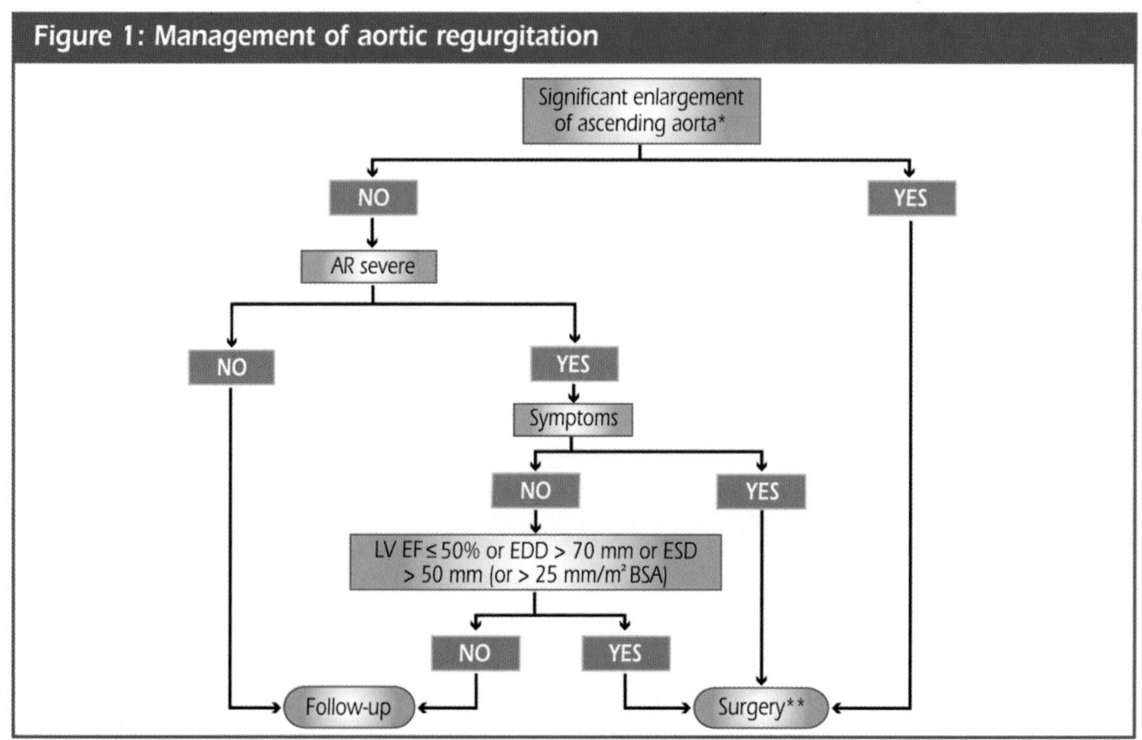

AR = aortic regurgitation, LV = left ventricle, EF = ejection fraction, EDD = end-diastolic dimension, ESD = end-systolic dimension, BSA = body surface area

* See Table 4 for definitions.

** Surgery must also be considered if significant changes occur during follow-up.

Medical therapy

The role of vasodilators in asymptomatic patients without hypertension or congestive heart failure is unproven. In patients with Marfan's syndrome beta-blockers should be given before and after the operation.

3.2 Aortic stenosis

Indications for surgery

Early valve replacement should be strongly considered in all symptomatic patients with severe AS who are otherwise candidates for surgery. As long as mean gradient is still >40 mmHg, there is virtually no lower EF limit for surgery. The management of patients with low-flow, low-gradient AS (severely reduced EF and mean gradient <40 mmHg) is more controversial. Surgery is advised in patients with evidence of contractile reserve. Conversely, in patients without contractile reserve surgery can, nonetheless, be performed but decision-making should take into account clinical condition, and feasibility of revascularization.

Balloon valvuloplasty

This can be considered as a bridge to surgery in haemodynamically unstable patients who are at high risk for surgery (*Recommendation class IIb level of evidence C*), or in patients with symptomatic severe AS who require urgent major non-cardiac surgery (*Recommendation class IIb level of evidence C*).

Medical therapy

Modification of atherosclerotic risk factors must be strongly recommended following the guidelines of secondary prevention in atherosclerosis.

Serial testing

Patients should be carefully educated about the importance of follow-up and reporting symptoms as soon as they develop.

In cases of moderate to severe calcification of the valve and peak aortic jet velocity >4 m/s at initial evaluation patients should be re-evaluated every 6 months for the occurrence of symptoms, change in exercise tolerance or in echo-parameters. If peak aortic jet velocity has increased since the last visit (>0.3 m/sec. per year), surgery should be considered. If no change has occurred and the patient remains asymptomatic, 6 monthly clinical and 6-12 monthly clinical and echocardiographic re-evaluations are recommended.

In patients who do not meet these criteria, a clinical yearly follow-up is necessary, follow-up being closer in those with borderline values.

Table 5: Indications for aortic valve replacement in aortic stenosis

	Class
Patients with severe AS and any symptoms	IB
Patients with severe AS undergoing coronary artery bypass surgery, surgery of the ascending aorta, or on another valve	IC
Asymptomatic patients with severe AS and systolic LV dysfunction (LVEF <50%) unless due to other cause	IC
Asymptomatic patients with severe AS and abnormal exercise test showing symptoms on exercise	IC
Asymptomatic patients with severe AS and abnormal exercise test showing fall in blood pressure below baseline	IIaC
Patients with moderate AS* undergoing coronary artery bypass surgery, surgery of the ascending aorta or another valve	IIaC
Asymptomatic patients with severe AS and moderate to severe valve calcification, and a rate of peak velocity progression ≥0.3 m/sec per year	IIaC
AS with low gradient (<40 mmHg) and LV dysfunction with contractile reserve	IIaC
Asymptomatic patients with severe AS and abnormal exercise test showing complex ventricular arrhythmias	IIbC
Asymptomatic patients with severe AS and excessive LV hypertrophy (≥15 mm) unless this is due to hypertension	IIbC
AS with low gradient (<40 mmHg) and LV dysfunction without contractile reserve	IIbC

* Moderate AS is defined as valve area 1.0 to 1.5 cm^2 (0.6 cm^2/m^2 to 0.9 cm^2/m^2 BSA) or mean aortic gradient 30 to 50 mmHg in the presence of normal flow conditions. However, clinical judgment is required.

AS = aortic stenosis, LV = left ventricular, EF = ejection fraction, BSA = body surface area

Figure 2: Management of severe aortic stenosis

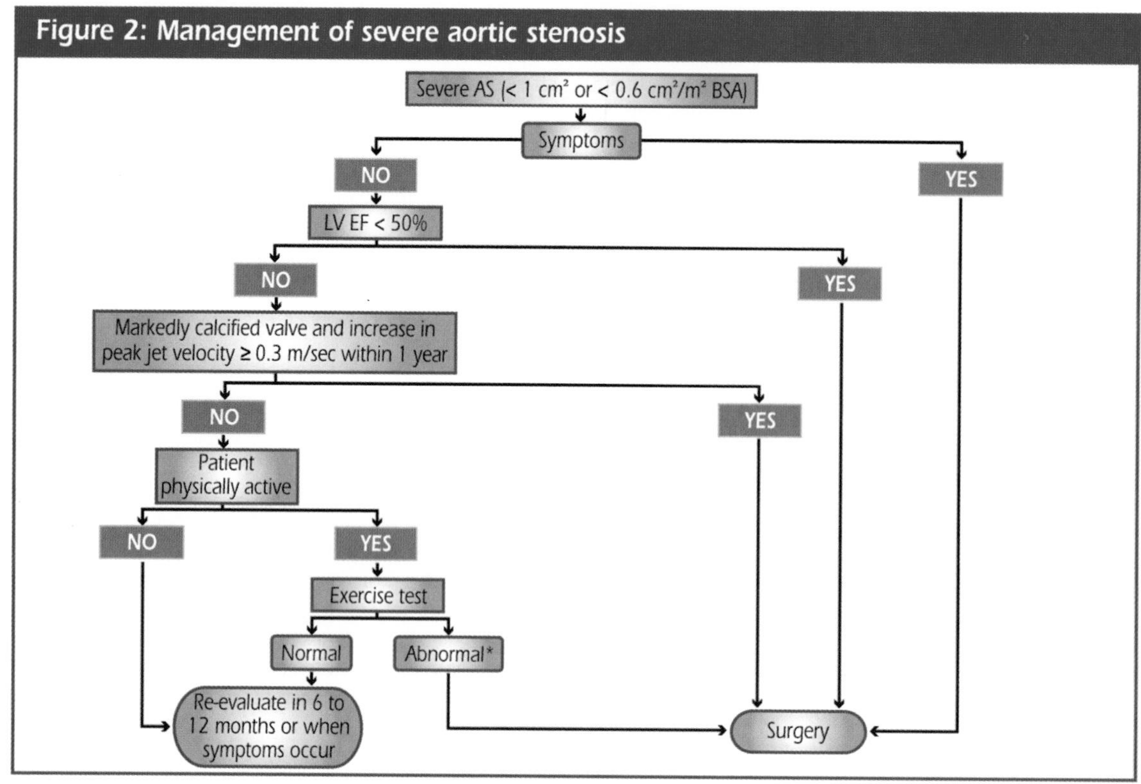

AS = aortic stenosis, LV = left ventricle, EF = ejection fraction, BSA = body surface area

* See Table 5 for definitions.

Note: The management of patients with low gradient and low ejection fraction is detailed in the text.

3.3 Mitral regurgitation

Organic mitral regurgitation

Organic MR covers all aetiologies in which leaflet abnormality is the primary cause of the disease, in opposition to ischaemic and functional MR, in which MR is the consequence of LV disease.

Indications for surgery

Valve repair, when feasible and durable results can be expected, is the optimal surgical treatment in patients with severe MR.

Table 6: Indications for surgery in severe chronic organic mitral regurgitation

	Class
Symptomatic patients with LVEF >30% and ESD <55 mm*	IB
Asymptomatic patients with LV dysfunction (ESD >45 mm* and/or LVEF ≤60%)	IC
Asymptomatic patients with preserved LV function and atrial fibrillation or pulmonary hypertension (systolic pulmonary artery pressure >50 mmHg at rest)	IIaC
Patients with severe LV dysfunction (LVEF <30% and/or ESD >55 mm*) refractory to medical therapy with high likelihood of durable repair and low comorbidity	IIaC
Asymptomatic patients with preserved LV function, high likelihood of durable repair, and low risk for surgery	IIbB
Patients with severe LV dysfunction (LVEF <30% and/or ESD >55 mm*) refractory to medical therapy with low likelihood of repair and low comorbidity	IIbC

Severity is based on clinical and echocardiographic assessment.

* Lower values can be considered for patients of small stature.

ESD = end systolic dimension, EF = ejection fraction, LV = left ventricular

Figure 3: Management of severe chronic organic mitral regurgitation

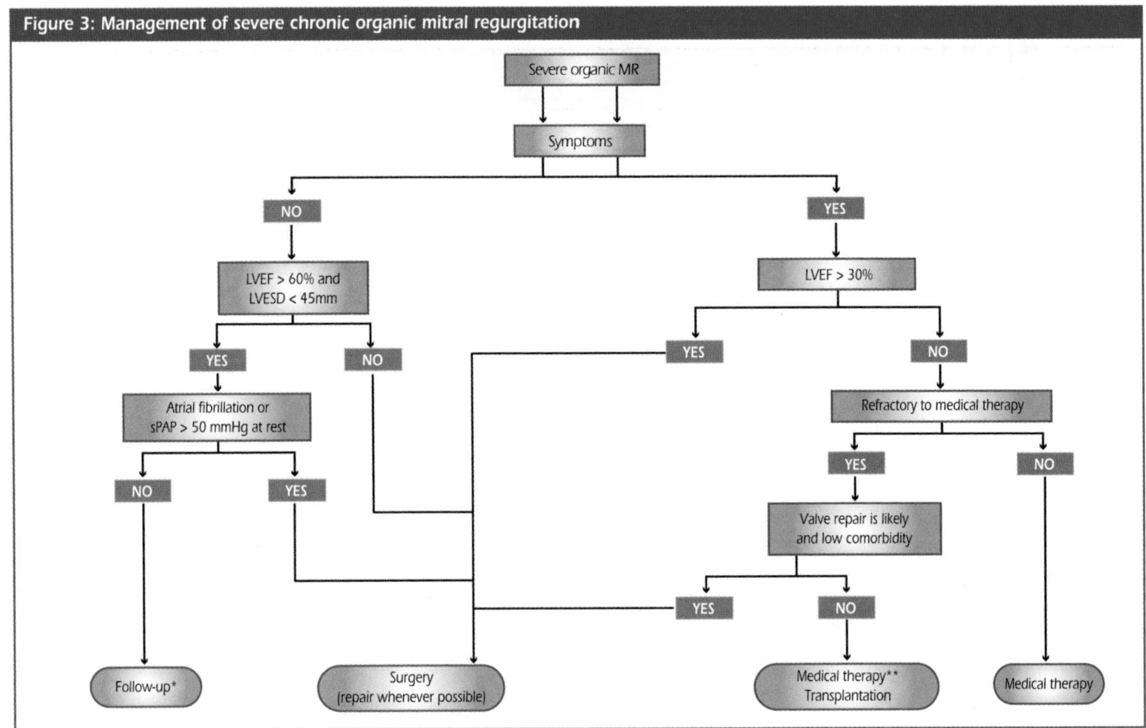

LV = left ventricle, EF = ejection fraction, sPAP = systolic pulmonary artery pressure, ESD = end-systolic dimension

* Valve repair can be considered when there is a high likelihood of durable valve repair at a low risk.

** Valve replacement can be considered in selected patients with low comorbidity.

The management of asymptomatic patients is an area of controversy where the indications for surgery depend on risk stratification, the possibility of valve repair, and the preference of the informed patient.

Medical therapy

Anticoagulant therapy, with a target International Normalised Ratio (INR) range between 2 and 3, should be given in patients with MR and permanent or paroxysmal atrial fibrillation or whenever there is a history of systemic embolism or evidence of left atrial thrombus, and during the first 3 months following mitral valve repair. Vasodilators, including ACE-inhibitors, are not recommended in patients with chronic MR without heart failure or hypertension.

Serial testing

Asymptomatic patients with moderate MR and preserved LV function can be clinically followed-up on a yearly basis and echocardiography should be performed every 2 years.

Asymptomatic patients with severe MR and preserved LV function should be seen every 6 months and echocardiography performed every year, the follow-up being closer if no previous evaluation is available, and in patients with borderline values, or significant changes since the last visit.

Ischaemic mitral regurgitation

Ischaemic MR is common, however, it is frequently overlooked in the setting of acute or chronic coronary disease.

Indications for surgery

The limited data in the field of ischaemic MR results in less evidence-based management.

Functional mitral regurgitation

This includes MR observed in cardiomyopathy and in ischaemic disease with severe LV dysfunction. Isolated mitral valve surgery in combination with LV reconstruction techniques, may be considered in selected patients with severe functional MR and severely depressed LV function, including those with coronary disease where bypass surgery is not indicated, who remain symptomatic despite optimal medical therapy, and if comorbidity is low, the aim being to avoid, or postpone transplantation.

Table 7: Indications for surgery in chronic ischaemic mitral regurgitation

	Class
Patients with severe MR, LVEF >30%, undergoing CABG	IC
Patients with moderate MR undergoing CABG if repair is feasible	IIaC
Symptomatic patients with severe MR, LVEF <30% and option for revascularization	IIaC
Patients with severe MR, LVEF >30%, no option for revascularization, refractory to medical therapy, and low comorbidity	IIbC

CABG = coronary artery bypass grafting, MR = mitral regurgitation, EF = ejection fraction, LV = left ventricular

Medical therapy is the preferred treatment which should be used before considering surgical correction of functional MR. ACE-inhibitors and beta-blockers are indicated. Nitrates and diuretics are also useful.

Resynchronization therapy and implantable cardioverter defibrillators should be used according to the appropriate recommendations.

3.4 Mitral stenosis

Indications for intervention

Intervention should be performed in symptomatic patients. In the PMC era, most symptomatic patients with favourable valve anatomy undergo PMC. Indications are a matter of debate for patients with unfavourable anatomy

Table 8: Indications for percutaneous mitral commissurotomy in mitral stenosis with valve area < 1.5 cm²

	Class
Symptomatic patients with favourable characteristics* for PMC	IB
Symptomatic patients with contra-indications or high risk for surgery	IC
As initial treatment in symptomatic patients with unfavourable anatomy but otherwise favourable clinical characteristics*	IIaC
Asymptomatic patients with favourable characteristics* and high thromboembolic risk or high risk of haemodynamic decompensation:	
• previous history of embolism	IIaC
• dense spontaneous contrast in the left atrium	IIaC
• recent or paroxysmal atrial fibrillation	IIaC
• systolic pulmonary pressure >50 mmHg at rest	IIaC
• need for major non-cardiac surgery	IIaC
• desire of pregnancy	IIaC

PMC = percutaneous mitral commissurotomy

* Favourable characteristics for PMC can be defined by the absence of several of the following unfavourable characteristics:

• Clinical characteristics: old age, history of commissurotomy, NYHA class IV, atrial fibrillation, severe pulmonary hypertension.

• Anatomic characteristics: echo score > 8, Cormier score 3 (Calcification of mitral valve of any extent, as assessed by fluoroscopy), very small mitral valve area, severe tricuspid regurgitation.

Table 9: Contra-indications to percutaneous mitral commissurotomy

• Mitral valve area >1.5 cm²
• Left atrial thrombus
• More than mild mitral regurgitation
• Severe or bicommissural calcification
• Absence of commissural fusion
• Severe concomitant aortic valve disease, or severe combined tricuspid stenosis and regurgitation
• Concomitant coronary artery disease requiring bypass surgery

Figure 4: Management of severe mitral stenosis

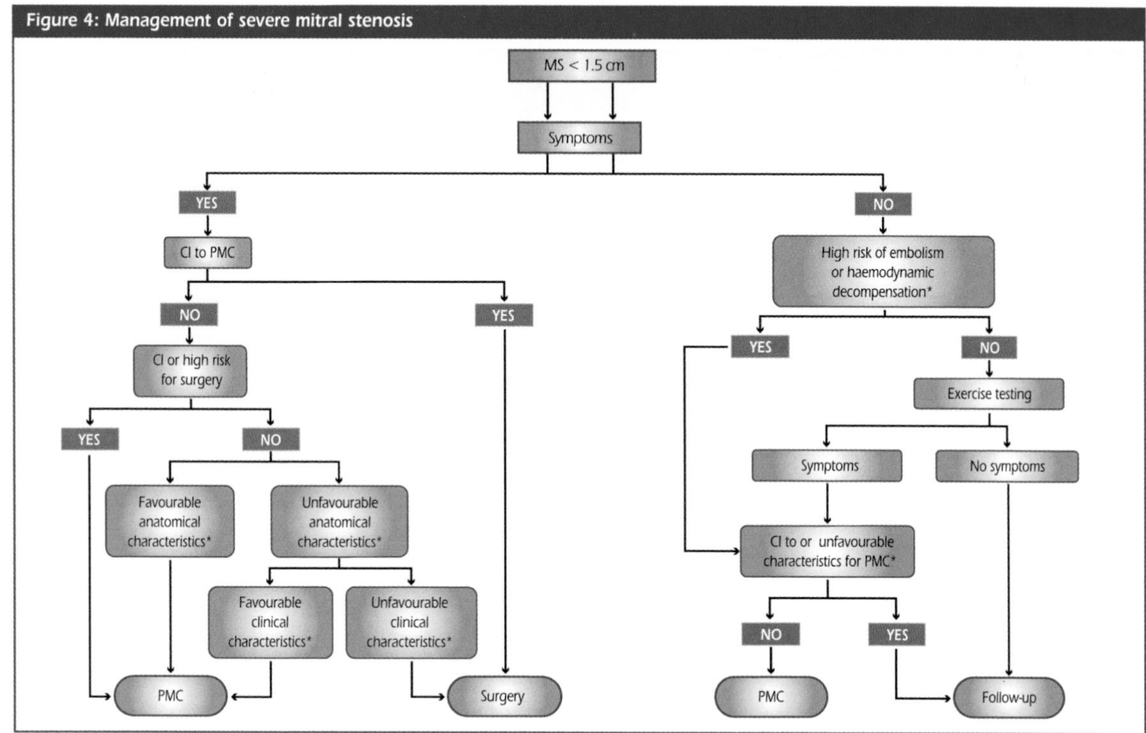

MS = mitral stenosis, CI = contra-indication, PMC = percutaneous mitral commissurotomy

* See Table 8 for definitions.

where decision-making must take into account the multifactorial nature of result prediction of PMC and the relative experience in PMC and surgery of the treating centre.

Because of the small but definite risk inherent in PMC, truly asymptomatic patients are not usually candidates for the procedure, except in the cases where there is increased risk of thromboembolism, or of haemodynamic decompensation such as severe pulmonary hypertension or a desire of pregnancy. In such patients, PMC should only be performed if they have favourable characteristics and by experienced operators. In asymptomatic patients with MS, surgery is very seldom considered and is limited to the rare patients at high risk of complication and with contra-indications for PMC.

Medical therapy

Diuretics, beta-blockers or heart-rate regulating calcium channel blockers are useful. Anticoagulant therapy with a target INR in the upper half of the range 2 to 3 is indicated in patients with either permanent or paroxysmal atrial fibrillation. In patients in sinus rhythm anti-coagulation is mandatory when there has been prior embolism or a thrombus is present in the left atrium (*Recommendation class I level of evidence C*), and recommended when TEE shows dense spontaneous echo contrast or in patients who have an enlarged left atrium (diameter >50 mm) (*Recommendation class IIa level of evidence C*).

Cardioversion is not indicated before intervention in patients with severe MS as it does not usually restore sinus rhythm in the medium- or long-term. If atrial fibrillation is of recent onset and the left atrium only moderately enlarged, cardioversion should be performed soon after successful intervention.

Serial testing

Asymptomatic patients with clinically significant MS who have not undergone intervention should be followed up yearly, by means of clinical and echocardiographic examinations and at longer intervals in cases with stenosis of a lesser degree.

Special patient populations

When PMC is not successful and symptoms persist, surgery should be considered early unless there are definite contra-indications. When re-stenosis with symptoms occurs after surgical commissurotomy PMC can be considered if the patient has favourable characteristics and no contra-indications and if the predominant mechanism of re-stenosis is commissural re-fusion. Similarly, repeat PMC can be proposed in selected

Table 10: Indications for intervention in tricuspid valve disease

	Class
Severe TR in a patient undergoing left-sided valve surgery	IC
Severe primary TR and symptoms despite medical therapy without severe right ventricular dysfunction	IC
Severe TS (± TR), with symptoms despite medical therapy*	IC
Severe TS (± TR) in a patient undergoing left-sided valve intervention*	IC
Moderate organic TR in a patient undergoing left-sided valve surgery	IIaC
Moderate secondary TR with dilated annulus (>40 mm) in a patient undergoing left-sided valve surgery	IIaC
Severe TR and symptoms, after left-sided valve surgery, in the absence of left-sided myocardial, valve, or right ventricular dysfunction and without severe pulmonary hypertension (systolic pulmonary artery pressure > 60 mmHg)	IIaC
Severe isolated TR with mild or no symptoms and progessive dilation or deterioration of right ventricular function	IIbC

* Percutaneous technique can be attempted as a first approach if TS is isolated.

TR = tricuspid regurgitation, TS = tricuspid stenosis

patients with the same characteristics as above if re-stenosis occurs several years after an initially successful PMC. In patients with MS combined with moderate aortic valve disease PMC can be performed as a means of postponing the surgical treatment of both valves.

3.5 Tricuspid disease

Detection requires careful evaluation, as it is almost always associated with left-sided valve lesions that dominate the presentation.

Indications for surgery

If technically possible, conservative surgery is preferable to valve replacement, for which bioprostheses are preferred. Surgery should be carried out early enough to avoid irreversible right ventricular dysfunction.

4. Prosthetic valves

4.1 Choice of prosthetic valve

There is no perfect valve substitute. All involve some compromise and all introduce new disease processes, whether they are mechanical or biological. The decision should be based on the integration of several factors.

4.2 Management after valve replacement

Baseline assessment and modalities of follow-up

A complete baseline assessment should ideally be performed 6 to 12 weeks after surgery, or failing that at the end of the postoperative stay. This will include clinical assessment, chest X-ray, ECG, TTE, and blood testing.

Table 11: Choice of the prosthesis: In favour of mechanical prosthesis

	Class
Desire of the informed patient and absence of contra-indication for long-term anti-coagulation	IC
Patients at risk of accelerated structural valve deterioration*	IC
Patient already on anti-coagulation because of other mechanical prosthesis	IC
Patients already on anti-coagulation because at high risk for thromboembolism**	IIaC
Age <65-70 and long life expectancy***	IIaC
Patients for whom future redo valve surgery would be at high risk (due to left ventricular dysfunction, previous CABG, multiple valve prosthesis)	IIaC

* Young age, hyperparathyroidism.

** Risk factors for thromboembolism: severe left ventricular dysfunction, atial fibrillation, previous thrombo embolism, hypercoagulable state.

*** According to age, gender, the presence of comorbidity, and country-specific life expectancy.

CABG = coronary artery bypass grafting

Table 12: Choice of the prosthesis: In favour of bioprosthesis

	Class
Desire of the informed patient	IC
Unavailability of good quality anti-coagulation (contra-indication or high risk, unwillingness, compliance problems, life style, occupation)	IC
Re-operation for mechanical valve thrombosis in a patient with proven poor anticoagulant control	IC
Patient for whom future redo valve surgery would be at low risk	IIaC
Limited life expectancy*, severe comorbidity, or age >65-70	IIaC
Young woman contemplating pregnancy	IIbC

* According to age, gender, the presence of comorbidity, and country-specific life expectancy.

Clinical assessment should be performed yearly or as soon as possible if new cardiac symptoms occur. TTE should be performed if any new symptoms occur after valve replacement or if complications are suspected. Yearly echocardiographic examination is recommended after the 5th year in patients with bioprosthesis. Transprosthetic gradients during follow-up are best interpreted in comparison to the patient's baseline values, rather than in comparison to theoretical values for a given prosthesis.

TEE should be considered if TTE is of poor quality and in all cases of suspected prosthetic dysfunction or endocarditis. Cinefluoroscopy can provide useful additional information if valve thrombus or pannus is suspected.

Antithrombotic management

Oral anti-coagulation is recommended for the following situations:

- lifelong for all patients with mechanical valves and for patients with bioprostheses who have other indications for anti-coagulation,
- for the first 3 months after insertion in all patients with bioprostheses with a target INR of 2.5.

Target INR

The choice of optimum INR should take into account patient risk factors and the thrombogenicity of the prosthesis (Table 13).

Antiplatelet drugs

Indications for the addition of an antiplatelet agent to anti-coagulation include concomitant arterial disease, in particular coronary disease and other significant atherosclerotic disease. Antiplatelet agents can also be added after recurrent or one definite embolic episode with adequate INR.

Addition of antiplatelet agents should be associated with a full investigation and treatment of identified risk factors and optimisation of anti-coagulation management (*Recommendation class IIa level of evidence C*). The use of drug-eluting stents should be restricted in patients with mechanical prostheses to shorten as much as possible the use of triple antithrombotic therapy. During this period, weekly monitoring of INR is advised.

Table 13: Target International Normalised Ratio (INR) for mechanical prostheses

	Patient-related risk factors**	
Prosthesis thrombogenicity*	No risk factor	≥1 risk factor
Low	2.5	3.0
Medium	3.0	3.5
High	3.5	4.0

* Prosthesis thrombogenicity: Low = Carbomedics (aortic position), Medtronic Hall, St. Jude Medical (without Silzone); Medium = Bjork-Shiley, other bileaflet valves; High = Lillehei-Kaster, Omniscience, Starr-Edwards

** Patient-related risk factors: • mitral, tricuspid, or pulmonary valve replacement; • previous thromboembolism; • atrial fibrillation; • left atrial diameter >50 mm; • left atrial dense spontaneous contrast; • mitral stenosis of any degree; • left ventricular ejection fraction < 35%; • hypercoagulable state

Interruption of anticoagulant therapy

Anti-coagulation during subsequent non-cardiac surgery requires very careful management based on risk assessment according to prosthesis- and patient-related prothrombotic factors (Table 13). For very high-risk patients, anticoagulation interruption should be avoided, if at all possible. Many minor surgical procedures (including dental extraction) and those where bleeding is easily controlled do not require anti-coagulation interruption. The INR should be lowered to a target of 2 (*Recommendation class I level of evidence B*).

For major surgical procedures, in which anticoagulant interruption is considered essential (INR <1.5), patients should be admitted to hospital in advance and transferred to intravenous unfractionated heparin (*Recommendation class IIa level of evidence C*).

Heparin is stopped 6 hours before surgery and resumed 6-12 hours after. Low molecular weight heparin (LMWH) can be given subcutaneously as an alternative preoperative preparation for surgery (*Recommendation class IIb level of evidence C*).

When LMWHs are used, they should be administered twice-a-day using therapeutic rather than prophylactic doses, adapted to body weight and if possible according to monitoring of anti-Xa activity. Effective anti-coagulation should be resumed as soon as possible after the surgical procedure and maintained until the INR is once again in the therapeutic range.

Management of valve thrombosis

Obstructive valve thrombosis should be promptly suspected in any patient with any type of prosthetic valve who presents with a recent increase in shortness of breath or embolic event. The analysis of risk and benefits of fibrinolysis should be adapted to patient characteristics and local resources.

Urgent or emergency valve replacement is the treatment of choice for obstructive thrombosis in critically ill patients without serious comorbidity, (*Recommendation class I level of evidence C*). Fibrinolysis should be considered in:

- critically ill patients unlikely to survive surgery,
- situations in which surgery is not immediately available on site,
- thrombosis of tricuspid or pulmonary valve replacement.

Figure 5: Management of left-sided obstructive prosthetic thrombosis

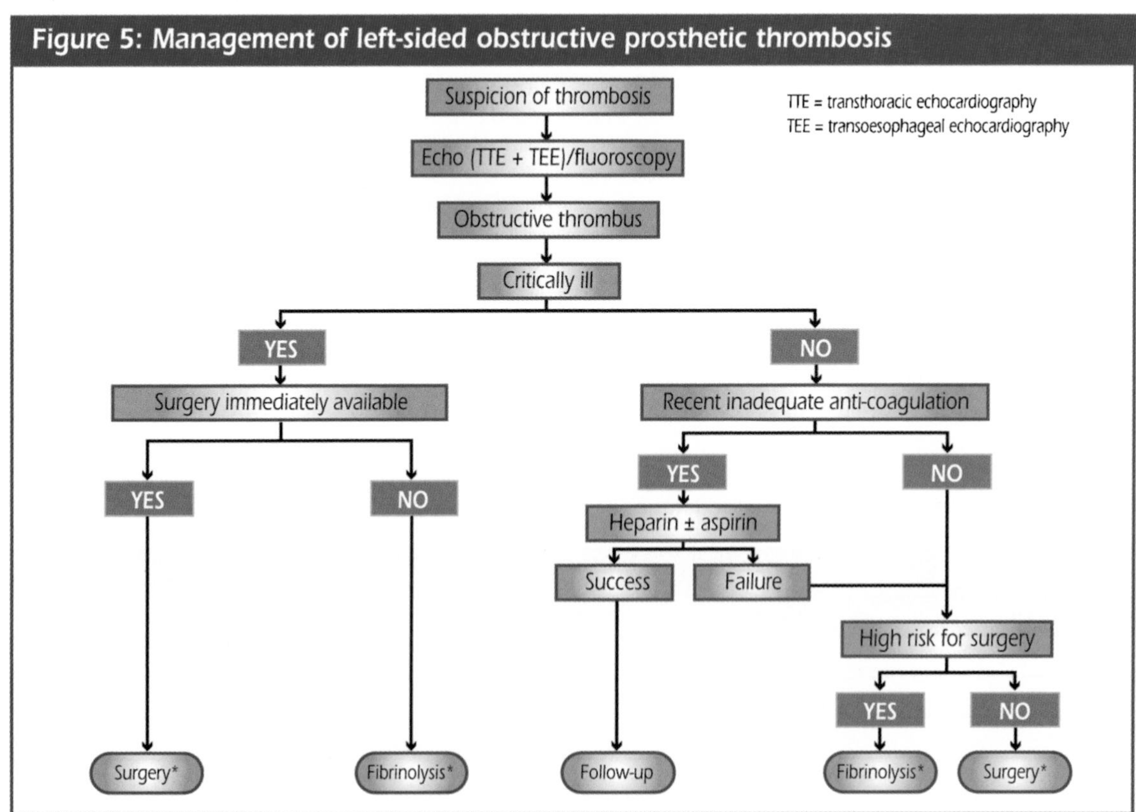

* Risk and benefits of both treatments should be individualised. The presence of a first-generation prosthesis is an incentive to surgery.

The management of patients with *non-obstructive prosthetic thrombosis* depends mainly on the occurrence of a thromboembolic event and the size of the thrombosis. Close monitoring by echocardiography and/or cinefluoroscopy is mandatory. The prognosis is favourable with medical therapy in most cases of small thrombosis (length <10 mm). A good response with gradual resolution of the thrombus obviates the need for either surgery or fibrinolysis. Conversely, surgery is recommended for large (>10 mm) non-obstructive prosthetic thrombosis complicated by embolism (*Recommendation class IIa level of evidence C*) or which persist despite optimal anti-coagulation. Fibrinolysis may be considered as an alternative if surgery is high risk. However, the use of fibrinolysis for non-obstructive prosthetic thrombosis raises serious concerns regarding the risk of bleeding and thromboembolism and should therefore be very limited.

Thorough investigation of each episode of thromboembolism is essential to allow for appropriate management. Prevention of further thromboembolic events involves: treatment or reversal of remediable risk factors, and optimisation of anticoagulation control, if possible with patient self-management. Aspirin should be added, at a low dose formulation (≥100 mg daily), if not previously prescribed.

Management of haemolysis and paravalvular leak (PVL)

Re-operation is advised if PVL is related to endocarditis or if PVL causes haemolysis needing repeated blood transfusions or leading to severe symptoms (*Recommendation class I level of evidence C*). In patients where surgery is contraindicated, medical therapy includes iron supplementation, beta-blockers and erythropoietin, if haemolysis is severe.

Management of bioprosthetic failure

Re-operation is advised in symptomatic patients with significant prosthetic dysfunction (significant increase in trans-prosthetic gradient or severe regurgitation) (*Recommendation class I level of evidence C*) and in asymptomatic patients with any significant prosthetic dysfunction, if they are at low risk for re-operation (*Recommendation class IIa level of evidence C*).

Prophylactic replacement of a bioprosthesis implanted > 10 years ago, without structural deterioration, could be considered during an intervention on another valve or coronary artery.

Heart failure

Heart failure after valve surgery should lead to a search for prosthetic-related complications, deterioration of repair, LV dysfunction (in particular after correction of regurgitation), or progression of another valve disease. Non-valvular related causes such as coronary disease, hypertension or sustained arrhythmias should also be considered.

5. Management during non-cardiac surgery

Before non-cardiac surgery, severe VHD should be identified and the clinical status of the patient carefully evaluated and agreement reached after a full discussion with cardiologists, anaesthesiologists, ideally with a particular skill in cardiology, and surgeons. The management of patients with *AS* is as indicated in figure 6.

In asymptomatic patients with significant *MS* and a systolic pulmonary artery pressure <50 mmHg non-cardiac surgery can be performed at low risk. In symptomatic patients or in patients with systolic pulmonary artery pressure >50 mmHg correction of MS, by means of PMC whenever possible, should be attempted before non-cardiac surgery. In asymptomatic patients with severe *MR* or *AR*, and preserved LV function, non-cardiac surgery can be performed at low risk. In symptomatic patients or in patients with depressed LV function (EF < 30%) non-cardiac surgery should only be performed if strictly needed.

6. Management during pregnancy

Ideally, valve disease should be evaluated before pregnancy and treated if necessary.

Echocardiographic examination should be performed in any pregnant patient presenting with a more than trivial heart murmur, dyspnoea, or who has a prosthetic valve.

When the first visit occurs during pregnancy, early termination may be considered in the following situations: severe LV dysfunction (EF <40%); Marfan's syndrome with aneurysm of ascending aorta >40 mm; or severe symptomatic stenotic valve disease, which cannot be treated using percutaneous procedures. During pregnancy, clinical and echocardiographic follow-up should be performed at 3 and 5 months, and every month thereafter in pregnant patients with severe valve stenosis. Symptomatic *MS* should be treated using bed rest, beta-blockers, possibly associated with diuretics. Beta-agonist agents are contra-indicated. PMC should be considered in patients with severe symptoms or pulmonary artery systolic pressure > 50 mmHg despite medical therapy. In patients with severe *AS* who remain symptomatic despite diuretics, balloon aortic valvuloplasty

Figure 6: Severe aortic stenosis and elective non-cardiac surgery

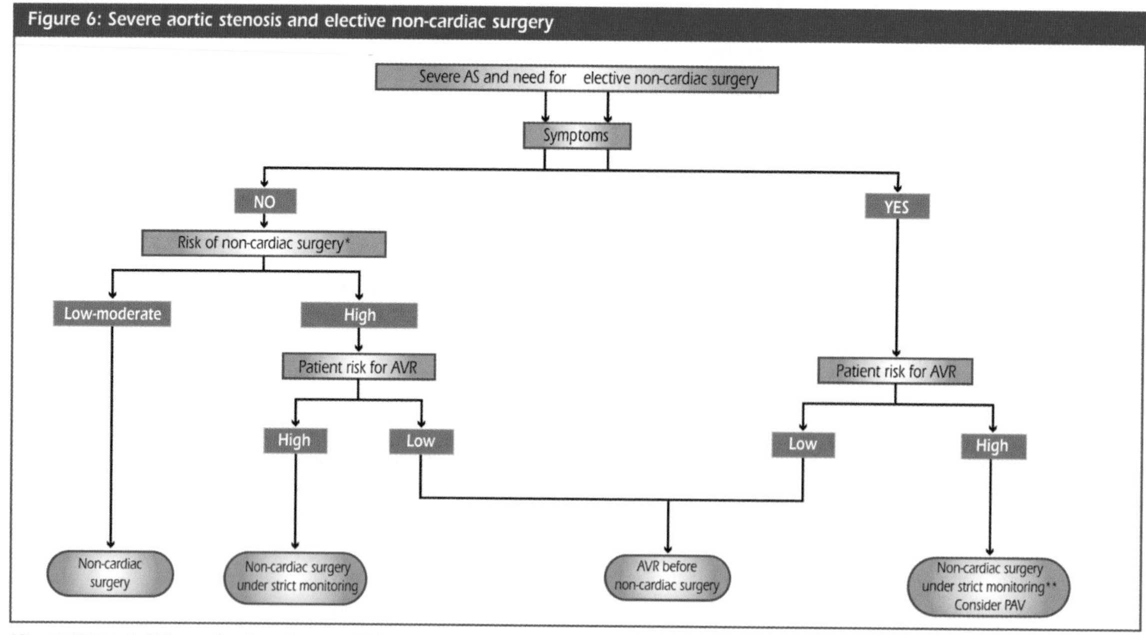

AS = aortic stenosis, AVR = aortic valve replacement, PAV = percutaneous aortic valvuloplasty

* Assessment of the risk of cardiac complications for non-cardiac surgery (from Eagle KA et al. Guideline Update for Perioperative Cardiovascular Evaluation for Non-cardiac Surgery—Executive Summary: a report of the ACC/AHA. J Am Coll Cardiol 2002;39:542–553).

** Non-cardiac surgery performed only if strictly needed.

- High risk (>5%): Emergent major operations, particularly in the elderly; Aortic and other major vascular surgery; Peripheral vascular surgery; Anticipated prolonged surgical procedures associated with large fluid shifts and /or blood loss
- Intermediate risk (1 to 5%): Carotid endarterectomy; Head and neck surgery; Intraperitoneal and intrathoracic surgery; Orthopedic surgery; Prostate surgery
- Low risk (< 1%): Endoscopic procedures; -Superficial procedure; Cataract surgery; Breast surgery

can be considered during pregnancy. Patients with *AR* or *MR* who become symptomatic should be treated medically using diuretics and vasodilators avoiding ACE-inhibitors and angiotensin receptors blockers. In most cases, surgery can be postponed until the postoperative period. Beta-blockers should be used throughout pregnancy in patients with *Marfan's syndrome* to avoid aortic dissection.

In patients with a *mechanical prosthesis*, vitamin K antagonists are favoured during the second and third trimester until the 36th week when they are replaced by unfractionated heparin. During the first trimester, the choice should take into account patient wishes after information, adherence to treatment, and the possibility to use low-dose warfarin which is the safest regimen for the mother. The use of warfarin throughout pregnancy until the 36th week is recommended when warfarin dose is <5 mg/day during the first trimester. The use of LMWH cannot be recommended based on the information currently available.

Surgery under extracorporeal circulation should be performed during pregnancy only in situations that threaten the mother's life and are not amenable to percutaneous treatment. If valve replacement is necessary during pregnancy a bioprosthesis is the preferred valve substitute.

The mode of delivery should be discussed and planned by cardiologists, obstetricians, anaesthetists and the patient before delivery, even more so for the patients who need to interrupt oral anti-coagulation. Caesarean section is considered in patients who have Marfan's syndrome with an aortic diameter > 40 mm, those in whom haemodynamic conditions are unstable, in particular in the presence of AS, or in case of premature delivery under oral anti-coagulation.

Vaginal delivery is recommended whenever possible in the other cases. Haemodynamic monitoring is recommended in women with severe MS, AS, or LV dysfunction.

When valvular surgery is required during pregnancy, Caesarean section should be performed first if the foetus is viable.

Section X:
Infective Endocarditis

1. Infective Endocarditis

Chapter 1

Infective Endocarditis*
2004

Chairperson:
Dieter Horstkotte, MD, PhD, FESC
Department of Cardiology
Heart Center North Rhine-Westphalia
Ruhr University Bochum
Georgstrasse 11
D-32545 Bad Oeynhausen, Germany
Tel: +49 5731 97 1258
Fax: +49 5731 97 2194
Email: akohlstaedt@hdz-nrw.de

Task Force Members:
1. Ferenc Follath, Zurich, Switzerland
2. Erno Gutschik, Copenhagen, Denmark
3. Maria Lengyel, Budapest, Hungary
4. Ali Oto, Ankara, Turkey
5. Alain Pavie, Paris, France
6. Jordi Soler-Soler, Barcelona, Spain
7. Gaetano Thiene, Padua, Italy
8. Alexander von Graevenitz, Zurich, Switzerland

ESC Staff:
1. Keith McGregor, Sophia Antipolis, France
2. Veronica Dean, Sophia Antipolis, France
3. Catherine Després, Sophia Antipolis, France
4. Xue Li, Sophia Antipolis, France

Introduction

If untreated, Infective Endocarditis (IE) is a fatal disease. Major diagnostic (first of all echocardiography) and therapeutic progress (mainly surgery during active IE) have contributed to some prognostic improvement. However, if the diagnosis is delayed or appropriate therapeutic measures postponed, mortality is still high. In this respect, it is of utmost importance that:

(a) IE is considered early in every patient with fever or septicaemia and cardiac murmurs;
(b) echocardiography is applied without delay in suspected IE;
(c) cardiologists, microbiologists and cardiac surgeons cooperate closely if IE is suspected or definite.

Definitions

IE is an endovascular, microbial infection of intracardiac structures facing the blood including infections of the large intrathoracic vessels and of intracardiac foreign bodies. The early characteristic lesion is a variably sized vegetation, although destruction, ulceration or abscess formation may be seen earlier by echocardiography.

Terminology

Terminology (Table 1) should give the following information:

(a) activity of the disease;
(b) recurrence;
(c) diagnostic status;
(d) pathogenesis;
(e) anatomical site;
(f) microbiology.

*Adapted from the Guidelines on Prevention, Diagnosis and Treatment of Infective Endocarditis (European Heart Journal 2004; 25(3): 267-276).

Classes of Recommendations and Levels of Evidence

Class I	Evidence and/or general agreement that a given diagnostic procedure/treatment is beneficial, useful and effective
Class II	Conflicting evidence and/or divergence of opinion about the usefulness/efficacy of a procedure or treatment
Class IIa	Weight of evidence/opinion is in favour of usefulness/efficacy
Class IIb	Usefulness/efficacy is less well established by evidence/opinion
Class III*	Evidence or general agreement that the treatment is not useful/effective and in some cases may be harmful

Level of Evidence A	Data derived from multiple randomised clinical trials or meta-analyses
Level of Evidence B	Data derived from a single randomised trial or large non-randomised studies
Level of Evidence C	Consensus of opinion of experts and/or small studies, retrospective studies, registries

*Use of Class III is discouraged by the ESC

Table 1. Terminology for Infective Endocarditis (IE). Examples: active mitral valve IE due to Enterococcus faecalis; healed recurrent prosthetic aortic valve endocarditisdue to Staphylococcus epidermidis; suspected culture-negative late prosthetic mitralvalve endocarditis

	Activity	Recurrence	Diagnostic terminology	Pathology	Anatomical site	Microbiology
	active healed				mitral aortic, tricuspid mural, etc	microorganism culture-negative, serologically negative, PCR[3] negative, histologically negative
first episode[1]	→	relapsing recurrent				
definite[1]	→	→	suspected possible			
native[1]	→	→	→	early prosthetic late prosthetic IVDA[2]		

[1] If the columns "Recurrence", "Diagnostic terminology", and/or "Pathology" are without text, they signify the first episode of IE (not relapsing or recurrent), "definite" (not suspected or possible) IE and involvement of a native cardiac valve
[2] IVDA = Intravenous Drug Abusers
[3] PCR = Polymerase Chain Reaction

Prevention of Infective Endocarditis

For prophylactic reasons, antibiotics should be given before a bacteraemia is expected. If antibiotic prophylaxis is not given prior to this event, antibiotics may help late clearance if administered intravenously within 2-3 hours.

Cardiac conditions/patients at risk

A previous history of IE, the presence of prosthetic heart valves or other foreign material, surgically created conduits, and complex cyanotic congenital abnormalities are considered high-risk situations. Only patients with high or moderate risk (Table 2) should receive prophylaxis. This is a class I recommendation based on level C evidence.

Table 2. Cardiac conditions in which antimicrobial prophylaxis is indicated

HIGH RISK
- Prosthetic heart valves
- Complex congenital cyanotic heart diseases
- Previous infective endocarditis
- Surgically constructed systemic or pulmonary conduits

MODERATE RISK
- Acquired valvular heart diseases
- Mitral valve prolapse with valvular regurgitation or severe valve thickening
- Non-cyanotic congenital heart diseases (except for secundum type ASD*) including bicuspid aortic valves
- Hypertrophic cardiomyopathy

* ASD = Atrial Septal Defect

Patient-related non-cardiac conditions

Older age, and the following conditions:
(a) promoting non-bacterial thrombotic vegetation;
(b) compromising host defense;
(c) compromising local non-immune defense mechanisms; and
(d) increased risk/frequency/amount of bacteraemia are considered patient related, non-cardiac risk conditions.

Predisposing diagnostic and therapeutic interventions

Procedures which may cause bacteraemia and for which antimicrobial prophylaxis is recommended are given in Table 3. Prophylaxis is not recommended for cardiac catheterization.

Dental hygiene is of major importance for the prevention of IE.

Table 3. Diagnostic and therapeutic interventions likely to produce bacteraemia

- bronchoscopy (rigid instrument)
- cystoscopy during urinary tract infection
- biopsy of urinary tract/prostate
- dental procedures with the risk of gingival/mucosal trauma
- tonsillectomy and adenoidectomy
- oesophageal dilation / sclerotherapy
- instrumentation of obstructed biliary tracts
- transurethral resection of prostate
- urethral instrumentation / dilation
- lithotripsy
- gynaecologic procedures in the presence of infection

Prophylactic antibiotic regimens

Prophylaxis aims primarily at Viridans Streptococci and HACEK organisms before dental, oral, respiratory and oesophageal procedures, and at Enterococci and Streptococcus bovis before gastrointestinal and genitourinary procedures. Despite a lack of convincing evidence, antibiotic prophylaxis (Table 4) is a class I recommendation based on level C evidence.

Table 4. Prophylactic antibiotic regimens

- Dental, oral, respiratory, and oesophageal procedures (P).
    - Patient not allergic to penicillin.
        - amoxicillin 2.0 g (children 50 mg/kg) p.o. 1 h before P.
        - **unable to take oral** medication: amoxicillin or ampicillin 2.0 g (children 50 mg/kg) i.v. within 1/2 - 1 h before P.
    - Patient allergic to penicillin.
        - clindamycin 600 mg (children 20 mg/kg) or azithromycin/clarithromycin 500 mg (children 15 mg/kg) 1 h before P.
- Genitourinary and gastrointestinal procedures (P).
    - Patient not allergic to penicillin.
        - **high-risk group**: ampicillin or amoxicillin 2.0 g i.v. plus gentamicin 1.5 mg/kg i.v. within 1/2 - 1 h before P; 6 h later, ampicillin or amoxicillin 1.0 g p.o.
        - moderate-risk group: ampicillin or amoxicillin 2.0 g i.v. (children 50 mg/kg) within 1/2 - 1 h before P; or amoxicillin 2.0 g (children 50 mg/kg) p.o. 1 h before P.
    - Patient allergic to penicillin.
        - **high-risk group**: vancomycin 1.0 g (children 20 mg/kg) over 1-2 h before P plus gentamicin 1.5 mg/kg i.v. or i.m.
        - moderate-risk group: vancomycin (see above) without gentamicin.

For patients undergoing cardiac surgery or procedures involving infected tissues, a first-generation cephalosporin, clindamycin or vancomycin (for methicillin-resistant S. aureus) would be the drug of choice.

Diagnosis

History, symptoms, signs and laboratory tests

The diagnosis of IE is established (definite IE) if, during a systemic infection, involvement of the endocardium is demonstrated. If in addition, bacteraemia (positive blood cultures) or bacterial DNA on a valve are found, IE is definite and culture/microbiologically positive, otherwise IE is definite but culture/microbiologically negative (Table 5), Duke or modified Duke criteria may be used to make the diagnosis.

Table 5. Criteria that should raise suspicion of IE

- High clinical suspicion (urgent indication for echocardiographic screening and possibly hospital admission)
  - new valve lesion / (regurgitant) murmur
  - embolic event(s) of unknown origin (esp. cerebral and renal infarction)
  - sepsis of unknown origin
  - haematuria, glomerulonephritis, and suspected renal infarction
  - "fever" plus
    - prosthetic material inside the heart
    - other high predispositions for IE
    - newly developed ventricular arrhythmias or conduction disturbances
    - first manifestation of chronic heart failure
    - positive blood cultures (if the organism identified is typical for NVE/PVE)
    - cutaneous (Osler, Janeway) or ophthalmic (Roth) manifestations
    - multifocal/rapid changing pulmonary infiltrations (right heart IE)
    - peripheral abscesses (renal, splenic, spine) of unknown origin
    - predisposition and recent diagnostic/therapeutic interventions known to result in significant bacteraemia
- Low clinical suspicion
  - fever plus none of the above

Echocardiography

Any patient suspected of having Native Valve Endocarditis (NVE) by clinical criteria should be screened by Transthoracic Echocardiography (TTE). When images are of good quality and prove to be negative and there is only a low clinical suspicion of IE, endocarditis is unlikely and other diagnoses are to be considered.

If suspicion of IE is high, TransoEsophageal Echocardiography (TEE) should be performed in all TTE-negative cases, in suspected Prosthetic Valve Endocarditis (PVE), and if TTE is positive but complications are suspected or likely and before cardiac surgery during active IE.

If TEE remains negative and there is still suspicion, it should be repeated within one week. A repeatedly negative study should virtually exclude the diagnosis (Fig. 1). These class I recommendations are based on level B evidence.

Three echocardiographic findings are considered to be major criteria in the diagnosis of IE:

(a) a mobile, echodense mass attached to the valvular or the mural endocardium or to implanted prosthetic material;

(b) demonstration of abscesses or fistulas;

(c) a new dehiscence of a valve prosthesis, especially when occurring late after implantation.

Figure 1. Algorithm for the use of TransThoracic Echocardiography (TTE) and TransoEsophageal Echocardiography (TEE) in suspected IE. TTE "positive" indicates findings typical of IE (e.g. fresh vegetation or abscess formation)

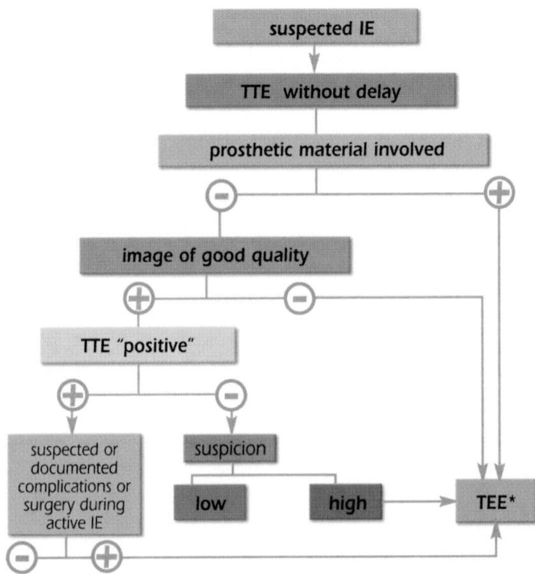

*If TEE is negative and suspicion is high, repeat TEE after 48h but within 7 days

Standard blood culture techniques

If IE is suspected, three or more Blood Cultures (BCs) should be taken irrespective of body temperature within the first 24 h. If initiation of antibiotic treatment is urgent, at least 3 BCs should be taken 1 h apart. If the patient has been on short-term antibiotics, one should wait, if possible, at least for three days after discontinuing antibiotic treatment before new BCs are taken. Blood cultures after long-term antibiotic treatment may not become positive after treatment has been discontinued for 6-7 days. One BC consists of one aerobic and one anaerobic bottle, each containing approx. 50 ml of medium (less in paediatric BC bottles). Venous blood, minimally 5 ml and better 10 ml in adults and 1-5 ml in children should be added to each bottle. Minimum inhibitory concentrations should be determined for the drugs of choice.

Culture-Negative Endocarditis (CNE)

The most frequent cause of CNE is previous antimicrobial treatment. If traditional (non-automatic) BC systems are used, longer incubation periods (> 6 days) are required when organisms of the HACEK group, *Propionibacterium* spp., *Neisseria* spp., *Brucella* spp., *Abiotrophia* spp., or *Campylobacter* spp. are suspected. Especially in CNE, all material excised during cardiac surgery for active IE should also be cultured and examined.

The value of serology has been proven for IE due to *Bartonella, Legionella, Chlamydia* (immunofluorescence) and *Coxiella burnetii.*

The use of broad-spectrum Polymerase Chain Reaction (PCR) provides a significant improvement in the capability to detect difficult-to-culture organisms and even dead bacteria.

Treatment and management

Antimicrobial therapy

For treatment strategies refer to Tables 6-9.

All patients with streptococcal IE should be treated for at least 2 weeks in hospital and observed for cardiac and non-cardiac complications. Patients may then be candidates for outpatient and home parenteral antibiotic therapy. Treatment recommendations for streptococcal IE are based on consistent results of a large number of studies (class I recommendation based on level B evidence).

Table 6. Decision making for antibiotic treatment of Native Valve Endocarditis (NVE) and Prosthetic Valve Endocarditis (PVE) due to streptococci

Regimen A	**NVE; full susceptibility to penicillin (MIC ≤ 0.1 mg/L)**
• Patients ≤ 65 years, normal serum creatinine levels	Penicillin G 12-20 million units/24 h i.v., divided into 4-6 doses for 4 weeks plus gentamicin 3 mg/kg/24h i.v. (maximum 240 mg/day), divided into 2-3 doses for 2 weeks
• Same conditions as above with uncomplicated courses and rapid clinical response to therapy	Penicillin G 12-20 million units/24 h i.v., divided into 4-6 doses for 2 or 4 weeks with ambulatory treatment after 7 days treatment in hospital
• Patients ≥ 65 years and/or serum creatinine levels elevated or allergy to penicillin	Penicillin G adapted to renal function for 4 weeks or Ceftriaxone 2 g/24 h i.v.[1] or i.m.[3] as single dose for 4 weeks
• Patients allergic to penicillin and cephalosporins	Vancomycin 30 mg/kg/24 h i.v. divided into 2 doses for 4 weeks
Regimen B	**susceptibility to penicillin (MIC 0.1 mg /L - 0.5 mg/L) or PVE**
	Penicillin G 20-24 million units/24 h i.v. divided into 4-6 doses[2] or ceftriaxone 2 g/24 h i.v. or i.m.[3] as single dose both for 4 weeks plus gentamicin 3 mg/kg/24 h i.v., divided into 2-3 doses for 2 weeks[4], followed by ceftriaxone 2 g/24 h i.v.[1] or i.m.[3] for additional 2 weeks
	Vancomycin as single drug treatment for 4 weeks (dosage see above)
Regimen C	**resistance to penicillin (MIC > 0.5 mg/L[5])**
	Treatment as for IE due to enterococci

[1] For 2 weeks regimen see table 5 of the full version of these guidelines: on www.escardio.org or European Heart Journal 2004; 25 (3): 267-276.
[2] Especially for patients allergic to penicillin.
[3] Intramuscular injections should be avoided during active IE; if unavoidable in selected patients with access problems divide into 2 doses and inject into a large muscle.
[4] 2-3 mg/kg netilmicin once daily may be an alternative (peak serum level < 16 mg/L)
[5] High level resistance (HLR) to penicillin or ceftriaxone (MIC > 8 mg/L) and HLR to gentamicin (MIC > 500 mg/L) or resistance to vancomycin or teicoplanin (MIC ≥ 4 mg/L) are rare among strains of streptococci. In such situations, extended susceptibility testing and a close cooperation with the clinical microbiologist are mandatory.

Table 7. Decision-making for antibiotic treatment of IE due to staphylococci

Regimen A — Native valve endocarditis	
• MSSA[1] no allergy to penicillin	Oxacillin[2] 8-12 g/24 h i.v., divided into 3-4 doses for at least 4 weeks[3], plus gentamicin 3 mg/kg/24 h i.v. (maximum 240 mg/day), divided into 2-3 doses for the first 3-5 days of treatment
• MSSA[1] allergy to penicillin[4]	Vancomycin 30 mg/kg/24 h i.v. divided into 2 doses[5] for 4-6 weeks[6], plus gentamicin 3 mg/kg/24 h i.v. (maximum 240 mg/day) divided into 2-3 doses for the first 3-5 days of treatment
• MRSA[7]	Vancomycin 30 mg/kg/24 h i.v. divided into 2 doses[5] for 6 weeks
Regimen B — Endocarditis involving prosthetic material / cardiac valve prostheses	
• MSSA[1]	Oxacillin[2] 8-12 g/24 h i.v., divided into 3-4 doses, plus rifampicin 900 mg/24 h i.v. divided into 3 doses, both for 6-8 weeks, plus gentamicin 3 mg/kg/24 h i.v. (maximum 240 mg/day) divided into 2-3 doses for the first 2 weeks of treatment
• MRSA[7], CONS[8-9]	Vancomycin 30 mg/kg/24 h i.v. divided into 2 doses[5] for 6 weeks, plus rifampicin 300 mg/24 h i.v. divided into 3 doses, plus gentamicin[10] 3 mg/kg/24 h i.v. (maximum 240 mg/day) divided into 2-3 doses, all for 6-8 weeks

[1] Methicillin-susceptible S. aureus
[2] Or its congeners
[3] Except for drug addicts for whom a two-week regimen may be sufficient (see section on Treatment and Management of Infective Endocarditis (IE) in IntraVenous Drug Abusers (IVDAs) of the Full Guidelines: www.escardio.org or European Heart Journal 2004; 25(3): 267-276).
[4] For both, immediate (IgE) type and hypersensitivity reaction during treatment.
[5] Infusion over at least 60 min.
[6] Total treatment duration for patients initially treated with oxacillin should be at least 4 weeks. These patients should not have a second course of gentamicin treatment.
[7] Methicillin-resistant S. aureus.
[8] Coagulase-negative staphylococci. In oxacillin-susceptible CONS vancomycin should be replaced by oxacillin.
[9] For resistant staphylococci treatment with oxazolidinone may be an option but should be initiated only after advice from a reference centre has been taken.
[10] If gentamicin susceptibility has been shown in vitro, gentamicin is added in MRSA for the full course but for CoNS only for the first two weeks of treatment. If the organism is resistant to all aminoglycosides, gentamicin may be substituted by a fluoroquinolone.

Table 8. Decision-making for antibiotic treatment of IE due to enterococci and penicillin-resistant streptococci

Penicillin MIC ≤ 8 mg/L and for gentamicin MIC < 500 mg/L	Penicillin G, 16-20 million units in 4-6 divided doses plus gentamicin 3 mg/kg, i.v., divided in 2 doses for 4 weeks
Penicillin-allergic patients with penicillin/gentamicin susceptible enterococcal isolates	Vancomycin 30 mg/kg/day i.v. in two divided doses plus gentamicin (dosage as above) for 6 weeks
Penicillin-resistant strains MIC > 8 mg/L[1]	Vancomycin plus gentamicin (dosage as above) for 6 weeks
Vancomycin-resistant strains including strains with low resistance to vancomycin (MIC 4-16 mg/L) or high resistance to gentamicin[1]	Assistance of an experienced microbiologist is mandatory. If antimicrobial therapy fails, valve replacement should be considered early.

[1] For resistant enterococci, treatment with oxazolidinone may be an option but should be initiated only after advice from a reference centre has been taken.

IE caused by Methicillin-Resistant Staphylococcus Aureus (MRSA) is a therapeutic challenge as most strains are also resistant to most aminoglycosides. If the clinical course is complicated, treatment should be as for PVE.

Coagulase-Negative Species (CoNS) causing PVE within the first year after valve replacement are usually methicillin-resistant. Therapy of choice is a combination of vancomycin and rifampicin for at least 6 weeks with the addition of gentamicin for the initial 2 weeks.

Despite lacking randomized studies and thus level A evidence, the scientific material available is convincing and allows for a class I recommendation.

Enterococci are generally resistant to a wide range of antimicrobial agents including aminoglycosides (MIC for gentamicin 4-64 mg/L) (Table 8).

Duration of treatment should be at least 4 weeks for the combination and at least 6 weeks in complicated cases, in patients having symptoms for more than 3 months, and in patients with PVE. These class IIa recommendations are based on level B evidence.

Drug level monitoring

Gentamicin trough levels should be less than 1 mg/L to avoid renal or ototoxic effects.

Optimum vancomycin effects are achieved if serum concentrations are continuously kept at least 2-4 times above the MIC of the causative organism. Trough levels should be at least 10-15 mg/L. In patients with normal renal function, drug levels should be controlled once, but 2-3 times weekly if combined with aminoglycosides.

Empirical therapy

In cases complicated by sepsis, severe valvular dysfunction, conduction disturbances or embolic events, empirical antimicrobial therapy should be started after three blood cultures have been taken (see section on Standard blood culture techniques).

Recommendations for empirical antibiotic treatment (before microbiologic test results are available) and CNE are given in Table 9.

Special subsets

Antimicrobial therapy for infections of permanently implanted pacemakers or Implantable Cardiac Defibrillator (ICD) leads are based on culture and susceptibility results. Duration of therapy should be 4-6 weeks in most cases. Removal of the entire system is generally recommended.

In IntraVenous Drug Abusers (IVDAs), a Methicillin-susceptible *S. aureus* (MSSA) is the causative organism in about 60-70% of cases.

The tricuspid valve is affected in more than 70%. The most common organism (S. aureus) must always be covered by the antibiotic regimen. Treatment will include either penicillinase-resistant penicillins or vancomycin, depending on the local prevalence of MRSA. If the patient is a pentazocine addict, an antipseudomonas agent should be added. If IVDAs use brown sugar dissolved in lemon juice, candida should be considered and antifungal treatment added. In IVDAs with underlying valve lesions and/or left-sided involvement, antibiotic treatment against streptococci and enterococci must be added.

Management of complications

Rapid and effective antimicrobial treatment may help to prevent embolism. If the patient is on long-term oral anticoagulation, coumarin therapy should be discontinued and replaced by heparin immediately after the diagnosis of IE has been established.

After an embolic complication, the risk for recurrent episodes is high. After manifestation of a cerebral embolism, cardiac surgery to prevent a recurrent episode

Table 9. Antimicrobial treatment in CNE or if therapy is urgent and the causative organism unidentified

NVE		
Vancomycin + Gentamicin	15.0 mg/kg i.v. every 12 hours[1, 2] 1.0 mg/kg i.v. every 8 hours	4-6 weeks 2 weeks
PVE		
Vancomycin + Rifampicin + Gentamicin	15.0 mg/kg i.v. every 12 hours 300-450 mg p.o. every 8 hours 1.0 mg/kg i.v. every 8 hours	4-6 weeks 4-6 weeks 2 weeks

[1] Maximum 2 g/day; for drug level monitoring see text. [2] Aminopenicillin may be added

is not contraindicated if performed early (best within 72 hours) and cerebral haemorrhage has been excluded by cranial computed tomography immediately before the operation. If surgery is not performed early it is advisable to be postponed for 3-4 weeks.

Surgery for active NVE

The following indications for urgent valve surgery are accepted:

- Heart failure due to acute aortic regurgitation;
- Heart failure due to acute mitral regurgitation;
- Persistent fever and demonstration of bacteraemia for more than 8 days despite adequate antimicrobial therapy;
- Demonstration of abscesses, pseudoaneurysms, abnormal communications like fistulas or rupture of one or more valves, conduction disturbances, myocarditis or other findings indicating local spread (locally uncontrolled infection);
- Involvement of microorganisms which are frequently not cured by antimicrobial therapy (e.g. fungi; *Brucella* and *Coxiella*) or microorganisms which have a high potential for rapid destruction of cardiac structures (e.g. *S. lugdunensis*).

If vegetations are larger than 10 mm on the mitral valve or if they are increasing in size despite antibiotic therapy or if they represent mitral kissing vegetations, early surgery should also be considered.

The prognosis of right-sided IE is favourable. Surgery is necessary if tricuspid vegetations are larger than 20 mm after recurrent pulmonary emboli.

Surgery for active PVE

The following indications are accepted;

- Early PVE (less than 12 months after surgery);
- Late PVE complicated by prosthesis dysfunction including significant perivalvular leaks or obstruction, persistent positive blood cultures, abscess formation, conduction abnormalities, and large vegetations, particularly if staphylococci are the infecting agents.

Postoperative antibiotic treatment

Full course of antimicrobial treatment should be completed regardless of the duration of treatment prior to surgery.

List of Abbreviations

ASD	Atrial Septal Defect
BC	Blood Culture
CHF	Congestive Heart Failure
CNE	Culture-Negative Endocarditis
CoNS	Coagulase-Negative Staphylococci
HACEK	Group of bacteria consisting of Haemophilus spp., Actinobacillus actinomycetemcomitans, Cardiobacterium hominis, Eikenella corrodens, Kingella kingae
ICD	Implantable Cardioverter Defibrillator
IE	Infective Endocarditis
IVDA	Intravenous Drug Abuser
MIC	Minimal Inhibitory Concentration
MRSA	Methicillin-Resistant Staphylococcus Aureus
MSSA	Methicillin-Sensitive Staphylococcus Aureus
NVE	Native Valve Endocarditis
PCR	Polymerase Chain Reaction
PVE	Prosthetic Valve Endocarditis
Spp	Plural of "species"
TEE	TransoEsophageal Echocardiography
TTE	TransThoracic Echocardiography

Section XI:
Pulmonary Arterial Hypertension

1. Pulmonary Arterial Hypertension

Chapter 1

Pulmonary Arterial Hypertension*

2004

Co-chairperson:
Prof. Nazzareno Galiè, FESC
Institute of Cardiology
University of Bologna
Via Massarenti, 9
40138 Bologna - Italy
Phone: +39 051 349 858
Fax: +39 051 344 859
E-mail: nazzareno.galie@unibo.it

Co-chairperson:
Prof. Gérald Simonneau, FESC
Service de Pneumologie
Hôpital Antoine Béclère
157 rue de la Porte de Triveaux
92141 Clamart Cedex - France
Phone: +33 (1) 45 37 44 17
Fax: +33 (1) 46 30 38 24
E-mail: gerald.simonneau@abc.ap-hop-paris.fr

Task Force Members:
1. Adam Torbicki, Warsaw, Poland
2. Robyn Barst, New York, USA
3. Philippe Dartevelle, Le Plessis-Robinson, France
4. Sheila Haworth, London, UK
5. Tim Higenbottam, Waltham on the Wolds, UK
6. Horst Olschewski, Giessen, Germany
7. Andrew Peacock, Glasgow, UK
8. Guiseppe Pietra, Castagnola, Switzerland
9. Lewis J. Rubin, La Jolla, USA

ESC Staff:
1. Keith McGregor, Sophia Antipolis, France
2. Veronica Dean, Sophia Antipolis, France
3. Catherine Després, Sophia Antipolis, France
4. Karine Piellard, Sophia Antipolis, France

Recommendations are provided in Table 3 and are used as follows:

Class I	Evidence and/or general agreement that a given treatment or procedure is beneficial, useful and effective
Class II	Conflicting evidence and/or divergence of opinion about the usefulness/efficacy of the treatment or procedure
Class IIa	Weight of evidence/opinion is in favour of usefulness/efficacy
Class IIb	Usefulness/efficacy is less well established by evidence/opinion
Class III	Evidence or general agreement that the treatment or procedure is not useful or effective and in some cases may be harmful

Level of Evidence A	Data derived from multiple randomized clinical trials or meta-analyses
Level of Evidence B	Data derived from a single randomized clinical trial or large non-randomized studies
Level of Evidence C	Consensus of opinion of the experts and/or small studies, retrospective studies, registries

1. Definitions and classification

Pulmonary Hypertension (PH) is defined by a mean Pulmonary Artery Pressure (PAP) > 25 mmHg at rest or > 30 mmHg with exercise. Current classification of PH is presented in Table 1.

*Adapted from the ESC Guidelines on the Diagnosis and Treatment of Pulmonary Arterial Hypertension (European Heart Journal 2004;25:2243-2278)

Table 1. Clinical Classification of Pulmonary hypertension – Venice 2003

1. Pulmonary Arterial Hypertension (PAH)
    - 1.1. Idiopathic (IPAH)
    - 1.2. Familial (FPAH)
    - 1.3. Associated with (APAH):
        - 1.3.1. Connective tissue disease
        - 1.3.2. Congenital systemic to pulmonary shunts
        - 1.3.3. Portal Hypertension
        - 1.3.4. HIV infection
        - 1.3.5. Drugs and toxins
        - 1.3.6. Other (thyroid disorders, glycogen storage disease, Gaucher's disease, hereditary haemorrhagic telangiectasia, haemoglobinopathies, myeloproliferative disorders, splenectomy)
    - 1.4. Associated with significant venous or capillary involvement
        - 1.4.1. Pulmonary Veno-Occlusive Disease (PVOD)
        - 1.4.2. Pulmonary Capillary Haemangiomatosis (PCH)
    - 1.5. Persistent Pulmonary Hypertension of the Newborn (PPHN)
2. Pulmonary hypertension associated with left heart diseases
    - 2.1. Left-sided atrial or ventricular heart disease
    - 2.2. Left-sided valvular heart disease
3. Pulmonary hypertension associated with lung respiratory diseases and/or hypoxia
    - 3.1. Chronic obstructive pulmonary disease
    - 3.2. Interstitial lung disease
    - 3.3. Sleep disordered breathing
    - 3.4. Alveolar hypoventilation disorders
    - 3.5. Chronic exposure to high altitude
    - 3.6. Developmental abnormalities
4. Pulmonary hypertension due to chronic thrombotic and/or embolic disease
    - 4.1. Thromboembolic obstruction of proximal pulmonary arteries
    - 4.2. Thromboembolic obstruction of distal pulmonary arteries
    - t4.3. Non-thrombotic pulmonary embolism (tumour, parasites, foreign material)
5. Miscellaneous

    Sarcoidosis, histiocytosis X, lymphangiomatosis, compression of pulmonary vessels (adenopathy, tumour, fibrosing mediastinitis)

Pulmonary arterial hypertension (PAH, Class 1) is defined as a group of diseases characterized by a progressive increase of pulmonary vascular resistance (PVR) leading to right ventricular failure and premature death. The median life expectancy from the time of diagnosis in patients with idiopathic PAH (IPAH)), formerly termed primary pulmonary hypertension (PPH), before the availability of disease-specific (targeted) therapy was 2.8 years in the mid-1980's.

PAH includes IPAH and pulmonary hypertension associated with various conditions such as connective tissue diseases (CTD), congenital systemic-to-pulmonary shunts, portal hypertension and HIV infection.

All these conditions share equivalent obstructive pathologic changes of the pulmonary microcirculation suggesting shared pathobiological processes among the disease spectrum of PAH.

2. Diagnosis of pulmonary arterial hypertension

The diagnostic approach of PAH requires a series of investigations aimed to confirm the clinical suspicion of pulmonary hypertension, to clarify the clinical class and the specific underlying condition (Table 1) and to evaluate the functional and haemodynamic impairment (Figure 1). A sequential stage-by-stage approach can be adopted even if some investigations can provide concurrent information appropriate for different stages. For practical purposes the following four stages can be identified:

2.1 Clinical Suspicion of Pulmonary Hypertension
2.2 Detection of Pulmonary Hypertension
2.3 Pulmonary Hypertension Clinical Class Identification
2.4 Pulmonary Arterial Hypertension Evaluation (Type, Functional Capacity, Haemodynamics)

2.1

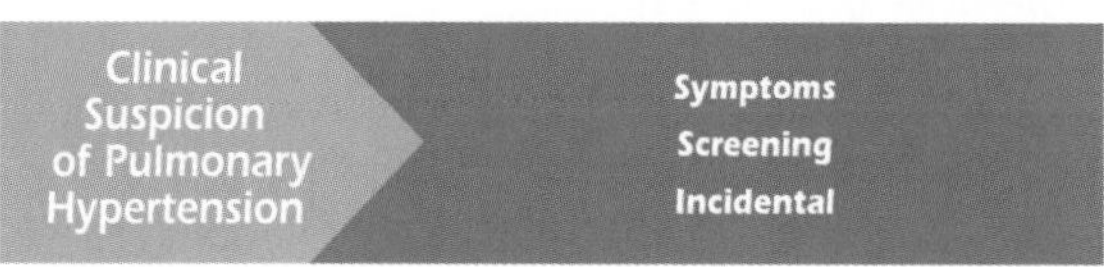

Symptoms

The clinical suspicion of pulmonary hypertension should arise in any case of compatible symptoms such as breathlessness, fatigue, weakness, angina, syncope, and abdominal distension. Symptoms at rest are reported only in very advanced cases.

Screening

Pulmonary hypertension can be identified also in asymptomatic patients who undergo screening programmes because they are known to be affected by conditions that can be associated to PAH such as connective tissue diseases, portal hypertension, HIV infection and congenital heart diseases with systemic-to-pulmonary shunts.

Incidental

Finally, pulmonary hypertension can be suspected in case of incidental abnormal electrocardiographic, chest X-ray or echocardiographic findings.

2.2

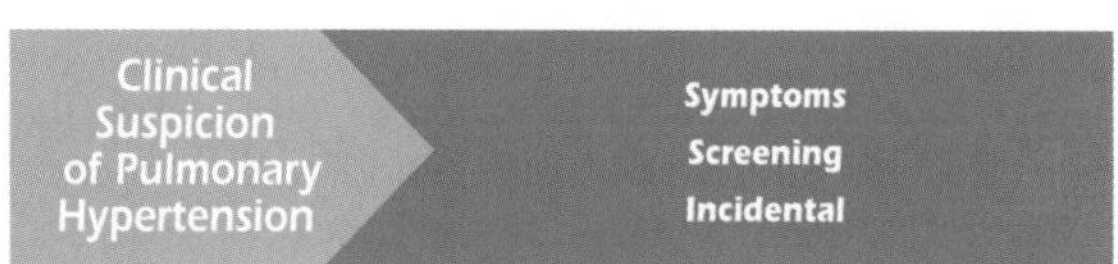

The detection of PH requires a few routine investigations such as clinical physical examination, ECG, chest X-ray and transthoracic Doppler echocardiography.

Physical signs

The initial physical signs of pulmonary hypertension include left parasternal lift, accentuated pulmonary component of second sound, pansystolic murmur of tricuspid regurgitation, diastolic murmur of pulmonary insufficiency and right ventricular third sound. Jugular vein distension, hepatomegaly, peripheral oedema, ascites and cool extremities characterize patients in a more advanced state with right ventricular failure at rest. Central and/or peripheral cyanosis may also be present. Lung sounds are usually normal.

ECG

The ECG may provide suggestive or supportive evidence of pulmonary hypertension by demonstrating right ventricular hypertrophy and strain, and right atrial dilation. However, normal ECG does not exclude the presence of severe pulmonary hypertension.

Chest X-ray

Chest X-ray is abnormal in 90% of cases and findings include central pulmonary arterial dilatation, which contrasts with 'pruning' (loss) of the peripheral blood vessels. Right atrial and ventricular enlargement may be seen. Concomitant conditions such as moderate-to-severe lung disease or pulmonary venous hypertension due to left heart abnormalities can be reasonably excluded by chest X-ray.

Transthoracic Doppler-echocardiography

Transthoracic Doppler-echocardiography is an excellent non-invasive screening test for the patient with suspected pulmonary hypertension by the assessment of the systolic regurgitant tricuspid flow velocity and the consequent estimation of right ventricular and pulmonary artery systolic pressures.

According to the normal ranges of Doppler-derived values of pulmonary artery pressures, mild pulmonary hypertension can be defined as a pulmonary artery systolic pressures of approximately 36–50 mmHg or a resting tricuspid regurgitant velocity of 2.8–3.4 m/sec (assuming a normal right atrial pressure of 5 mmHg). It should be noted that also with this definition a number of false positive diagnoses can be anticipated especially in elderly subjects and confirmation with right heart catheterization is required especially in symptomatic patients (NYHA functional class II–III).

In asymptomatic subjects (NYHA class I) concomitant connective tissue disease should be excluded and echocardiography should be repeated in six months. Also the possibility of false negative Dopplerechocardiographic results should be considered in case of high clinical suspicion. Additional echocardiographic and Doppler changes include right ventricular dilatation, reduced ventricular function, reduced size of left ventricle, inferior vena cava dilatation and pericardial effusion. Transthoracic echocardiography also allows a differential diagnosis with left heart valvular and myocardial diseases (Clinical class 2 e.g. Pulmonary Hypertension Associated with Left Heart Diseases, Table 1) and congenital heart diseases. The venous injection of contrast medium may help the identification of atrial septal defects that can be confirmed by transoesophageal echocardiography.

2.3

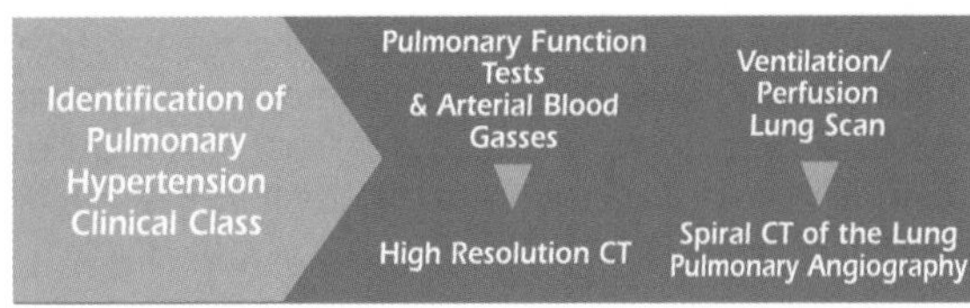

Pulmonary function tests

The identification of the clinical class (Table 1) requires additional examinations such as pulmonary function tests (including arterial blood gas sample) to recognize patients with parenchymal lung diseases (Clinical class 3, Table 1) namely chronic obstructive lung diseases and lung fibrosis. Patients with PAH usually have decreased lung diffusion capacity for carbon monoxide (DL_{CO}) [typically in the range of 40–80 % predicted] and mild to moderate reduction of lung volumes. The arterial oxygen tension (PaO_2) is normal or only slightly lower than normal and arterial carbon dioxide tension ($PaCO_2$) is decreased as a result of alveolar hyperventilation.

Ventilation and perfusion (V/Q) lung scan

Ventilation and perfusion (V/Q) lung scan is required to detect patients with chronic thromboembolic pulmonary hypertension (CTEPH, Clinical class 4, Table 1). In PAH the lung V/Q scans may be entirely normal however they may also show small peripheral non-segmental defects in perfusion. These are normally ventilated and thus represent V/Q mismatch. In CTEPH the normally ventilated perfusion defects are usually found in lobar and segmental regions. A caveat is that unmatched perfusion defects are also seen in pulmonary veno-occlusive disease. Such a patient requires careful further investigation (see section on high resolution CT). In patients with parenchymal lung disease the perfusion defects are matched by ventilation defects.

Chest high resolution CT

Chest High Resolution CT (HRCT) may be required in patients with parenchymal lung diseases (Clinical class 3, Table 1) to better characterize lung parenchymal changes. HRCT may be indicated in cases of the presence of interstitial markings on the chest X-ray without evidence of left ventricular failure. In these cases the confirmation of a diffuse central ground-glass opacification and thickening of interolobular septa suggest pulmonary veno-occlusive disease; additional findings are lymphadenopathy, pleural shadows and effusions.

Contrast enhanced spiral CT and pulmonary angiography (CTEPH)

Contrast enhanced spiral CT and pulmonary angiography are requested in patients with CTEPH (Clinical class 4, Table 1) to assess the indication for pulmonary endoarterectomy (or in case of inconclusive perfusion lung scan). CT features of chronic thromboembolic disease are complete occlusion of pulmonary arteries, eccentric filling defects consistent with thrombi, recanalization, and stenoses or webs. Traditional pulmonary angiography is still required in the work-up of CTEPH to better identify patients that can benefit from the intervention of endarterectomy. Pulmonary angiography may be more accurate in the identification of distal obstructions and it is indicated also in cases of inconclusive contrast-enhanced spiral CT in patients with clinical and lung scintigraphy suspicion of CTEPH.

2.4

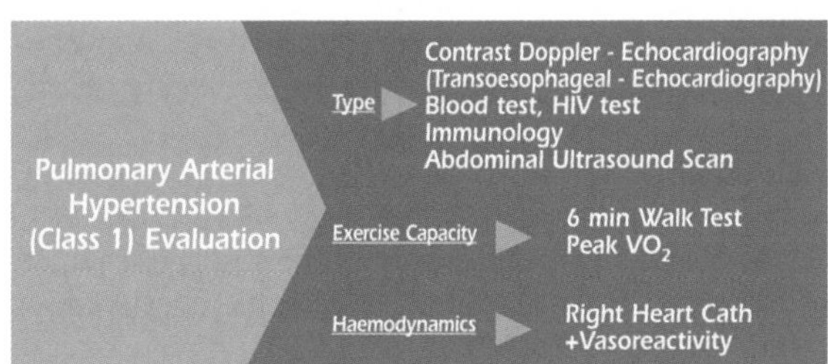

For the final evaluation of patients with PAH (Clinical class 1, Table 1), the ultimate definition of the underlying condition (type) and the assessment of the functional capacity and of the haemodynamic characteristics are needed. Additional examinations required to define the type include abdominal ultrasound scan, routine biochemistry, haematology, thyroid function, HIV and immunology tests. When no underlying condition is detected a diagnosis of idiopathic PAH is made.

PAH type

The venous injection of agitated saline as contrast medium at echocardiographic examination can help the identification of patent foramen ovale or sinus venosus type atrial septal defects that can be overlooked on the standard transthoracic examination. Transoesophageal echocardiography is rarely required and is usually used to confirm the presence and assess the exact size of small atrial septal defects.

Routine biochemistry, haematology and thyroid function tests are required. Connective tissue diseases (CTD) are diagnosed primarily on clinical and laboratory criteria and an autoimmune screen consists of Anti-Nuclear antibodies (ANA), including anti-centromere antibody, anti-SCL70 and RNP. About one third of patients with IPAH have positive but low anti-nuclear antibody titre (≥ 1:80 dilutions). Patients with a substantially elevated ANA and/or suspicious clinical features require further serologic assessment and rheumatology consultation. Finally all patients should be consented for and undertake a human immunodeficiency virus (HIV) serology test.

Liver cirrhosis and/or portal hypertension can be reliably excluded by the use of abdominal ultrasound scan. The use of contrast agents may improve the diagnosis. Portal hypertension can be confirmed by the detection of an increased gradient between free and occluded (wedge) hepatic vein pressure at the time of the Right Heart catheterization (RHC).

Exercise capacity

The objective assessment of exercise capacity in patients with PAH is an important instrument for evaluating disease severity and treatment effect. The most commonly used exercise tests for PH are the six-minute walk test (6MWT) and Cardio-Pulmonary Exercise Testing (CPET) with gas exchange measurement. The 6MWT is technically simple, is predictive of survival in IPAH and also correlates inversely with NYHA functional status severity. CPET allows measurement of ventilation and pulmonary gas exchange (VO_2) during exercise testing providing additional "pathophysiological" information to that derived from standard exercise testing. However, it is technically more difficult and it may fail to confirm improvements observed with 6MWT. A possible explanation may relate to a lack of sensitivity of CPET in measuring response to treatments which have less effect on maximal as opposed to submaximal exercise.

Haemodynamics

RHC is required to confirm the diagnosis of PAH, to assess the severity of the haemodynamic impairment and to test the vasoreactivity of the pulmonary circulation.

PAH is defined by a mean PAP > 25 mmHg at rest or > 30 mmHg with exercise, by a Pulmonary Wedge (occluded) Pressure (PWP) ≤ 15 mmHg and by pulmonary vascular resistance > 3 mmHg/l/min (Wood units). Left heart catheterization is required in the rare circumstances in which a reliable PWP cannot be measured. The assessment of PWP may allow the distinction between arterial and venous PH in patients with concomitant left heart diseases.

RHC is important also in patients with definite moderate-to-severe PAH because the haemodynamic variables have prognostic relevance. Elevated mean right atrial pressure, mean PAP and reduced cardiac output and central venous O_2 saturation identify IPAH patients with the worst prognosis.

Uncontrolled studies have suggested that long-term administration of calcium-channel blockers (CCBs) prolongs survival in the acutely responsive IPAH patients (10-15%) compared with unresponsive ones. It is generally accepted that patients who may benefit from long-term CCBs can be identified by an acute vasodilator challenge performed during RHC.

Acute vasodilator testing should only be done using short-acting pulmonary vasodilators at the time of the initial RHC in experienced centers to minimize the potential risks. Currently the agents used in acute testing are intravenous prostacyclin or adenosine and inhaled nitric oxide.

A positive acute vasoreactive response (positive acute responders) is defined as a reduction of mean PAP ≥ 10 mmHg to reach an absolute value of mean PAP ≤ 40 mmHg with an increase or unchanged cardiac output. Generally, only about 10 to 15% of IPAH patients will meet these criteria.

Positive acute responders are most likely to show a sustained response to long-term treatment with high doses of CCBs and are the only patients that can safely be treated with this type of therapy. Empirical treatment with CCBs without acute vasoreactivity test is strongly discouraged due to possible severe adverse effects.

Positive long-term responders to high dose CCB treatment are defined as patients being in NYHA functional class I or II with near normal haemodynamics after several months of treatment with CCB alone. Only about a half of IPAH positive acute responders are also positive long-term responders to CCBs and only in these cases is the continuation of CCB as single treatment warranted.

The usefulness of acute vasoreactivity tests and long-term treatment with CCB in patients with PAH associated with underlying processes, such as connective tissue diseases or congenital heart disease is less clear as compared to IPAH. However, experts suggest that these cases should also be listed to test patients for acute vasoreactivity and to look for a long-term response to CCB in the appropriate subjects.

3. Evaluation of severity

Multiple variables that have been shown to predict prognosis in IPAH when assessed at baseline or after targeted treatments are shown in Table 2. In clinical practice, the prognostic value of a single variable in the individual patient may be less than the value of multiple concordant variables (Table 2).

Very little information is available in other conditions such as PAH associated with CTD, congenital systemic-to-pulmonary shunts, HIV infection or portal hypertension. In these circumstances, additional factors may contribute to the overall outcome. In fact, PAH associated with CTD has a worse prognosis than IPAH patients, whereas patients with PAH associated with congenital systemic-to-pulmonary shunts have a slower progressive course than IPAH patients.

Table 2. Prognostic parameters in patients with Idiopathic Pulmonary Arterial Hypertension (IPAH)
Clinical parameters - Baseline NYHA functional class - NYHA functional class on chronic epoprostenol treatment - History of right heart failure
Exercise capacity - Baseline 6MWT distance - 6MWT distance on chronic epoprostenol treatment - Baseline Peak VO_2
Echocardiographic parameters - Pericardial effusion size - Right atrial size - Left ventricular eccentricity index - Doppler right ventricular (Tei) index - Colour Doppler tricuspid regurgitant area
Haemodynamics - Right atrial pressure - Mean PAP - Cardiac output - Mixed venous O_2 saturation - Positive acute response to vasoreactivity tests - Fall in pulmonary vascular resistance < 30% after 3 months of epoprostenol
Blood Tests - Hyperuricemia - Baseline brain natriuretic peptide - Brain natriuretic peptide after 3 months therapy - Troponin – detectable, especially persistent leakage - Plasma norepinephrine - Plasma endothelin-1

6MWT: Six-Minute Walk Test; NYHA: New York Heart Association

4. Treatment of pulmonary arterial hypertension

See Table 3 opposite.

General measures

Include adjustments (reduction) of daily activities, avoiding altitudes above 1500 meters, prevention of pulmonary infections, birth control, pregnancy termination, psychological assistance and appropriate management of elective general surgery. Pregnancy and delivery in PAH patients are associated with an increased rate of deterioration and death (30–50%) and an appropriate method of birth control is highly recommended in women with childbearing potential. There is a consensus among guidelines from the American Heart Association and the American College of Cardiology which recommends that pregnancy be avoided or terminated in women with cyanotic congenital heart disease, PH, and Eisenmenger syndrome.

Oral anticoagulants

The evidence for favorable effects of oral anticoagulant treatment in patients with IPAH or PAH associated to anorexigens is based on retrospective analysis of single center studies. The target INR in patients with IPAH varies somewhat being 1.5 to 2.5 in most centers in North America and 2.0 to 3.0 in European centers. The evidence supporting anticoagulation in patients with IPAH may be extrapolated to other patients with other forms of PAH provided that the risk/benefit ratio is carefully considered.

Diuretics

Patients with decompensated right heart failure develop fluid retention that lead to increased central venous pressure, abdominal organ congestion, peripheral oedema and in advanced cases also ascites. Appropriate diuretic treatment in case of right heart failure allows clear symptomatic and clinical benefits in patients with PAH even if specific Randomized Controlled Clinical Trials (RCTs) have not been performed. In the recent RCTs on new targeted treatments, 49% to 70% of patients were treated with diuretics.

Oxygen

Most patients with PAH (except those with associated congenital heart disease) present with only mild degrees

Table 3: Classes of Recommendations and Levels of Evidence for Efficacy of Treatments for Pulmonary Arterial Hypertension

Country-specific regulatory approval and labelling for PAH related therapeutic procedures are also reported in the table.

Treatment	Classes of Recommendations	Levels of Evidence	Country	Labelling	
				Aetiology	NYHA
General Measures	IIa	C	-	-	-
Oral Anticoagulants	IIa*	C	-	-	-
Diuretics	I	C	-	-	-
Digoxin	IIb	C	-	-	-
Oxygen †	IIa	C	-	-	-
Calcium-Channel Blockers	I ‡	C	-	-	-
Epoprostenol	I §	A	Europe**	IPAH	II-IV
			USA Canada	IPAH & PAH-CTD	III-IV
Treprostinil (subcutaneous)	IIa	B	USA	PAH	II-III-IV
			France	PAH	II
Treprostinil (intravenous)	IIa	B	USA	PAH	III-IV
Iloprost (inhalation)	IIa***	B***	European Union	IPAH	III
			Australia	IPAH, PAH-CTD and CTEPH	III-IV
			USA	PAH	III-IV
Iloprost (intravenous)	IIa	C	New Zealand	PAH	III-IV
Beraprost	IIb	B	Japan Korea	IPAH	II-III-IV
Bosentan	I ††	A***	European Union	PAH	III
			USA Canada	PAH	III-IV
Sitaxsentan ‡‡		B***	-	-	-
Ambrisentan ‡‡		C***	-	-	-
Sildenafil	I §§	A	European Union	PAH	III
			USA	PAH	-
Combination Therapy	IIb***	C***	-	-	-
Balloon Atrial Septostomy	IIa	C	-	-	-
Lung Transplantation	I	C	-	-	-

See abbreviations in the glossary at the end of the booklet

* IIa for IPAH, IIb for other PAH conditions.

† If arterial oxygen saturation 90%

‡ Only in patients responding to acute reactivity tests, I for IPAH, IIb for other PAH conditions

§ IIa C in conditions different from IPAH and PAH associated to CTD

** Epoprostenol in Europe has not been registered through the centralized procedure of the European Union (EMEA) but it is approved in different European countries on a national basis.

*** According to the results of new trials available since the publication of the first version of the Guidelines, the following changes of the grade of recommendations and of the levels of evidence are foreseen:

INHALED ILOPROST from grade of recommendations IIa, level of evidence B to grade of recommendations I, level of evidence A (new data from a second randomized study performed in the USA - STEP study - on the efficacy of inhaled iloprost combined with bosentan).

BOSENTAN from level of evidence C to level of evidence B in patients with PAH associated with congenital systemic-to-pulmonary shunt (new data from a randomized study - BREATHE 5)

SITAXSENTAN from level of evidence B to level of evidence A (new data from a second randomized study - STRIDE 2 - on the efficacy of sitaxsentan in PAH patients).

AMBRISENTAN from level of evidence C to level of evidence A (new data from two randomized studies - ARIES-1 and ARIES-2 - on the efficacy of ambrisentan in PAH patients).

COMBINATION THERAPY from grade of recommendation IIb, level of evidence C to grade of recommendation IIa, level of evidence B (new data from a first randomized study performed in the USA - STEP study - on the efficacy of inhaled iloprost combined with bosentan).

†† IIa B in NYHA class IV, IIa C in conditions different from IPAH and PAH associated to CTD or congenital systemic to pulmonary shunts

‡‡ These drugs are currently available only for patients enrolled in investigational studies and no classes of recommendations are given

§§ IIa C in conditions different from IPAH and PAH associated to CTD.

of arterial hypoxaemia at rest. In some patients with profound hypoxaemia a secondary opening of a patent foramen ovale can be found. In patients with PAH associated with congenital cardiac defects, hypoxaemia is related to reversal of left-to-right shunting and is refractory to increased inspired oxygen. No consistent data are currently available on the effects of long-term oxygen treatment in PAH. However, it is generally considered important to maintain oxygen saturations at greater than 90% at all times.

Digitalis and inotropic drugs

The use of digitalis in PAH patients with refractory right heart failure is based primarily on the judgment of the physician rather than on scientific evidence of efficacy. Digitalis may be used in the rare PAH patients with atrial fibrillation or atrial flutter to slow ventricular rate. Digoxin was administered in 18% to 53% of patients enrolled in recent RCTs in PAH. Patients with end stage PAH are treated with i.v. dobutamine in most expert centers. This treatment often results in clinical improvement that may persist for a variable period of time, like in advanced left heart failure.

Calcium-channel blockers

Treatment with high doses of CCBs is mandatory in responders to acute vasoreactivity tests (see definition in the diagnostic section). Careful titration to optimally tolerated doses (up to 120/240 mg/day for nifedipine and 240–720 mg/day for diltiazem) may be required. There are no reports on efficacy, tolerability and effective doses of new generation CCBs such as amlodipine and flodpine. Long-term response (after 3–6 months) need to be evaluated and subjects on NYHA class I-II and with marked haemodynamic improvement can continue calcium channel blockers as monotherapy.

ET-1 receptor antagonists

The evidence of the activation of the endothelin system (involved in vasoconstriction and proliferation) in PAH provides a sound rationale for testing endothelin antagonists in PAH patients. The most efficient way to antagonize the endothelin system is the use of endothelin receptor antagonists that can block either ET_A or both ET_A and ET_B-receptors.

At present, the only approved drug of this class is the orally active dual ET_A and ET_B-receptor antagonist bosentan. Bosentan has been evaluated in two randomized trials that have shown improvement in exercise capacity, functional class, haemodynamics, echocardiographic and Doppler variables, and time to clinical worsening. Additional long-term studies have shown persistent efficacy over time. Increases in hepatic aminotransferases occurred in 10% of the subjects treated with 125 mg BID, were found to be dose-dependent and reversible after dose reduction or discontinuation. For these reasons monthly assessments of hepatic aminotransferases are required.

Two selective orally active ET_A-receptor antagonists are currently under evaluation: sitaxsentan (100 mg OD) has been assessed in two phase III trials which have demonstrated efficacy on exercise capacity and haemodynamics and ambrisentan evaluated in a phase II and two phase III studies which have shown efficacy on exercise capacity, haemodynamics and time to clinical worsening. Incidence of abnormal liver function tests appears to be 3–4% with sitaxsentan and apparently even less with ambrisetan. Sitaxsentan interferes with warfarin metabolism.

Prostanoids

A dysregulation of the prostacyclin metabolic pathways, involved in vasodilatation and antiproliferative activities, has been shown in patients with PAH and this represents a convincing rationale for the therapeutic use of prostacyclin in PAH patients.

The efficacy of continuous i.v. administration of epoprostenol (the synthetic salt of prostacyclin) has been tested in 3 unblinded, clinical trials in idiopathic and associated with scleroderma PAH. Epoprostenol improves symptoms, exercise capacity and haemodynamics in both clinical conditions, and is the only treatment to be shown in clinical trials to improve survival in the idiopathic form. The optimal dose is variable between individual patients ranging in the majority between 20 and 40 ng/kg/min. Serious adverse events related to the delivery system include pump malfunction, local site infection, central venous catheter obstruction and sepsis. Epoprostenol may also be used in NYHA class III patients who are refractory to endothelin-receptor antagonists or other prostanoids. Some authors still use first-line epoprostenol in NYHA class III patients, due to its demonstrated survival benefits.

The clinical use of prostacyclin in patients with PAH has been extended by the synthesis of stable analogues that possess different pharmacokinetic properties but share similar pharmacodynamic effects.

Among prostanoids, treprostinil is administered subcutaneously by micro-infusion pumps and small subcutaneous catheters. The effects of treprostinil were studied in the largest worldwide study performed in this condition, and showed improvements in exercise capacity, haemodynamics and clinical events. Infusion site pain was the most common side-effect of treprostinil. Trials on the intravenous and inhaled use of this compound are ongoing.

Inhaled iloprost (6–9 daily repetitive inhalations) has been evaluated in one clinical trial, which demonstrated an increase in exercise capacity, symptoms, pulmonary vascular resistance and clinical events. A second study on patients already treated with bosentan has shown similar results.

Beraprost is the first chemically stable and orally active prostacyclin analogue. Two clinical studies have shown an improvement of exercise capacity that unfortunately persists only up to 3–6 months.

cGMP-phosphodiesterase type 5 inhibitors

cGMP-phosphodiesterase type 5 is selectively abundant in the pulmonary circulation and PDE-5 gene expression and activity are increased in chronic PH. cGMP- phosphodiesterase type 5 inhibition increases the intracellular concentration of cGMP that in turn induces relaxation and antiproliferative effects on vascular smooth muscle cells.

The orally-active form of cGMP- phosphodiesterase type 5 inhibitor sildenafil has been evaluated in a study on 278 patients (treated with sildenafil 20, 40 or 80 mg TID). An improvement in exercise capacity, functional class and haemodynamics was shown with the three doses. The dose of 20 mg TID has been approved by the FDA and EMEA for the treatment of PAH patients (Table 3).

A study on cGMP-phosphodiesterase type 5 inhibitor tadalafil in PAH patients is currently ongoing.

Combination therapy

Combination therapy can be pursued by the simultaneous initiation of two (or more) treatments or by the addition of a second (or third) treatment to a previous therapy that may be considered insufficient. The best choice between these two strategies is currently unknown.

Combination therapy may be considered for patients who fail to improve or deteriorate with first-line treatment, even though data on this specific strategy are currently limited to two clinical controlled trials combining respectively bosentan and epoprostenol (concurrent initiation) and inhaled iloprost to patients treated with bosentan. Different single-centre non-randomised studies with different combinations are also available.

Interventional procedures

Balloon atrial septostomy is performed in severely ill patients as a palliative bridge to lung transplantation. This procedure should be performed in experienced centres.

Double lung or heart-lung transplantation are indicated in patients with advanced NYHA class III and class IV symptoms that are refractory to available medical treatments. The 3 and 5 year survival after lung and heart-lung transplantation is approximately 55% and 45%, respectively.

5. Treatment algorithm (Figure 1)

- The treatment algorithm for PH is shown in Figure 1. The algorithm is appropriate for NYHA class III or IV idiopathic or patients with PAH associated with connective tissue diseases. Extrapolation of these

Figure 1: Treatment Algorithm of Pulmonary Arterial Hypertension

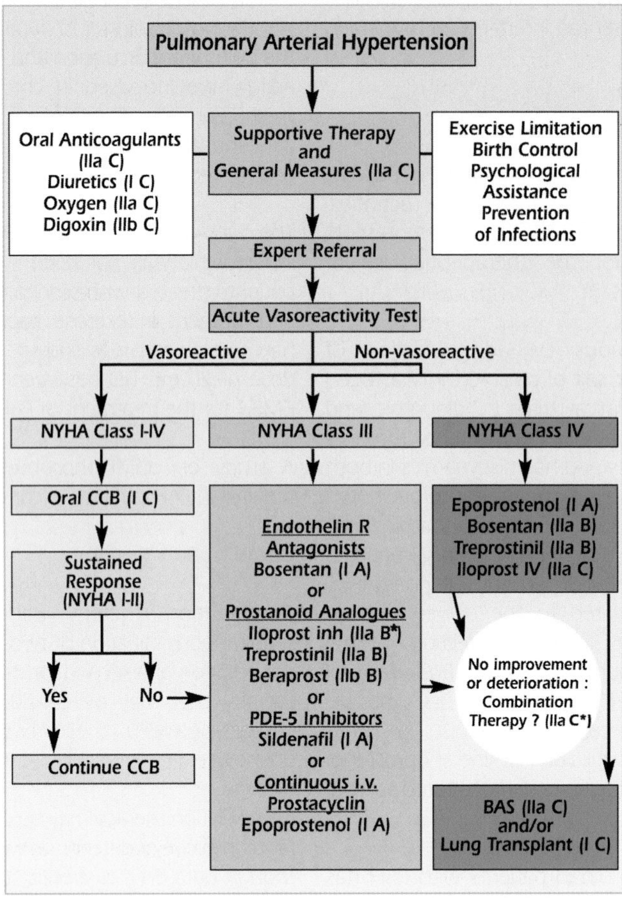

*See foreseen changes in grade of recommendation and level of evidence in Table 3 and see legend, page 232.

recommendations to the other PAH subgroups should be made with caution.

- The suggested initial approach is the adoption of the general measures and initiation of the supportive therapy.

Due to the complexity of the evaluation and the treatment options available, it is strongly recommended that PAH patients are then referred to a specialized centre.

- Oral anticoagulant treatment should be initiated in patients with idiopathic PAH. The proposed target INR varies somewhat being 1.5 to 3.0. The anticoagulation of other forms of PAH is also suggested if no bleeding-risk factors are present.

- Appropriate diuretic treatment in case of right heart failure allows clear symptomatic and clinical benefits.

- Despite the fact that no consistent data are currently available on long-term oxygen treatment in PAH, it is generally considered important to maintain oxygen saturation at greater than 90% at all times.

- The usefulness of digitalis is controversial and i.v. inotropes such as dobutamine may be used in end-stage right heart failure.

- Treatment with high doses of calcium-channel blockers is mandatory in responders to acute vasoreactivity tests. Long-term response (after 3-6 months) need to be evaluated and subjects in NYHA class I-II and with marked haemodynamic improvement can continue calcium channel blockers as monotherapy.

- Non-responders to acute vasoreactivity testing who are in NYHA functional class I and II and no signs of poor prognosis (Table 2) should continue with general measures and supportive therapy under close clinical follow-up.

- Non-responders to acute vasoreactivity testing, or responders who remain in NYHA functional class III should be considered candidates for treatment with either an endothelin-receptor antagonist, a cGMP-phosphodiesterase type 5 inhibitor or a prostanoid. Also, non-responders to acute vasoreactivity testing who are in NYHA functional class I and II and with multiple signs of poor prognosis (Table 2), should be treated with the same strategy.

- As no head-to-head comparisons between the three classes of drugs are available it is not possible to define the "first line compound" to be used. Therefore the choice of the drug is dependent on a variety of factors, including the approval status, route of administration, side-effect profile, patient's preferences, physician's experience and costs.

- Combination therapy may be considered for patients who fail to improve or deteriorate with first-line treatment, even though data on this specific strategy are limited. This strategy should be implemented only in experienced referral centres.

- Continuous i.v. epoprostenol, may be considered as first line therapy for patients in NYHA functional class IV because of the demonstrated survival benefit in this subset. However, these patients should be concurrently listed for lung transplantation and subsequently delisted in case of improvement. Although both bosentan and treprostinil are approved in NYHA class IV patients, most experts consider these treatments as a second line for severely ill patients. Although no controlled trials have been performed with the i.v. delivery of iloprost, this prostacyclin analogue has been approved in New Zealand*.

- Balloon atrial septostomy is performed in severely ill patients as a palliative bridge to lung transplantation. Double lung or heart-lung transplantation are indicated in patients with advanced NYHA class III and class IV symptoms that are refractory to available medical treatments.

6. Associated conditions

Pulmonary Arterial Hypertension associated to congenital heart defects involving systemic-to-pulmonary shunts and Eisenmenger's syndrome

- The persistent exposure of the pulmonary vasculature to increased blood flow as well as increased pressure may result in PAH.

- The more severe form, Eisenmenger's syndrome, is defined as a congenital heart defect that initially causes a large left-to-right shunt that induces severe pulmonary vascular disease and PAH, with resultant reversal of the direction of shunting.

- Survival of patients with Eisenmenger's syndrome is better than that of subjects with IPAH with comparable functional class.

- Phlebotomy with isovolumic replacement should be performed in patients with moderate or severe symptoms of hyperviscosity (e.g. headache and poor concentration) that usually are present when haematocrit is > 65%.

- The use of supplemental oxygen therapy is controversial and should be used in cases in which it produces a consistent increase in arterial oxygen saturation and/or improved clinical well being.

- In some centres, Eisenmenger's syndrome patients are anticoagulated similarly to other subjects with PAH in the absence of contraindication.

- Epoprostenol has been shown to improve haemodynamics and exercise capacity and the effects of subcutaneous treprostinil in Eisenmenger patients was not different from that on IPAH.

- A randomized controlled trial has shown that bosentan improves exercise capacity and haemodynamics in Eisenmenger patients.

- Combined heart-lung transplantation is an option in patients with markers of a poor prognosis (syncope, refractory heart failure, NYHA functional class III or IV, or severe hypoxaemia).

Porto-pulmonary hypertension

- PAH is a well-recognized complication of chronic liver disease. Portal hypertension rather than the hepatic disorder itself seems to be the main determining risk factor.

- The clinical picture of patients with porto-pulmonary hypertension may be indistinguishable from that of IPAH and include a combination of symptoms and signs of the underlying liver disease.

- Echocardiographic screening for the detection of PH in patients with liver diseases is appropriate in symptomatic patients and/or in candidates for liver transplantation.

*IV iloprast is used in countries where IV epoprostentol is not available. The notion that a regular agency has approved its use is important to be reported in international guidelines such as the present ones.

- Right heart catheterization should be performed in all cases with increased systolic PAP in order to clarify the underlying haemodynamic changes and define prognosis and treatment.

- Compared with patients with IPAH, patients with porto-pulmonary hypertension have a significantly higher cardiac output and significantly lower systemic vascular resistance and PVR.

- Patients with porto-pulmonary hypertension have a better rate of survival than patients with IPAH, although there is some debate on this issue.

- Anticoagulant therapy should be avoided in patients at increased risk of bleeding.

- Patients with porto-pulmonary hypertension seem to respond favourably to chronic i.v. epoprostenol. Despite preliminary short term favourable results the risk-to-benefit ratio of endothelin receptor antagonists in patients with liver disease needs to be carefully evaluated on a long-term basis.

- Significant PAH can substantially increase the risk associated with liver transplantation and usually PAH is a contraindication if mean PAP is ≥ 35 mmHg and/or PVR is ≥ 250 dynes·s·cm^{-5}.

Pulmonary Arterial Hypertension (PAH) associated with HIV infection

- PAH is a rare but well-documented complication of HIV infection.

- Echocardiographic screening in patients with HIV infection is required in symptomatic ones.

- A right heart catheterization is recommended in all cases of suspected PAH associated with HIV infection to confirm the diagnosis, determine severity, and rule out left-sided heart disease.

- PAH is an independent predictor of mortality in this patient population.

- Oral anticoagulation is often contraindicated because of bleeding risk factors.

- Epoprostenol seems to be effective in improving functional status and haemodynamics.

- Favorable clinical and haemodynamic results have been shown with the use of bosentan in an uncontrolled study.

Pulmonary Arterial Hypertension associated with Connective Tissue Diseases (CTD)

- PAH is a complication of systemic sclerosis, systemic lupus erythematosus, mixed CTD, and to a lesser extent, rheumatoid arthritis, dermatopolymyositis, and primary Sjögren's syndrome.

- In these patients, PAH may occur in association with interstitial fibrosis or as a result of an isolated lung arteriopathy. Pulmonary venous hypertension from left heart disease can also be present.

- The mortality was confirmed to be higher than that seen with IPAH.

- Echocardiographic screening should be performed yearly in asymptomatic patients with the scleroderma spectrum of diseases and only in presence of symptoms in other conditions.

- Right heart catheterization is recommended in all cases of suspected PAH associated with CTD to confirm the diagnosis, determine severity, and rule out left-sided heart disease.

- Immunosuppressive therapy seems to be effective on PAH only in a minority of patients mainly suffering from conditions other than scleroderma.

- The rate of acute vasoreactivity and of a long-term favourable response to CCB treatment is lower compared to IPAH.

- The risk-to-benefit ratio of oral anticoagulation is not well understood.

- Epoprostenol has been shown to improve exercise capacity, symptoms and haemodynamics in patients with the scleroderma spectrum of the disease but the efficacy is less than in IPAH.

- Subcutaneous treprostinil has been shown to increase exercise capacity and haemodynamics.

- Subgroup analysis of patients with scleroderma enrolled in trials performed with bosentan, sitaxsentan, ambrisentan and sildenafil have shown favourable effects with all these orally administered drugs. However, the efficacy of all these compounds in scleroderma patients appears to be reduced as compared to IPAH subjects.

Pulmonary Veno-occlusive Disease (PVOD) and Pulmonary Capillary Hemangiomatosis (PCH)

- PVOD and PCH are uncommon conditions that are increasingly recognized as causes for PAH.
- The pathological changes usually occur in the venules without involvement of the larger veins.
- Clinical presentation of these patients is often indistinguishable from that of patients with IPAH.
- Physical examination can demonstrate digital clubbing and/or basilar rales on chest auscultation.
- PVOD/PCH is associated with more severe hypoxaemia and reduction of single-breath DLCO.
- Haemodynamic data are similar between PVOD/PCH and IPAH and pulmonary wedge pressure is often normal despite the postcapillary involvement.
- On a standard chest X-ray roentgenogram the presence of Kerley B lines, pleural effusion and patchy irregularities may provide important clues that suggest the diagnosis.
- HRCT of the chest may show a patchy centrilobular pattern of ground-glass opacities, thickened septal lines, pleural effusion, and mediastinal adenopathy.
- Compared with IPAH, PVOD/PCH is characterized by significantly elevated broncho-alveolar lavage cell counts with an increased number of haemosiderin-laden macrophages.
- PVOD/PCH have a worse, with a more rapid downhill course as compared to IPAH.
- Epoprostenol has to be used with great caution because of the high risk of pulmonary oedema even if reports of sustained clinical improvement in individual patients are available.
- There are no data regarding the use of newer medical therapies in the treatment of PVOD/PCH.
- The only curative therapy for PVOD/PCH is lung transplantation.

7. Paediatric Pulmonary Arterial Hypertension (PPAH)

- The prevalence of congenital heart disease is higher amongst children with PAH than in adults.
- Persistent PH of the newborn is different from other forms of PAH because it is usually transient with infants either recovering completely without chronic medical therapy or dying during the neonatal period despite maximal cardiopulmonary therapeutic interventions.
- In the NIH registry a higher mortality was shown in children than adults with PAH if untreated.
- There is agreement on a less predictable course in children with PAH as compared to adults.
- Children with severe PH undergo a similar diagnostic evaluation as has been described in adults.
- Diagnosis needs to be confirmed by the right heart catheterization and the prevalence of acute vasoreactivity is higher in children with IPAH.
- The therapeutic algorithm for children who have PAH is similar to that used in adults.
- Children with PAH must be definitely treated by a physician experienced in this condition.
- Pneumonia requires hospitalization and aggressive medical treatment.
- More children than adults are acutely vasoreactive and are effectively treated with CCBs and they tolerate and appear to need a higher dose per kg than adults.
- The current approach of experts is to anticoagulate children with PAH and right heart failure.
- Bosentan, sildenafil and epoprostenol have also been shown to be effective in children even if dose requirements appear to be less established.
- Lung transplantation needs to be considered in case of unsatisfactory response to full medical therapy.

8. Glossary

ANA	Antinuclear Antibodies
BID	bis in die – two times a day
CCB	Calcium Channel Blocker
CT	Computerised Tomography
CTD	Connective Tissue Diseases
cGMP	Cyclic Guanosine 3′-5′ Monophosphate
CPET	Cardiopulmonary Exercise Testing
CTEPH	Chronic Thromboembolic Pulmonary Hypertension
DLco	Diffusion Capacity for Carbon Monoxide
ECG	Electrocardiogram
EMEA	European Agency for the Evaluation of the Medical Products
ET	Endothelin
HIV	Human Immunodeficiency Virus
HRCT	High Resolution Computerised Tomography
IPAH	Idiopathic Pulmonary Arterial Hypertension
INR	International Normalized Ratio
i.v.	intravenous
6MWT	Six Minute Walk Test
NYHA	New-York Heart Association
O_2	Oxygen
OD	Once Daily
PAH	Pulmonary Arterial Hypertension
$PaCO_2$	Arterial Carbon Dioxide Tension
PaO_2	Arterial Oxygen Tension
PAP	Pulmonary Arterial Pressure
PCH	Pulmonary Capillary Haemangiomatosis
PPH	Primary Pulmonary Hypertension
PVOD	Pulmonary Veno-Occlusive Disease
PVR	Pulmonary Vascular Resistance
PWP	Pulmonary Wedge Pressure
RHC	Right Heart Catheterization
VO_2	Oxygen Consumption
V/Q	Ventilation/Perfusion

Section XII: Arrhythmias

1. Supraventricular Arrhythmias (SVA)

2. Atrial Fibrillation (AF)

3. Management of Syncope

4. Ventricular Arrhythmias and the Prevention of Sudden Cardiac Death

5. Cardiac Pacing and Cardiac Resynchronization Therapy

Chapter 1

Supraventricular Arrhythmias (SVA)*
2003

Co-chairperson:
Carina Blomström-Lundqvist, MD, PhD, FESC
Representing: ESC
University Hospital in Uppsala
Department of Cardiology
S-751 85 Uppsala
Sweden

Phone: (46) 18 611 27 35
Fax: (46) 18 51 02 43
E-mail: carina.blomstrom-lundqvist@akademiska.se

Co-chairperson:
Melvin M. Scheinman, MD, FACC
Representing: ACC/AHA
Professor of Medicine
University of California San Francisco
MU East Tower, 4th Flr. S., Box 1354
500 Parnassus Ave
San Francisco, CA 94143-1354 - USA
Phone: (415) 476 5708
Fax: (415) 476 6260
E-mail: mels@medicine.ucsf.edu

Task Force Members:
1. Etienne M. Aliot, Nancy, France
2. Joseph S. Alpert, Tucson, USA
3. Hugh Calkins, New York, USA
4. A. John Camm, London, UK
5. W. Barton Campbell, Nashville, USA
6. David E. Haines, Charlottesville, USA
7. Karl H. Kuck, Hamburg, Germany
8. Bruce B. Lerman, New York, USA
9. D. Douglas Miller, Saint-Louis, USA
10. Charlie W. Shaeffer, Jr., Rancho Mirage, USA
11. William G. Stevenson, Boston, USA
12. Gordon F. Tomaselli, Baltimore, USA

ESC Staff:
1. Keith McGregor, Sophia-Antipolis, France
2. Veronica Dean, Sophia-Antipolis, France
3. Dominique Poumeyrol-Jumeau, Sophia-Antipolis, France
4. Catherine Després, Sophia-Antipolis, France

I. Introduction

Supraventricular arrhythmias (SVAs) include rhythms emanating from or involving the sinus node, atrial tissue (atrial tachycardias (ATs), atrial flutter), and junctional tissue (atrioventricular nodal reciprocating tachycardia (AVNRT)). Accessory pathway-mediated or atrioventricular reciprocating tachycardia (AVRT) are also included. Supraventricular arrhythmia occurs in all age groups and may be associated with minimal symptoms, such as palpitations, or may present with syncope. In some conditions (i.e. those associated with bypass tracts) arrhythmias may be life-threatening. The prevalence of paroxysmal supraventricular tachycardia (PSVT) is 2-3 per 1,000. Over the past decade, impressive advances in curative treatment modes (catheter ablation) have been made.

The purpose of this booklet is to summarize guidelines for use of drug and ablative procedures for patients with supraventricular tachycardia (SVT). Guidelines for treatment of atrial fibrillation were recently published, hence this subject is excluded in the present booklet. In addition, SVT in the paediatric population is excluded. The ACC/AHA/ESC Guidelines for the Management of Patients with Atrial Fibrillation (2) discuss antiarrhythmic drug doses and adverse effects, and therefore, this will not be repeated.

The guidelines outlined come from an expert committee selected by the European Society of Cardiology (ESC), American College of Cardiology (ACC), and American Heart Association (AHA). The ultimate judgment regarding care of a particular patient must be made by the physician and patient in light of all of the circumstances

* Adapted from the ACC/AHA/ESC Guidelines for the Management of Patients with Supraventricular Arrhythmias: Executive Summary (European Heart Journal 2003; 24 (20): 1857-1897) (1)

presented by that patient. In some circumstances deviations from these guidelines may be appropriate.

Recommendations are provided in tables and use the following classification outline, summarizing both the evidence and expert opinion:

Class I:	Conditions for which there is evidence for and/or general agreement that the procedure or treatment is useful and effective.
Class II:	Conditions for which there is conflicting evidence and/or a divergence of opinion about the usefulness/efficacy of a procedure or treatment.
Class IIa:	The weight of evidence or opinion is in favor of the procedure or treatment.
Class IIb:	Usefulness/efficacy is less well established by evidence or opinion.
Class III:	Conditions for which there is evidence and/or general agreement that the procedure or treatment is not useful/effective and in some cases may be harmful.

II. General evaluation and management of :

A. Patients without documented arrhythmia (Figure 1)

Clinical History

Distinguish whether palpitations are regular or irregular.

- Pauses or dropped beats followed by a sensation of a strong heartbeat support presence of premature beats.
- Irregular palpitations may be due to premature extra beats, atrial fibrillation or multifocal atrial tachycardia.
- Regular and recurrent palpitations with abrupt onset and termination are designated as paroxysmal (also referred to as PSVT). Termination by vagal manoeuvres suggests a re-entrant tachycardia involving atrioventricular (AV) nodal tissue (e.g. AVNRT, AVRT).
- Sinus tachycardia is non-paroxysmal and accelerates and terminates gradually.

B. Patients with documented arrhythmia

1. Narrow QRS-complex tachycardia

If the ventricular action (QRS) is narrow (less than 120 milliseconds [ms]), then the tachycardia is almost always supraventricular and the differential diagnosis relates to its mechanism (Figure 2). The clinician must determine the relationship of the P waves to the ventricular complex (Figure 3). Responses of narrow QRS-complex tachycardias to adenosine (Figure 4) or carotid massage may aid in the differential diagnosis.

2. Wide QRS-complex tachycardia (Figure 5)

At times, the patient will present with rapid wide QRS-complex tachycardia (greater than 120 ms) and the clinician must decide whether the patient has :

a) SVT with bundle branch block (BBB) (or aberration),

b) SVT with AV conduction over an accessory pathway,

c) ventricular tachycardia (VT).

This categorization depends not only on the relation of P wave to QRS but also on specific morphological findings, especially in the precordial leads (Figure 5).

3. Management

If the diagnosis of SVT cannot be proven, the patient should be treated as if VT were present. Medications for SVT (verapamil or diltiazem) may precipitate haemodynamic collapse in a patient with VT. Special circumstances (i.e., pre-excited tachycardias and VT due to digitalis toxicity) may require alternative therapy. Immediate direct current (DC) cardioversion is the treatment of choice for any haemodynamically unstable tachycardia.

Indications for referral to a cardiac arrhythmia specialist:

- All patients with Wolff-Parkinson-White (WPW) syndrome (pre-excitation + arrhythmias).
- All patients with severe symptoms during palpitations, such as syncope or dyspnea.
- Wide QRS-complex tachycardia of unknown origin.
- Narrow QRS-complex tachycardias with drug resistance, drug intolerance or desire to be free of drug therapy.

Recommendations for acute management of haemodynamically stable and regular tachycardia

ECG	Recommendation*	Class	Level of evidence
Narrow QRS-complex tachycardia (SVT)	Vagal manoeuvres	I	B
	Adenosine	I	A
	Verapamil, diltiazem	I	A
	Beta-blockers	II b	C
	Amiodarone	II b	C
	Digoxin	II b	C
Wide QRS-complex tachycardia • SVT and BBB • Pre-excited SVT/AF †	See above		
	Flecainide ‡	I	B
	Ibutilide ‡	I	B
	Procainamide ‡	I	B
	DC cardioversion	I	C
• Wide QRS-complex tachycardia of unknown origin	Procainamide ‡	I	B
	Sotalol ‡	I	B
	Amiodarone	I	B
	Lidocaine	II b	B
	Adenosine §	II b	C
	Beta-blockers ¶	III	C
	Verapamil**	III	B
	DC cardioversion	I	B
Wide QRS-complex tachycardia of unknown origin in patients with poor LV function	Amiodarone	I	B
	Lidocaine		
	DC cardioversion	I	B

The order in which treatment recommendations appear in this table within each class of recommendation does not necessarily reflect a preferred sequence of administration. Please refer to text for details. For pertinent drug dosing information, please refer to the ACC/AHA/ESC Guidelines for the Management of Patients with Atrial Fibrillation (2). * All listed drugs are administered intravenously. † See Section IIID, specific section in reference 1. ‡ Should not be taken by patients with reduced LV function. § Adenosine should be used with caution in patients with severe coronary artery disease because vasodilation of normal coronary vessels may produce ischaemia in vulnerable territory. It should be used only with full resuscitative equipment available. ¶ Beta-blockers may be used as first-line therapy for those with catecholamine-sensitive tachycardias, such as right ventricular outflow tachycardia. ** Verapamil may be used as first-line therapy for those with LV fascicular VT. AF = atrial fibrillation ; BBB = bundle-branch block; DC = direct current; ECG = electrocardiogram; LV = left ventricular; QRS = ventricular activation on ECG; SVT = supraventricular tachycardia.

III. Specific arrhythmias

A. Inappropriate sinus tachycardia

Inappropriate sinus tachycardia refers to a persistent increase in resting heart rate unrelated to the level of physical, emotional, pathological or pharmacological stress. Approximately 90% are female. The degree of disability can vary from asymptomatic to individuals who are totally incapacitated.

The diagnosis is based on the following criteria:

- Persistent sinus tachycardia (heart rate > 100 bpm) during the day with excessive rate increase in response to activity and nocturnal normalization of rate as confirmed by a 24 hour Holter recording.
- The tachycardia and its symptoms are not paroxysmal.
- P-wave morphology is identical to sinus rhythm.
- Exclusion of a secondary systemic cause (hyperthyroidism, pheochromocytoma, physical deconditioning).

Treatment

The treatment is predominantly symptom driven. The long-term success rate of sinus node modification by catheter ablation has been reported to be around 66%. The diagnosis of Postural Orthostatic Tachycardia Syndrome (POTS) must be excluded before considering ablation.

Recommendations for treatment of inappropriate sinus tachycardia

Treatment	Recommendation	Class	Level of evidence
Medical	Beta-blockers	I	C
	Verapamil, diltiazem	II a	C
Interventional	Catheter ablation - sinus node modification/elimination*	II b	C

The order in which treatment recommendations appear in this table within each class of recommendation does not necessarily reflect a preferred sequence of administration. Please refer to text for details. For pertinent drug dosing information, please refer to the ACC/AHA/ESC Guidelines for the Management of Patients with Atrial Fibrillation (2). *Used as a last resort.

B. Atrioventricular Nodal Reciprocating Tachycardia (AVNRT)

AVNRT is a re-entry tachycardia involving the AV node as well as perinodal atrial tissue. One pathway (fast) is located near the superior portion of the AV node and the other (slow) along the septal margin of the tricuspid annulus. During typical AVNRT (85-90%), antegrade conduction occurs over the slow pathway with a turnaround point in the AV junction, and retrograde conduction occurs over the fast pathway. The converse is found during atypical AVNRT, resulting in a long R-P tachycardia with negative P waves in III and aVF inscribed prior to the QRS.

Treatment

Standard treatment is use of drugs that primarily block AV nodal conduction (beta-blockers, calcium channel blockers, adenosine). Another treatment option that has been shown to be effective and safe involves catheter ablation to destroy the slow pathway. Indications for ablation depend on clinical judgement and are often predicated on patient preference. Factors that contribute to the decision include tachycardia frequency, tolerance of symptoms, and patient inclination relative to chronic drug therapy vs. ablation. The patient must accept the risk, albeit small (< 1%), of AV block and pacemaker insertion.

Recommendations for long-term treatment of patients with recurrent AVNRT

Clinical presentation	Intervention	Class	Level of evidence
Poorly tolerated AVNRT with haemodynamic intolerance	Catheter ablation	I	B
	Verapamil, diltiazem, beta-blockers, sotalol, amiodarone	II a	C
	Flecainide*, propafenone*	IIa	C
Recurrent symptomatic AVNRT	Catheter ablation	I	B
	Verapamil	I	B
	Diltiazem, beta-blockers	I	C
	Digoxin †	II b	C
Recurrent AVNRT unresponsive to beta-blockade or calcium-channel blocker and patient not desiring RF ablation	Flecainide*, propafenone*, sotalol	II a	B
	Amiodarone	II b	C
AVNRT with infrequent or single episode in patients who desire complete control of arrhythmia	Catheter ablation	I	B
Documented PSVT with only dual AV-nodal pathways or single echo beats demonstrated during electrophysiological study and no other identified cause of arrhythmia	Verapamil,diltiazem, beta-blockers, flecainide*, propafenone*	I	C
	Catheter ablation ‡	I	B
Infrequent, well-tolerated AVNRT	No therapy	I	C
	Vagal manoeuvres	I	B
	«Pill-in-the-pocket»	I	B
	Verapamil,diltiazem, beta-blockers	I	B
	Catheter ablation	I	B

The order in which treatment recommendations appear in this table within each class of recommendation does not necessarily reflect a preferred sequence of administration. Please refer to text for details. For pertinent drug dosing information, please refer to the ACC/AHA/ESC Guidelines for the Management of Patients with Atrial Fibrillation (2). * Relatively contraindicated for patients with coronary artery disease, LV dysfunction, or other significant heart disease. † Digoxin is often ineffective because pharmacological effects can be overridden by enhanced sympathetic tone. ‡ Decision depends on symptoms. AV = atrioventricular; AVNRT = atrioventricular nodal reciprocating tachycardia; LV = left ventricular; PSVT = paroxysmal supraventricular tachycardia; RF = radiofrequency.

C. Focal and nonparoxysmal junctional tachycardia

1. Focal junctional tachycardia

The unifying feature of focal junctional tachycardia, also known as automatic or junctional ectopic tachycardia, is their origin from the AV node or His bundle. The ECG features of focal junctional tachycardia include heart rates of 110–250 bpm and a narrow complex or typical BBB conduction pattern with AV dissociation. Occasionally the junctional rhythm is quite erratic, suggesting AF. This is a rare arrhythmia seen in young adults and if persistent, it may produce congestive heart failure. Drug therapy has been associated with only variable success and catheter ablative procedures are associated with a 5–10% risk of AV block.

2. Nonparoxysmal junctional tachycardia

Nonparoxysmal junctional tachycardia is a benign arrhythmia that is characterized by a narrow complex tachycardia with rates of 70–120 bpm. The arrhythmia is thought to be due to abnormal automaticity or triggered rhythms and serves as a marker for underlying problems including digitalis toxicity, postcardiac surgery, hypokalemia, or myocardial ischaemia. Treatment is most often directed at the underlying condition.

Recommendations for treatment of focal and nonparoxysmal junctional tachycardia syndromes

Clinical presentation	Recommendation	Class	Level of evidence
Focal junctional tachycardia	Beta-blockers	II a	C
	Flecainide	II a	C
	Propafenone *	II a	C
	Sotalol *	II a	C
	Amiodarone *	II a	C
	Catheter ablation	II a	C
Nonparoxysmal junctional tachycardia	Reverse digitalis toxicity	I	C
	Correct hypokalemia	I	C
	Treat myocardial ischaemia	I	C
	Beta-blockers, calcium-channel blockers	II a	C

The order in which treatment recommendations appear in this table within each class of recommendation does not necessarily reflect a preferred sequence of administration. Please refer to text for details. For pertinent drug dosing information, please refer to the ACC/AHA/ESC Guidelines for the Management of Patients with Atrial Fibrillation (2). *Data available for paediatric patients only.

D. Atrioventricular reciprocating re-entry tachycardia (extranodal accessory pathways)

Typical accessory pathways are extranodal pathways that connect the myocardium of the atrium and the ventricle across the AV groove. Accessory pathways that are capable of only retrograde conduction are referred to as "concealed", whereas those capable of anterograde conduction are "manifest", demonstrating pre-excitation on a standard ECG. The term WPW syndrome is reserved for patients who have both pre-excitation and tachyarrhythmias.

Several forms of tachycardias may occur:

- Orthodromic AVRT (most common, 95%) involves anterograde conduction over the AV node and retrograde conduction over the accessory pathway.
- Antidromic AVRT anterograde conduction over the accessory pathway and retrograde conduction over the AV node (or rarely over a second accessory pathway) resulting in pre-excited QRS-complexes during tachycardia.
- Pre-excited tachycardias in patients with AT or atrial flutter with a bystander (not a critical part of tachycardia circuit) accessory pathway.
- Pre-excited atrial fibrillation, the most feared arrhythmia, occurs in 30% of patients with the WPW syndrome.
- PJRT (permanent form of junctional reciprocating tachycardia) - a rare clinical syndrome with a slowly conducting concealed posteroseptal accessory pathway characterized by an incessant, long RP tachycardia with negative P waves in leads II, III, and aVF.

Sudden Cardiac Death in WPW syndrome and risk stratification

Markers that identify patients at increased risk include: 1) a shortest pre-excited R-R interval < 250 ms during AF, 2) a history of symptomatic tachycardia, 3) multiple accessory pathways, and 4) Ebstein's anomaly. The risk for sudden cardiac death is estimated at between 0.15 - 0.39% of patients with WPW syndrome over 3 to 10 year follow-up.

Asymptomatic patients with accessory pathways

The positive predictive value of invasive electrophysiologic testing is too low to justify routine use in asymptomatic patients. The decision to ablate pathways in individuals with high risk occupations such as school bus drivers, pilots, and athletes, is made on individual clinical considerations.

Treatment

Acute treatment of patients with pre-excited tachycardias

AV nodal blocking agents are not effective and adenosine may produce AF with a rapid ventricular rate. Antiarrhythmic drugs preventing rapid conduction through the pathway (flecainide, procainamide, or ibutilide), are preferable, even if they may not convert the atrial arrhythmia.

Long term therapy

Antiarrhythmic drugs represent one therapeutic option for management of patients with accessory pathway-mediated arrhythmias, but they have been increasingly replaced by catheter ablation. A regimen designed for use of drug(s) at the onset of an episode should only be used for patients with infrequent, well-tolerated episodes.

Some patients with infrequent episodes of tachycardia may be managed with the single-dose "pill-in-the-pocket" approach: taking an antiarrhythmic drug only at the onset of a tachycardia episode. This approach to treatment is reserved for patients without pre-excitation and with uncommon and haemodynamically tolerated tachycardia.

Catheter ablative techniques are successful in approximately 95% of cases and have sufficient efficacy and low risk to be used for symptomatic patients, either as initial therapy or for patients experiencing side effects or arrhythmia recurrence during drug therapy. The type of possible complications varies depending on the site of the pathway. The incidence of inadvertent complete AV block ranges from 0.17 - 1.0%, and relates to septal and posteroseptal accessory pathways. Significant adverse effects range from 1.8 to 4% including 0.08 to 0.13% risk of death.

Recommendations for long-term therapy of accessory pathway-mediated arrhythmias

Arrhythmia	Recommendation	Class	Level of evidence
WPW syndrome (pre-excitation and symptomatic arrhythmias), well tolerated	Catheter ablation	I	B
	Flecainide, propafenone	II a	C
	Sotalol, amiodarone, beta-blockers	II a	C
	Verapamil, diltiazem, digoxin	III	C
WPW syndrome (with AF and rapid-conduction or poorly tolerated AVRT)	Catheter ablation	I	B
AVRT, poorly tolerated (no pre-excitation)	Catheter ablation	I	B
	Flecainide, propafenone	II a	C
	Sotalol, amiodarone	II a	C
	Beta-blockers	II b	C
	Verapamil, diltiazem, digoxin	III	C
Single or infrequent AVRT episode(s) (no pre-excitation)	None	I	C
	Vagal manoeuvres	I	B
	«Pill-in-the-pocket» Verapamil, diltiazem, beta-blockers	I	B
	Catheter ablation	II a	B
	Sotalol, amiodarone	II b	B
	Flecainide, propafenone	II b	C
	Digoxin	III	C
Pre-excitation, asymptomatic	None	I	C
	Catheter ablation	II a	B

The order in which treatment recommendations appear in this table within each class of recommendation does not necessarily reflect a preferred sequence of administration. Please refer to text for details. For pertinent drug dosing information, please refer to the ACC/AHA/ESC Guidelines for the Management of Patients with Atrial Fibrillation (2). AF = atrial fibrillation; AVRT = atrioventricular reciprocating tachycardia; WPW = Wolff-Parkinson-White.

E. Focal atrial tachycardia (FAT)

Focal ATs are characterized by radial spread of activation from a focus, with endocardial activation not extending through the entire atrial cycle. They are usually manifest by atrial rates between 100 and 250 bpm (rarely at 300 bpm). The mechanism has been attributed to abnormal or enhanced automaticity, triggered activity (due to delayed after depolarization), or micro-re-entry. A progressive increase in atrial rate with tachycardia onset ("warm-up") and/or progressive decrease before tachycardia termination ("cool-down") suggests an automatic mechanism. Approximately 10% of patients have multiple foci. Focal AT may be incessant leading to tachycardia-induced cardiomyopathy.

Treatment

Therapeutic options include use of drugs for rate control (beta-blockers, calcium-channel blockers, or digoxin) or for suppression of the arrhythmic focus. In addition, class Ia or Ic (flecainide and propafenone) drugs may prove effective.

The available studies suggest use of IV adenosine, beta-blockers or calcium-channel blockers for either acute termination (unusual) or more frequently to achieve rate control. Adenosine will terminate FAT in a significant number of patients. DC cardioversion seldom terminates automatic ATs but may be successful for ATs based on micro-re-entry or triggered automaticity, and should be attempted in patients with drug-resistant arrhythmia.

Chronic control involves initial use of AV nodal blocking drugs since they may prove effective and have minimal side effects. Other more potent agents should be reserved for after failure of an AV nodal blocker. Focal AT is ablated by targeting the site of origin of the AT. Catheter ablation has a success rate of 80% to 90% for right atrial foci and 70% to 80% for left atrial foci. The incidence of significant complications is low (1–2%). Ablation of AT from the atrial septum or Koch's triangle may produce AV block.

F. Multifocal Atrial Tachycardia (MAT)

The tachycardia is characterized by finding three or more different P wave morphologies at different rates. The rhythm is always irregular and frequently confused with AF. It is most commonly associated with underlying pulmonary disease, but may result from metabolic or electrolyte derangements. Therapy includes correction of underlying abnormalities, but often requires use of calcium channel blockers as there is no role for DC cardioversion, antiarrhythmic drugs or ablation.

G. Macro-re-entrant atrial tachycardia

Atrial flutter is defined as an organized rapid (250–350 bpm) macroreentrant atrial rhythm. The most common forms relate to reentrant rhythms that circulate around the tricuspid annulus. Isthmus-dependent flutter refers to circuits in which the arrhythmia involves the cavotricuspid isthmus (CTI). They are most frequently manifest as counterclockwise (negative flutter deflections in inferior leads) but can be clockwise (positive deflections in the inferior leads).

Non-isthmus dependent atrial flutter is less frequent and is often caused by surgical scars that produce a central obstacle for reentry. For patients with non-isthmus dependent flutter, large areas of atrial scar are found (with cardiac mapping) and are often associated with multiple reentrant circuits. Atrial flutter may cause insidious symptoms such as exercise-induced fatigue, worsening heart failure or pulmonary disease. Patients often present with a 2:1 AV conduction which, if left untreated, may promote cardiomyopathy.

Treatment

Acute therapy depends on the clinical status of the patient as well as underlying cardio-respiratory problems. If the arrhythmia is attended by heart failure, shock, or myocardial ischaemia then prompt DC cardioversion is in order. Rapid atrial (or esophageal pacing) as well as low energy DC cardioversion are all very effective in termination of atrial flutter. In most instances, however, patients with flutter are stable and trials of AV-nodal-blocking drugs for rate control are in order.

This is especially important if the subsequent use of antiarrhythmic drugs is planned, since slowing of the flutter rate by antiarrhythmic drugs (especially Class Ic drugs) may result in a paradoxical increase in the ventricular rate. If the atrial flutter persists for longer than 48 hours then either a 3–4 week course of anticoagulant therapy or a negative (Absence of clots) T.E.E. (Trans-esophageal Echocardiogram) is advisable prior to attempting electrical or drug conversion. These recommendations are identical to those used for management of atrial fibrillation. Neither atrioventricular (AV) nodal drugs nor amiodarone are effective for conversion of atrial flutter. Intravenous ibutilide appears to be the most effective agent for acute drug termination of flutter with an efficacy between 38% and 76%, and is more effective than intravenous class Ic agents.

Class III drugs, especially dofetilide appear to be quite effective chronic therapy for patients with flutter (73% response rate). Chronic therapy is usually not required after sinus rhythm is restored if atrial flutter occurs as part of an acute disease process.

Recommendations for treatment of focal atrial tachycardia*

Clinical situation	Recommendation	Class	Level of evidence
Acute treatment †			
A. Conversion			
Haemodynamically unstable patient	DC cardioversion	I	B
Haemodynamically stable patient	Adenosine	II a	C
	Beta-blockers	II a	C
	Verapamil, diltiazem	II a	C
	Procainamide	II a	C
	Flecainide, propafenone	II a	C
	Amiodarone, sotalol	II a	C
B. Rate regulation (in absence of digitalis therapy)	Beta-blockers	I	C
	Verapamil, diltiazem	I	C
	Digoxin	II b	C
Prophylactic therapy			
Recurrent symptomatic AT	Catheter ablation	I	B
	Beta-blockers, calcium-channel blocker	I	C
	Disopyramide ‡	II a	C
	Flecainide, propafenone ‡	II a	C
	Sotalol, amiodarone	II a	C
Asymptomatic or symptomatic incessant ATs	Catheter ablation	I	B
Nonsustained and asymptomatic	No therapy	I	C
	Catheter ablation	III	C

The order in which treatment recommendations appear in this table within each class of recommendation does not necessarily reflect a preferred sequence of administration. Please refer to text for details. For pertinent drug dosing information, please refer to the ACC/AHA/ESC Guidelines for the Management of Patients with Atrial Fibrillation (2). * Excluded are patients with MAT in whom beta-blockers and sotalol are often contraindicated due to pulmonary disease. † All listed drugs for acute treatment are taken intravenously. ‡ Flecainide, propafenone, and disopyramide should not be used unless they are combined with an AV-nodal-blocking agent. AT = atrial tachycardia; DC = direct current; MAT = multifocal atrial tachycardia.

Catheter ablation of the CTI is a safe and effective cure for patients with CTI dependent flutter. For those patients with non-isthmus dependent flutter referral to a specialized center is in order, since multiple complex circuits are frequently found. Success rates vary from 50 to 88% depending on lesion complexity.

Recommendations for acute management of atrial flutter

Clinical status/Proposed therapy	Recommendation	Class	Level of evidence
Poorly tolerated			
• Conversion	DC cardioversion	I	C
• Rate control	Beta-blockers	II a	C
	Verapamil, diltiazem	II a	C
	Digitalis †	II b	C
	Amiodarone	II b	C
Stable flutter			
• Conversion	Atrial or transesophageal pacing	I	A
	DC cardioversion	I	C
	Ibutilide ‡	II a	A
	Flecainide §	II b	A
	Propafenone §	II b	A
	Sotalol	II b	C
	Procainamide §	II b	A
	Amiodarone	II b	C
• Rate control	Diltiazem or Verapamil	I	A
	Beta-blockers	I	C
	Digitalis †	II b	C
	Amiodarone	II b	C

The order in which treatment recommendations appear in this table within each class of recommendation does not necessarily reflect a preferred sequence of administration. Please refer to text for details. For pertinent drug dosing information, please refer to the ACC/AHA/ESC Guidelines for the Management of Patients with Atrial Fibrillation (2). Cardioversion should be considered only if the patient is anticoagulated (INR equals 2 to 3), the arrhythmia is less than 48 hours in duration, or the TEE shows no atrial clots. All listed drugs are taken intravenously. † Digitalis may be especially useful for rate control in patients with heart failure. ‡ Ibutilide should not be used in patients with reduced LV function. § Flecainide, propafenone, and procainamide should not be used unless they are combined with an AV-nodal-blocking agent. AV = atrioventricular; DC = direct current; INR = international normalized ratio; LV = left ventricular; TEE = transesophageal echocardiography.

Recommendations for long-term management of atrial flutter

Clinical status/Proposed therapy	Recommendation	Class	Level of evidence
First episode and well-tolerated atrial flutter	Cardioversion alone	I	B
	Catheter ablation*	II a	B
Recurrent and well-tolerated atrial flutter	Catheter ablation*	I	B
	Dofetilide	II a	C
	Amiodarone, Sotalol, Flecainide †‡, quinidine †‡, propafenone †‡, procainamide †‡, disopyramide †‡	II b	C
Poorly tolerated atrial flutter	Catheter ablation*	I	B
Atrial flutter appearing after use of class Ic agentsor amiodarone for treatment of AF	Catheter ablation*	I	B
	Stop current drug and use another	II a	C
Symptomatic non-CTI-dependant flutter after failed antiarrhythmic drugtherapy	Catheter ablation*	II a	B

The order in which treatment recommendations appear in this table within each class of recommendation does not necessarily reflect a preferred sequence of administration. Please refer to text for details. For pertinent drug dosing information, please refer to the ACC/AHA/ESC Guidelines for the Management of Patients with Atrial Fibrillation (2). * Catheter ablation of the AV junction and insertion of a pacemaker should be considered if catheter ablative cure is not possible and the patient fails drug therapy. † These drugs should not be taken by patients with significant structural cardiac disease. Use of anticoagulants is identical to that described for patients with AF. ‡ Flecainide, propafenone, procainamide, quinidine, and disopyramide should not be used unless they are combined with an AV-nodal-blocking agent. AF = atrial fibrillation; AV = atrioventricular; CTI = cavotricuspid isthmus.

H. Special circumstances

1. Pregnancy

SVT occurring during pregnancy may be a particularly difficult problem. There is concern for the haemodynamic effects on the mother and foetus as well as for the possible adverse drug effects on the foetus. Certain principles should be emphasized. 1) Arrhythmias curable by ablation should be seriously considered prior to planned pregnancy. 2) Most arrhythmias consist of isolated atrial or ventricular premature beats and do not require therapy. 3) Acute therapy of arrhythmias should be directed at use of non-pharmacological approaches (i.e. vagal manoeuvres). IV adenosine and DC cardioversion have been shown to be safe. The major concern with antiarrhythmic drug treatment during pregnancy is the potential for adverse effects on the foetus. The first 8 weeks after conception is associated with the greatest teratogenic risk. Adverse effects on foetal growth/development are the major risks during the 2nd and 3rd trimester. Antiarrhythmic drug therapy should only be used if symptoms are intolerable or if the tachycardia causes haemodynamic compromise.

Recommendations for treatment strategies for SVT during pregnancy

Treatment strategy	Recommendation	Class	Level of evidence
Acute conversion of PSVT	Vagal manoeuvres	I	C
	Adenosine	I	C
	DC cardioversion	I	C
	Metoprolol, propranolol	II a	C
	Verapamil	II b	C
Prophylactic therapy	Digoxin	I	C
	Metoprolol *	I	B
	Propranolol *	II a	B
	Sotalol*, flecainide †	II a	C
	Quinidine, propafenone †, Verapamil	II b	C
	Procainamide	II b	B
	Catheter ablation	II b	C
	Atenolol ‡	III	B
	Amiodarone	III	C

The order in which treatment recommendations appear in this table within each class of recommendation does not necessarily reflect a preferred sequence of administration. Please refer to text for details. For pertinent drug dosing information, please refer to the ACC/AHA/ESC Guidelines for the Management of Patients with Atrial Fibrillation (2). * Beta-blocking agents should not be taken in the first trimester, if possible. † Consider AV-nodal-blocking agents in conjunction with flecainide and propafenone for certain tachycardias (see Section V). ‡ Atenolol is categorized in class C (drug classification for use during pregnancy) by legal authorities in some European countries. AV = atrioventricular; DC = direct current; PSVT = paroxysmal supraventricular tachycardia.

2. Adults with congenital heart disease

The treatment of SVT in adult patients with repaired or unrepaired congenital heart disease is often complicated and should be managed at experienced centers. Supraventricular arrhythmias are an important cause of morbidity and, in some patients, mortality. These patients often have multiple atrial circuits or mechanisms responsible for arrhythmias. Atrial arrhythmias can indicate deteriorating haemodynamic function, which in some cases warrants specific investigation and operative treatment. Coexistent sinus node dysfunction is common, requiring pacemaker implantation to allow management of SVTs. Cardiac malformations often increase the difficulty of pacemaker implantation and catheter ablation procedures. In addition, arrhythmia therapy by either drugs or catheter ablation must be properly coordinated within the context of surgical repair.

Recommendations for treatment of SVTs in adults with congenital heart disease

Condition	Recommendation	Class	Level of evidence
Failed antiarrhythmic drugs and symptomatic:			
• Repaired ASD:	Catheter ablation in an experienced center	I	C
• Mustard or Senning repair of transposition of the great vessels:	Catheter ablation in an experienced center	I	C
Unrepaired haemodynamically significant ASD with atrial flutter*	Closure of the ASD combined with ablation of the flutter isthmus	I	C
PSVT and Ebstein's anomaly with haemodynamic indications for surgical repair	Catheter or surgical ablation of accessory pathways since there may be one or more pathways at the time of operative repair of the malformation at an experienced center	I	C

*Conversion and antiarrhythmic drug therapy initial management as described for atrial flutter. ASD = atrial septal defect; PSVT = paroxysmal supraventricular tachycardia.

Figure 1. Initial evaluation of patients with suspected tachycardia

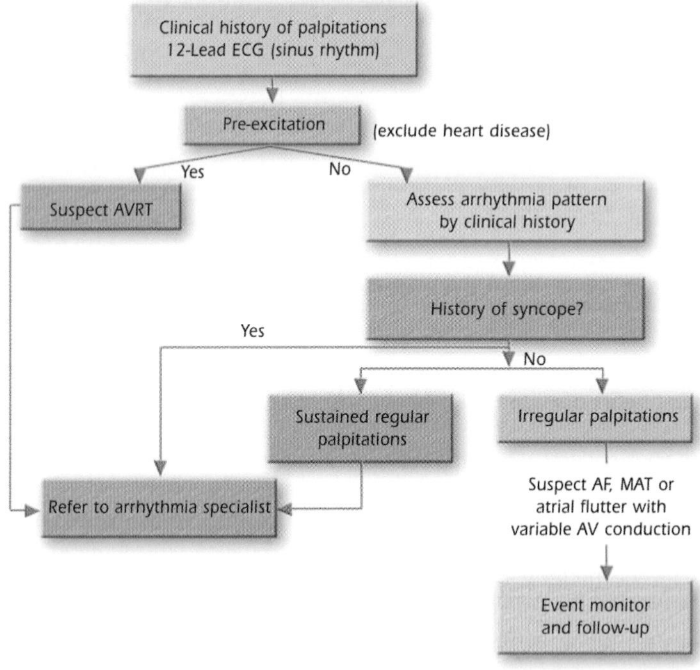

AVRT = atrioventricular reciprocating tachycardia; ECG = electrocardiogram; AF = atrial fibrillation; MAT = multifocal atrial tachycardia; AV = atrioventricular.

Figure 2. Differential diagnosis for narrow QRS tachycardia

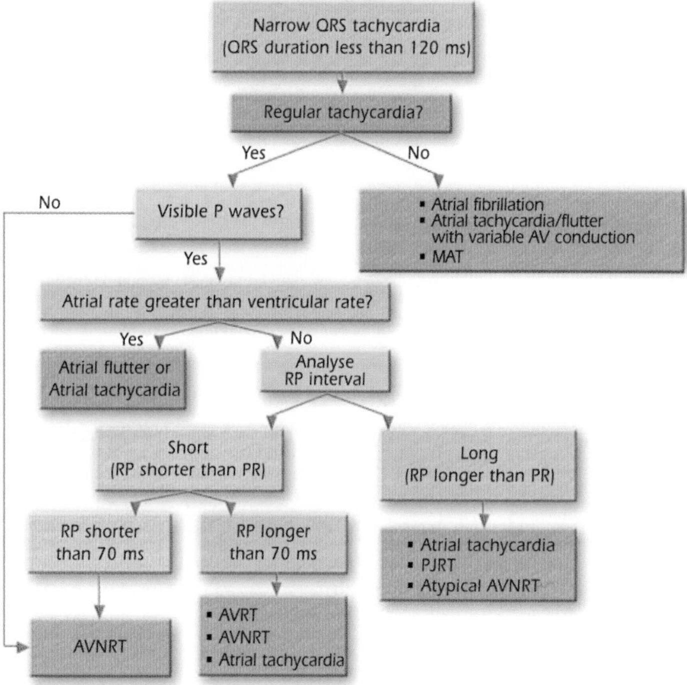

Patients with focal junctional tachycardia may mimic the pattern of slow-fast AVNRT and may show AV dissociation and/or marked irregularity in the junctional rate. AV = atrioventricular; AVNRT = atrioventricular nodal reciprocating tachycardia; AVRT = atrioventricular reciprocating tachycardia; MAT = multifocal atrial tachycardia; ms = milliseconds; PJRT = permanent form of junctional reciprocating tachycardia; QRS = ventricular activation on electrocardiogram.

Figure 3. ECG tracing with limb leads I, II, and III, showing an RP (initial R to initial P) interval longer than the PR interval

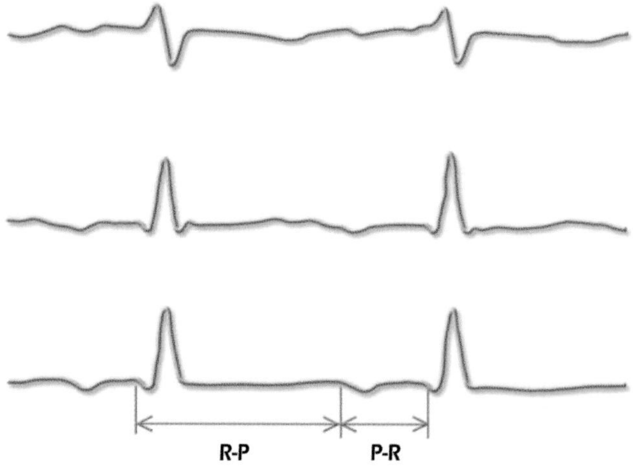

The P wave differs from the sinus P wave. ECG = electrocardiogram.

Figure 4. Responses of narrow complex tachycardias to adenosine

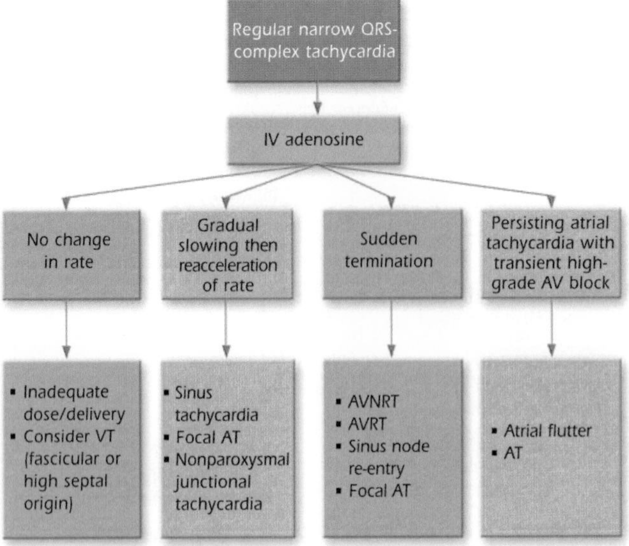

AT = atrial tachycardia; AV = atrioventricular; AVNRT = atrioventricular nodal reciprocating tachycardia; AVRT = atrioventricular reciprocating tachycardia; IV = intravenous; QRS = ventricular activation on electrocardiogram; VT = ventricular tachycardia.

Figure 5. Differential diagnosis for wide QRS-complex tachycardia (greater than 120 ms)

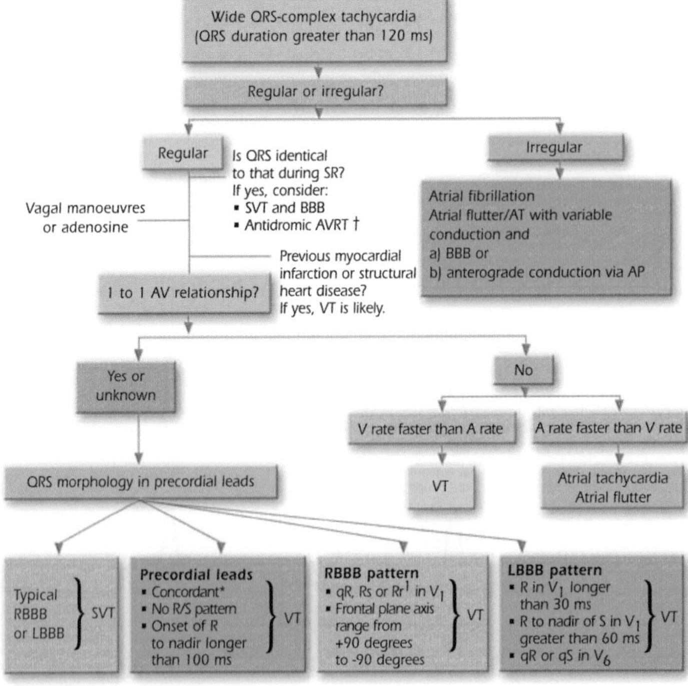

A QRS conduction delay during sinus rhythm, when available for comparison, reduces the value of QRS morphology analysis. Adenosine should be used with caution when the diagnosis is unclear because it may produce VF in patients with coronary artery disease and AF with a rapid ventricular rate in pre-excited tachycardias. Various adenosine responses are shown in Fig. 6. * Concordant indicates that all precordial leads show either positive or negative deflections. Fusion complexes are diagnostic of VT. † In pre-excited tachycardias, the QRS is generally wider (ie, more pre-excited) compared with sinus rhythm. A = atrial; AF = atrial fibrillation; AP = accessory pathway; AT = atrial tachycardia; AV = atrioventricular; AVRT = atrioventricular reciprocating tachycardia; BBB = bundle-branch block; LBBB = left bundlebranch block; ms = milliseconds; QRS = ventricular activation on ECG; RBBB = right bundle-branch block; SR = sinus rhythm; SVT = supraventricular tachycardias; V = ventricular; VF = ventricular fibrillation; VT = ventricular tachycardia.

Figure 6. Acute management of patients with haemodynamically stable and regular tachycardia

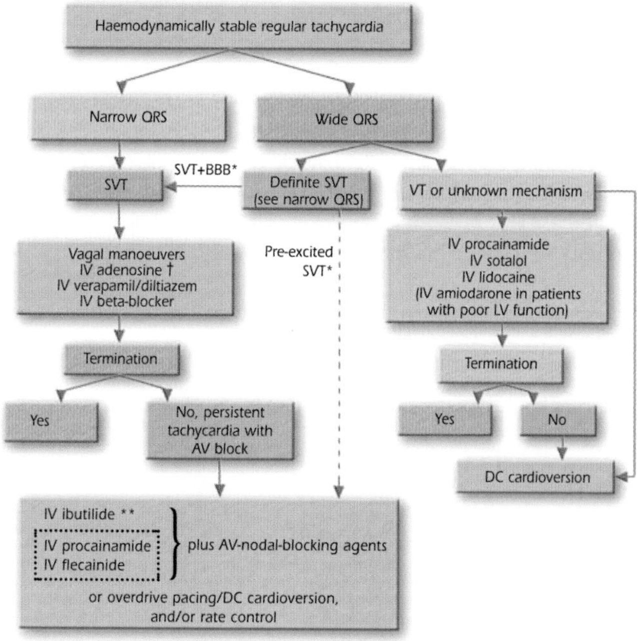

*A 12-lead ECG during sinus rhythm must be available for diagnosis. † Adenosine should be used with caution in patients with severe coronary artery disease and may produce AF, which may result in rapid ventricular rates for patients with pre-excitation. **Ibutilide is especially effective for patients with atrial flutter but should not be used in patients with EF less than 30% due to increased risk of polymorphic VT. AF = atrial fibrillation; AV = atrioventricular; BBB = bundle-branch block; DC = direct current; ECG = electrocardiogram; IV = intravenous; LV = left ventricle; QRS = ventricular activation on ECG; SVT = supraventricular tachycardia; VT = ventricular tachycardia.

Figure 7. Management of atrial flutter depending on haemodynamic stability

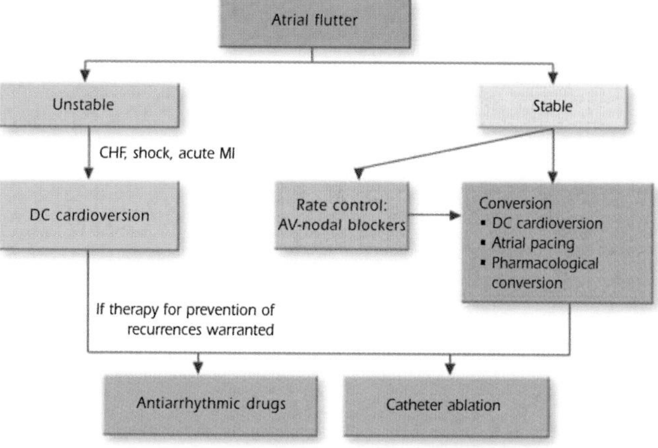

Attempts to electively revert atrial flutter to sinus rhythm should be preceded and followed by anticoagulant precautions, as per AF. AF = atrial fibrillation; AV = atrioventricular; CHF = congestive heart failure; DC = direct current; MI = myocardial infarction.

IV. References

(1) Adapted from the ACC/AHA/ESC Guidelines for the Management of Patients with Supraventricular Arrhythmias : Executive Summary
C. Blomström-Lundqvist and M. M. Scheinman (Chairpersons), E. M. Aliot, J. S. Alpert, H. Calkins, A. J. Camm, W. B. Campbell, D. E. Haines, K. H. Kuck, B. B. Lerman, D. D. Miller, C. W. Shaeffer Jr., W. G. Stevenson, G. F. Tomaselli
European Heart Journal 2003; 24 (20): 1857-1897.

(2) ACC/AHA/ESC Guidelines for the Management of Patients with Atrial Fibrillation Report from the Joint Task Force of the ESC, ACC and AHA
V. Fuster (Chairperson), L.E. Rydén (Co-Chair), R.W. Asinger, D.S. Cannom, H.J. Crijns, R.L. Frye, J.L. Halperin, G.N. Kay, W.W. Klein, S. Lévy, R.L. McNamara, E.N. Prystowsky, L.S. Wann, D.G. Wyse
European Heart Journal 2001; 22 (20): 1852-1923.

Chapter 2

Atrial Fibrillaton (AF)*
2006

Co-chairperson:
Prof. Lars Rydén
Representing: ESC
Dept. of Cardiology
Karolinska Hospital
SE-171 76 Stockholm
Sweden

Phone: +46(8) 5177 2171
Fax: +46(8) 31 10 40
E-mail: lars.ryden@medks.ki.se

Co-chairperson:
Prof. Valentin Fuster
Representing: ACC/AHA
Cardiovascular Institute
Mount Sinai Medical Center
One Gustave Levy Place
Box 1030
New York, NY 10029-6500, USA
Phone: +1(212) 241 7911
Fax: +1(212) 423 9488
E-mail: valentin.fuster@mssm.edu

Task Force Members:
1. David S. Cannom, MD, FACC
2. Harry J. Crijns, MD, FACC, FESC
3. Anne B. Curtis, MD, FACC, FAHA
4. Kenneth A. Ellenbogen, MD, FACC
5. Jonathan L. Halperin, MD, FACC, FAHA
6. Jean-Yves Le Heuzey, MD, FESC
7. G. Neal Kay, MD, FACC
8. James E. Lowe, MD, FACC
9. S. Bertil Olsson, MD, PhD, FESC
10. Eric N. Prystowsky, MD, FACC
11. Juan Luis Tamargo, MD, FESC
12. Samuel Wann, MD, FACC, FESC

ESC Staff:
1. Keith McGregor, Sophia Antipolis, France
2. Veronica Dean, Sophia Antipolis, France
3. Catherine Després, Sophia Antipolis, France
4. Karine Piellard, Sophia Antipolis, France

1. Introduction

Atrial fibrillation is a supraventricular tachyarrhythmia characterized by uncoordinated atrial activation with consequent deterioration of mechanical function. Atrial fibrillation (AF) is the most common sustained cardiac rhythm disturbance, increasing in prevalence with age. AF is often associated with structural heart disease although a substantial proportion of patients with AF have no detectable heart disease, haemodynamic impairment and thromboembolic events related to AF result in significant morbidity, mortality, and cost.

Accordingly, the American College of Cardiology (ACC), the American Heart Association (AHA), and the European Society of Cardiology (ESC) created a committee to establish Guidelines for optimum management of this frequent and complex arrhythmia.

The Pocket Guidelines are derived from the full text of the ACC/ AHA/ESC Guidelines for the Management of Patients With Atrial Fibrillation. These Guidelines were first published in 2001 and then revised in 2006. This text provides a more detailed explanation of the management of atrial fibrillation, along with appropriate caveats and levels of evidence. Both the full-text Guidelines and the executive summary are available online, at http://www.acc.org, http://www.americanheart.org or http://www.escardio.org. Users of these Pocket Guidelines should consult those documents for additional information.

*Adapted from the ACC/AHA/ESC Guidelines for the Management of Patients with Atrial Fibrillation, Executive Summary (European Heart Journal, 2006; 27: 1979-2030) and Full Text (Europace 2006 doi:10.1093/europace/eul097)

1.1 Scope of the Pocket Guidelines

The 2006 Guidelines for the Management of Patients With Atrial Fibrillation cannot be reproduced in their entirety in a pocket Guidelines format. For this reason, these Pocket Guidelines focus on issues most frequently encountered in clinical practice:

- Newly Discovered AF
- Recurrent Paroxysmal AF
- Recurrent Persistent AF
- Permanent AF
- Maintenance of Sinus Rhythm

1.2 Classification of recommendations

A classification of recommendation and a level of evidence have been assigned to each recommendation. Classifications of recommendations and levels of evidence are expressed in the ACC/AHA format as described in more detail in Figure 1.

2. Classification of AF

Various classification systems have been proposed for AF based on the ECG pattern, epicardial or endocavitary recordings, mapping of atrial electrical activity or clinical features. Although the pattern of AF can change over time, it may be helpful to characterize the arrhythmia at a given moment. The classifications scheme recommended here represents a consensus driven by a desire for simplicity and clinical relevance.

- **First detected AF**
  The clinician should distinguish a first-detected episode of AF, whether or not symptomatic or self-limited, recognizing the uncertainty about the actual duration of the episode and about previous undetected episodes (Figure 2).
- **Recurrent AF**
  After two or more episodes, AF is considered recurrent.
  - Paroxysmal
    If the arrhythmia terminates spontaneously, recurrent AF is designated paroxysmal; when sustained beyond 7 days, it is termed persistent.

Figure 1. Applying Classification of Recommendations and Level of Evidence

Size of Treatment Effect →

Estimate of Certainty (Precision) of Treatment Effect ↓

	CLASS I Benefit >>> Risk Procedure/Treatment SHOULD be performed/ administered	CLASS IIA Benefit >> Risk Additional studies with focused objectives needed IT IS REASONABLE to perform procedure/administer treatment	CLASS IIB Benefit ≥ Risk Additional studies with broad objectives needed; additional registry data would be helpful Procedure/Treatment MAY BE CONSIDERED	CLASS III Risk ≥ Benefit No additional studies needed Procedure/ Treatment should NOT be performed/administered SINCE IT IS NOT HELPFUL AND MAY BE HARMFUL
LEVEL A Multiple (3-5) population risk strata evaluated* General consistency of direction and magnitude of effect	- Recommendation that procedure or treatment is useful/effective - Sufficient evidence from multiple randomized trials or meta-analyses	- Recommendation in favour of treatment or procedure being useful/effective - Some conflicting evidence from multiple randomized trials or meta-analyses	- Recommendation's usefulness/efficacy less well established - Greater conflicting evidence from multiple randomized trials or meta-analyses	- Recommendation that procedure or treatment is not useful/effective and may be harmful - Sufficient evidence from multiple randomized trials or meta-analyses
LEVEL B Limited (2-3) population risk strata evaluated*	- Recommendation that procedure or treatment is useful/effective - Limited evidence from single randomized trial or non-randomized studies	- Recommendation in favour of treatment or procedure being useful/effective - Some conflicting evidence from single randomized trial or non-randomized studies	- Recommendation's usefulness/efficacy less well established - Greater conflicting evidence from single randomized trial or non-randomized studies	- Recommendation that procedure or treatment is not useful/effective and may be harmful - Limited evidence from single randomized trial or non-randomized studies
LEVEL C Very limited (1-2) population risk strata evaluated*	- Recommendation that procedure or treatment is useful/effective - Only expert opinion, case studies, or standard-of-care	- Recommendation in favour of treatment or procedure being useful/effective - Only diverging expert opinion, case studies, or standard-of-care	- Recommendation's usefulness/efficacy less well established - Only diverging expert opinion, case studies, or standard-of-care	- Recommendation that procedure or treatment is not useful/effective and may be harmful - Only expert opinion, case studies, or standard-of-care

* Data available from clinical trials or registries about the usefulness/efficacy in different subpopulations, such as gender, age, history of diabetes, history of prior myocardial infarction, history of heart failure, and prior aspirin use. A recommendation with Level of Evidence B or C does not imply that the recommendation is weak. Many important clinical questions addressed in the guidelines do not lend themselves to clinical trials. Even though randomized trials are not available, there may be a very clear clinical consensus that a particular test or therapy is useful or effective.

Figure 2. Patterns of Atrial Fibrillation

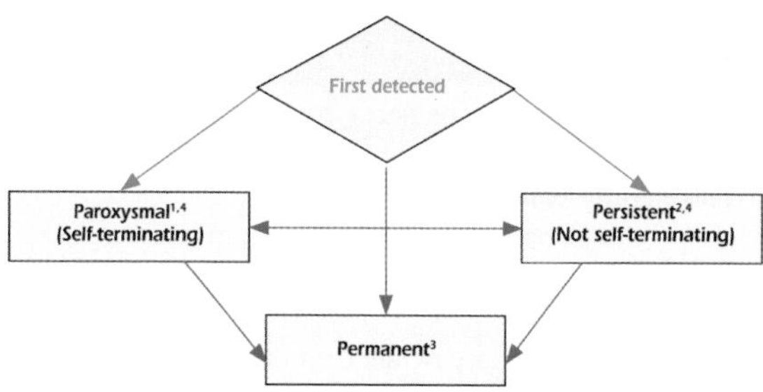

[1]Episodes that generally last less than or equal to 7 days (most less than 24 h); [2]usually more than 7 days; [3]cardioversion failed or not attempted; and [4]both paroxysmal and persistent AF may be recurrent.

- Persistent
  Termination with pharmacological therapy or direct current cardioversion does not alter the designation. First detected AF may be either paroxysmal or persistent.

- **Permanent AF**
  The category of persistent AF also includes cases of long-standing AF (e.g. greater than one year), usually leading to permanent AF, in which cardioversion has failed or has been foregone.

These categories are not mutually exclusive. One patient may have several episodes of paroxysmal AF and occasional persistent AF, or the reverse. It is practical to categorize a given patient by their most frequent presentation. The definition of permanent AF is often arbitrary, and the duration refers both to individual episodes and to how long the diagnosis has been present in a given patient. Thus, in a patient with paroxysmal AF, episodes lasting seconds to hours may occur repeatedly for years.This terminology applies to episodes lasting more than 30 seconds without a reversible cause.

Secondary AF in the setting of acute myocardial infarction (MI), cardiac surgery, pericarditis, myocarditis, hyperthyroidism, or acute pulmonary disease is considered separately. In these settings AF is not the primary problem, and treatment of the underlying disorder usually terminates the arrhythmia without recurrence. Conversely, when AF occurs in the course of a concurrent disorder like well-controlled hypothyroidism, the general principles for management of the arrhythmia apply.

The term lone AF applies to individuals under 60 years old without clinical or echocardiographic evidence of cardiopulmonary disease, including hypertension. These patients have a favourable prognosis with respect to thromboembolism and mortality. Over time, patients move out of the lone AF category due to aging or development of cardiac abnormalities such as enlargement of the left atrium, and the risks of thromboembolism and mortality rise. The term nonvalvular AF refers to cases without rheumatic mitral valve disease, prosthetic heart valve or valve repair.

3. Epidemiology and prognosis

AF is the most common arrhythmia in clinical practice, accounting for approximately one-third of hospitalizations for cardiac rhythm disturbances. An estimated 2.3 million people in North America and 4.5 million in the European Union have paroxysmal or persistent AF. During the last 20 years, hospital admissions for AF have increased by 66% due to the aging of the population, a rising prevalence of chronic heart disease, more frequent diagnosis through use of ambulatory monitoring devices and other factors.

4. Clinical evaluation

4.1 Clinical history and physical examination

The diagnosis of AF requires confirmation by ECG, sometimes in the form of bedside telemetry or ambulatory Holter recordings. The initial evaluation involves characterizing the pattern of the arrhythmia as paroxysmal or persistent, determining its cause, and defining associated cardiac and extracardiac factors pertinent to the etiology, tolerability and management. The workup and therapy can usually be accomplished in a single outpatient encounter (Table 1), unless the rhythm has not been specifically documented and additional monitoring is necessary.

5. Proposed management strategies

5.1 Strategic objectives

Management of patients with AF involves three, not mutually exclusive, objectives:

- Rate control;
- Prevention of thromboembolism;
- Correction of the rhythm disturbance.

The initial management involves primarily a rate or rhythm control strategy. Under the rate control strategy, the ventricular rate is controlled with no commitment to restore or maintain sinus rhythm while the rhythm control strategy attempts restoration and/or maintenance of sinus rhythm. The latter strategy also requires attention to rate control. Depending on the patient's course, the strategy initially chosen may prove unsuccessful and the alternate strategy is then adopted. Regardless of whether the rate control or rhythm control strategy is pursued, attention must also be directed to antithrombotic therapy for prevention of thromboembolism.

Table 1. Clinical Evaluation in Patients with AF

Minimum evaluation	Additional testing
1. History and physical examination, to define - Presence and nature of symptoms associated with AF - Clinical type of AF (first episode, paroxysmal, persistent, or permanent) - Onset of the first symptomatic attack or date of discovery of AF -Frequency, duration, precipitating factors, and modes of termination of AF - Response to any pharmacological agents that have been administered - Presence of any underlying heart disease or other reversible conditions (e.g. hyperthyroidism or alcohol consumption) **2. Electrocardiogram, to identify** - Rhythm (verify AF) - LV hypertrophy - P-wave duration and morphology or fibrillatory waves - Pre-excitation - Bundle-branch block - Prior MI - Other atrial arrhythmias - To measure and follow the R-R, QRS, and QT intervals in conjunction with antiarrhythmic drug therapy **3. Transthoracic echocardiogram, to identify** - Valvular heart disease - LA and RA atrial size - LV size and function - Peak RV pressure (pulmonary hypertension) - LV hypertrophy - LA thrombus (low sensitivity) - Pericardial disease **4. Blood tests of thyroid, renal, and hepatic function** - For a first episode of AF, when the ventricular rate is difficult to control	One or several tests may be necessary. **1. Six-minute walk test** - If the adequacy of rate control is in question **2. Exercise testing** - If the adequacy of rate control is in question (permanent AF) - To reproduce exercise-induced AF - To exclude ischaemia before treatment of selected patients with a type IC antiarrhythmic drug **3. Holter monitoring or event recording** - If diagnosis of the type of arrhythmia is in question - As a means of evaluating rate control **4. Transesophageal echocardiography** - To identify LA thrombus (in the LA appendage) - To guide cardioversion **5. Electrophysiological study** - To clarify the mechanism of wide-QRScomplex tachycardia - To identify a predisposing arrhythmia such as atrial flutter or paroxysmal supraventricular tachycardia - To seek sites for curative ablation or AV conduction block/modification **6. Chest radiograph, to evaluate** - Lung parenchyma, when clinical findings suggest an abnormality - Pulmonary vasculature, when clinical findings suggest an abnormality

Type IC refers to the Vaughan Williams classification of antiarrhythmic drugs (see Table 13 in the executive summary). AF = atrial fibrillation; AV = atrioventricular; LA = left atrial; LV = left ventricular; MI = myocardial infarction; RA = right atrial; and RV = right ventricular.

5.2 Overview of algorithms for management of patients with AF

Management of patients with AF requires knowledge of its pattern of presentation (paroxysmal, persistent, or permanent) underlying conditions and decisions about restoration and maintenance of sinus rhythm, control of the ventricular rate, and antithrombotic therapy. These issues are addressed in the various management algorithms for each presentation of AF (see Figures 3, 4, 5, and 6).

Due to scarcity of data from randomized trials of antiarrhythmic medications for treatment of patients with AF, the drug-selection algorithms were developed by consensus and are subject to revision as additional evidence emerges.

Figure 3. Pharmacological Management of Patients with Newly Discovered Atrial Fibrillation

Figure 4. Pharmacological Management of Patients with Recurrent Paroxysmal Atrial Fibrillation

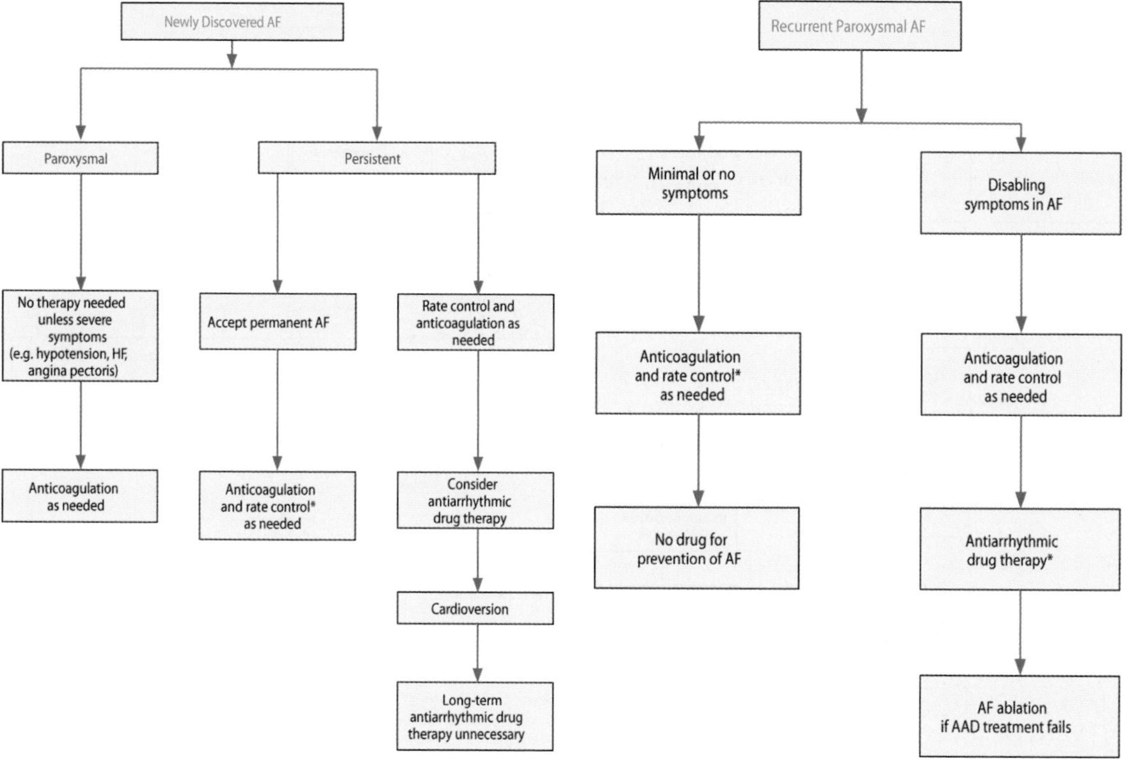

AF = atrial fibrillation; HF= heart failure.

*See Figure 6

AAD = antiarrhythmic drugs; AF = atrial fibrillation.

*See Figure 6

Figure 5. Pharmacological Management of Patients with Recurrent Persistent or Permanent Atrial Fibrillation

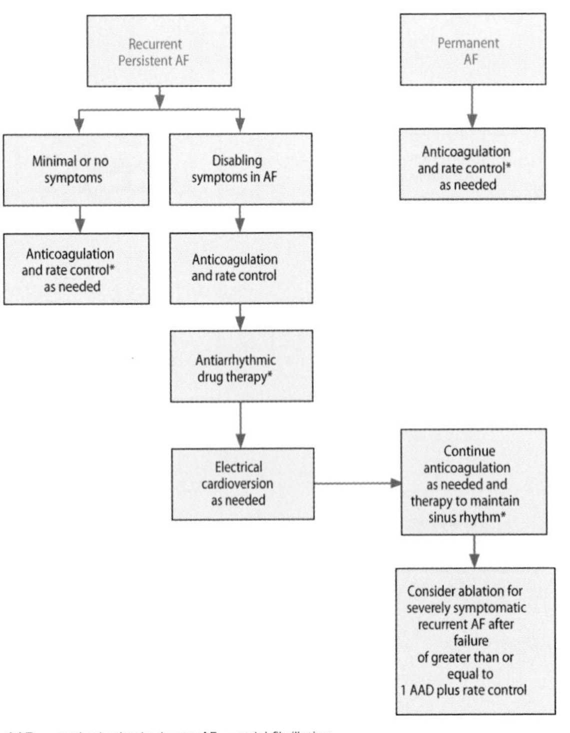

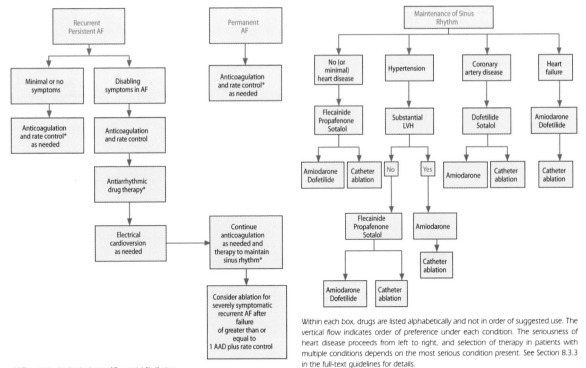

AAD = antiarrhythmic drugs; AF = atrial fibrillation.

*See Figure 6. Initiate drug therapy before cardioversion to reduce the likelihood of early recurrence of AF.

Figure 6. Antiarrhythmic Drug Therapy to Maintain Sinus Rhythm in Patients with Recurrent Paroxysmal or Persistent Atrial Fibrillation

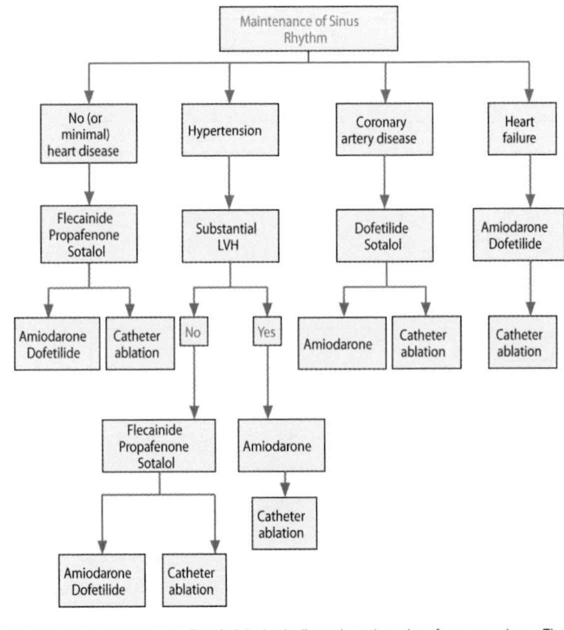

Within each box, drugs are listed alphabetically and not in order of suggested use. The vertical flow indicates order of preference under each condition. The seriousness of heart disease proceeds from left to right, and selection of therapy in patients with multiple conditions depends on the most serious condition present. See Section 8.3.3 in the full-text guidelines for details.

LVH = left ventricular hypertrophy.

5.3 Pharmacological cardioversion

A summary of recommendations concerning the use of pharmacological agents for cardioversion of AF is presented in Tables 2, 3, 4, and 5. Table 6 lists dosages and adverse effects. Algorithms for pharmacological management of AF are given in Figures 3, 4, 5 and 6. Throughout this document, reference is made to the Vaughan Williams classification of antiarrhythmic drugs, modified to include drugs that became available after the original classification was developed (Table 19 in the full text and 14 in the executive summary.) The recommendations given in this document are based on published data and do not necessarily adhere to the regulations and labeling requirements of governmental agencies.

Table 2. Recommendations for Pharmacological Cardioversion of Atrial Fibrillation of up to 7 Days Duration

Drug*	Route of Administration	Class of Recommendation	Level of Evidence
Agents with Proven Efficacy			
Dofetilide	Oral	I	A
Flecainide	Oral or intravenous	I	A
Ibutilide	Intravenous	I	A
Propafenone	Oral or intravenous	I	A
Amiodarone	Oral or intravenous	IIa	A
Less effective or incompletely studied agents			
Disopyramide	Intravenous	IIb	B
Procainamide	Intravenous	IIb	B
Quinidine	Oral	IIb	B
Should not be administered			
Digoxin	Oral or intravenous	III	A
Sotalol	Oral or intravenous	III	A

* The doses of medications used in these studies may not be the same as those recommended by the manufacturers. Drugs are listed alphabetically within each category of recommendation and level of evidence.

Table 3. Recommendations for Pharmacological Cardioversion of Atrial Fibrillation Present for more than 7 Days Duration

Drug*	Route of Administration	Class of Recommendation	Level of Evidence
Agents with Proven Efficacy			
Dofetilide	Oral	I	A
Amiodarone	Oral or intravenous	IIa	A
Ibutilide	Intravenous	IIa	A
Less effective or incompletely studied agents			
Disopyramide	Intravenous	IIb	B
Flecainide	Oral	IIb	B
Procainamide	Intravenous	IIb	C
Propafenone	Oral or intravenous	IIb	B
Quinidine	Oral	IIb	B
Should not be administered			
Digoxin	Oral or intravenous	III	B
Sotalol	Oral or intravenous	III	B

* The doses of medications used in these studies may not be the same as those recommended by the manufacturers. Drugs are listed alphabetically within each category of recommendation and level of evidence.

Table 4. Recommended Doses of Drugs Proven Effective for Pharmacological Cardioversion of Atrial Fibrillation

Drug*	Route of Administration	Dosage**	Potential Adverse Effects
Amiodarone	Oral	Inpatient: 1.2 to 1.8 g per day in divided dose until 10 g total, then 200 to 400 mg per day maintenance or 30 mg/kg as single dose Outpatient: 600 to 800 mg per day divided dose until 10 g total, then 200 to 400 mg per day maintenance	Hypotension, bradycardia, QT prolongation, torsades de pointes (rare), GI upset, constipation, phlebitis (IV)
	Intravenous/oral	5 to 7 mg/kg over 30 to 60 min, then 1.2 to 1.8 g per day continuous IV or in divided oral doses until 10 g total, then 200 to 400 mg per day maintenance	
Dofetilide	Oral	Creatinine clearance (mL/min) — Dose (mcg BID) >60 — 500 40 to 60 — 250 20 to 40 — 125 <20 — Contraindicated	QT prolongation, torsades de pointes; adjust dose for renal function, body size and age
Flecainide	Oral	200 to 300 mg†	Hypotension, atrial flutter with high ventricular rate
	Intravenous	1.5 to 3.0 mg/kg over 10 to 20 min†	
Ibutilide	Intravenous	1 mg over 10 min; repeat 1 mg when necessary	QT prolongation, torsades de pointes
Propafenone	Oral	600 mg	Hypotension, atrial flutter with high ventricular rate
	Intravenous	1.5 to 2.0 mg/kg over 10 to 20 min†	
Quinidine‡	Oral	0.75 to 1.5 g in divided doses over 6 to 12 h, usually with a rate-slowing drug	QT prolongation, torsades de pointes, GI upset, hypotension

GI = gastrointestinal; IV = intravenous; BID = twice a day.

* Drugs are listed alphabetically

** Dosages given in the table may differ from those recommended by the manufacturers.

† Insufficient data are available on which to base specific recommendations for the use of one loading regimen over another for patients with ischaemic heart disease or impaired left ventricular function, and these drugs should be used cautiously or not at all in such patients.

‡ The use of quinidine loading to achieve pharmacological conversion of atrial fibrillation is controversial and safer methods are available with the alternative agents listed in the table. Quinidine should be used with caution.

Table 5. Pharmacological Treatment Before Cardioversion in Patients with Persistent AF: Effects of Various Antiarrhythmic Drugs on Immediate Recurrence, Outcome of Transthoracic Direct-Current Shock, or Both

	Enhance Conversion by DC Shock and Prevent IRAF*	Class of Recommendation	Level of Evidence	Suppress SRAF and Maintenance Therapy Class
Effective	Amiodarone Flecainide Ibutilide Propafenone Sotalol	IIa	B	All drugs in recommendation Class I (except ibutilide) plus beta-blockers
Uncertain/unknown	Beta-blockers Diltiazem Disopyramide Dofetilide Procainamide Verapamil	IIb	C	Diltiazem Dofetilide Verapamil

All drugs (except beta-blockers and amiodarone) should be initiated in the hospital.

IRAF = immediate recurrence of atrial fibrillation; SRAF = subacute recurrence of atrial fibrillation; and DC = direct current.

*Drugs are listed alphabetically within each class of recommendation.

Table 6. Typical Doses of Drugs Used to Maintain Sinus Rhythm in Patients with Atrial Fibrillation*

Drug**	Daily Dosage	Potential Adverse Effects
Amiodarone†	100-400 mg	Photosensitivity, pulmonary toxicity, polyneuropathy, GI upset, bradycardia, torsades de pointes (rare), hepatic toxicity, thyroid dysfunction, eye complications
Disopyramide	400-750 mg	Torsades de pointes, HF, glaucoma, urinary retention, dry mouth
Dofetilide‡	500-1000 mcg	Torsades de pointes
Flecainide	200-300 mg	Ventricular tachycardia, HF, conversion to atrial flutter with rapid conduction through the AV node
Propafenone	450-900 mg	Ventricular tachycardia, HF, conversion to atrial flutter with rapid conduction through the AV node
Sotalol‡	160-320 mg	Torsades de pointes, HF, bradycardia, exacerbation of chronic obstructive or bronchospastic lung disease

GI = gastrointestinal; AV = atrioventricular; HF = heart failure.

*The drugs and doses given here have been determined by consensus based on published studies.

**Drugs are listed alphabetically.

† A loading dose of 600 mg per day is usually given for one month or 1000 mg per day for 1 week. ‡ Dose should be adjusted for renal function and QT-interval response during in-hospital initiation phase.

When rapid control of the ventricular response of AF is required or oral administration is not feasible, medication may be administered intravenously. In haemodynamically stable patients negative chronotropic medication may be administered orally (See Table 7).

Table 7. Intravenous and Orally Administered Pharmacological Agents for Heart Rate Control in Patients with Atrial Fibrillation

Drug	Class/LOE Recommendation	Loading Dose	Onset
Acute Setting			
Heart Rate Control in patients without accessory pathway			
Esmolol†	Class I, LOE C	500 mcg/kg IV over 1 min	5 min
Metoprolol†	Class I, LOE C	2.5 to 5 mg IV bolus over 2 min; up to 3 doses	5 min
Propranolol†	Class I, LOE C	0.15 mg/kg IV	5 min
Diltiazem	Class I, LOE B	0.25 mg/kg IV over 2 min	2-7 min
Verapamil	Class I, LOE B	0.075 to 0.15 mg/kg IV over 2 min	3-5 min
Heart Rate Control in patients with accessory pathway§			
Amiodarone‡||	Class IIa, LOE C	150 mg over 10 min	Days
Heart Rate Control in patients with heart failure and without accessory pathway			
Digoxin	Class I, LOE B	0.25 mg IV each 2 h, up to 1.5 mg	60 min or more§
Amiodarone‡	Class IIa, LOE C	150 mg over 10 min	Days
Non-Acute Setting and Chronic Maintenance Therapy¶			
Heart Rate Control			
Metoprolol†	Class I, LOE C	Same as maintenance dose	4-6 h
Propranolol†	Class I, LOE C	Same as maintenance dose	60-90 min
Diltiazem	Class I, LOE B	Same as maintenance dose	2-4 h
Verapamil	Class I, LOE B	Same as maintenance dose	1-2 h
Heart Rate Control in patients with heart failure and without accessory pathway			
Digoxin	Class I, LOE C	0.5 mg by mouth daily	2 days
Amiodarone‡	Class IIb, LOE C	800 mg daily for 1 wk, orally 600 mg daily for 1 wk, orally 400 mg daily for 4 to 6 wk, orally	1-3 wk

*Onset is variable and some effect occurs earlier.

†Only representative members of the type of beta-adrenergic antagonist drugs are included in the table, but other, similar agents could be used for this indication in appropriate doses. Beta-blockers are grouped in an order preceding the alphabetical listing of drugs.

‡Amiodarone can be useful to control the heart rate in patients with atrial fibrillation (AF) when other measures are unsuccessful or contraindicated.

§Conversion to sinus rhythm and catheter ablation of the accessory pathway are generally recommended; pharmacological therapy for rate control may be appropriate in certain patients.

5.4 Pharmacological enhancement of direct current cardioversion

When given in conjunction with direct-current cardioversion, the primary aims of antiarrhythmic medication therapy are to increase the likelihood of success and prevent early recurrence of AF. The risks of pharmacological treatment include the possibility of inducing ventricular arrhythmias.

5.5 Echocardiography and risk stratification

The relative risk of ischaemic stroke associated with specific clinical features, derived from a collaborative

Maintenance Dose	Major Side Effects
60 to 200 mcg/kg/min IV	↓BP, HB, ↓HR, asthma, HF
NA	↓BP, HB, ↓HR, asthma, HF
NA	↓BP, HB, ↓HR, asthma, HF
5 to 15 mg/h IV	↓BP, HB, HF
NA	↓BP, HB, HF
0.5 to 1 mg/min IV	↓BP, HB, Pulmonary toxicity, skin discolouration, hypothyroidism, hyperthyroidism, corneal deposits, optic neuropathy, warfarin interaction, sinus bradycardia
0.125 to 0.375 mg daily IV or orally	Digitalis toxicity, HB, HR
0.5 to 1 mg/min IV	↓BP, HB, Pulmonary toxicity, skin discolouration, hypothyroidism, hyperthyroidism, corneal deposits, optic neuropathy, warfarin interaction, sinus bradycardia
25 to 100 mg twice a day, orally	↓BP, HB, ↓HR, asthma, HF
80 to 240 mg daily in divided doses, orally	↓BP, HB, ↓HR, asthma, HF
120 to 360 mg daily in divided doses; slow release available, orally	↓BP, HB, HF
120 to 360 mg daily in divided doses; slow release available, orally	↓BP, HB, HF, digoxin interaction
0.125 to 0.375 mg daily, orally	Digitalis toxicity, HB, ↓HR
200 mg daily, orally	↓BP, HB, Pulmonary toxicity, skin discolouration, hypothyroidism, hyperthyroidism, corneal deposits, optic neuropathy, warfarin interaction, sinus bradycardia

||If rhythm cannot be converted or ablated and rate control is needed, intravenous (IV) amiodarone is recommended.

¶Adequacy of heart rate control should be assessed during physical activity as well as at rest.

BP = hypotension; HR = bradycardia; HB = heart block; HF = heart failure; LOE = level of evidence; and NA = not applicable.

analysis of participants given no antithrombotic therapy in the control groups of five randomized trials is displayed in Table 8 of the executive summary.

The $CHADS_2$ (Cardiac Failure, Hypertension, Age, Diabetes, Stroke [Doubled]) stroke risk index integrates elements from several of these schemes. It is based on a point system in which two points are assigned for a history of stroke or transient ischaemic attack (TIA), and one point each for age over 75 years, a history of hypertension, diabetes, or recent heart failure (HF) (Table 8).

In patients with nonvalvular AF, prior stroke or TIA is the strongest independent predictor of stroke, significantly

Table 8. Stroke Risk in Patients with Nonvalvular AF Not Treated with Anticoagulation According to the $CHADS_2$ Index

$CHADS_2$ Risk Criteria and Scoring		
Prior stroke or TIA .... 2 points Age >75 years .... 1 point Hypertension .... 1 point Diabetes mellitus .... 1 point Heart Failure .... 1 point		
Patients (N=1733)	**Adjusted Stroke Rate (%/year)* (95% CI)**	**$CHADS_2$ Score**
120	1.9 (1.2-3.0)	0
463	2.8 (2.0-3.8)	1
523	4.0 (3.1-5.1)	2
337	5.9 (4.6-7.3)	3
220	8.5 (6.3-11.1)	4
65	12.5 (8.2-17.5)	5
5	18.2 (10.5-27.4)	6

*The adjusted stroke rate was derived from multivariate analysis assuming no aspirin usage. Data from van Walraven C, Hart RG, Wells GA, et al. A clinical prediction rule to identify patients with atrial fibrillation and a low risk for stroke while taking aspirin. Arch Intern Med 2003; 163:936-43, et al. and Gage BF, Waterman AD, Shannon W, Boechler M, Rich MW, Radford MJ. Validation of clinical classification schemes for predicting stroke: results from the National Registry of Atrial Fibrillation. JAMA 2001; 285:2864-70.

TIA = transient ischaemic attack.

Table 9. Antithrombotic Therapy for Patients with Atrial Fibrillation

Risk Category	Recommended Therapy
No risk factors	Aspirin, 81-325 mg daily
One moderate risk factor	Aspirin, 81-325 mg daily or Warfarin (INR 2.0-3.0, target 2.5)
Any high risk factor or more than 1 moderate risk factor	Warfarin (INR 2.0-3.0, target 2.5)*

Less validated or weaker risk factors	Moderate risk factors	High risk factors
• Female gender	• Age ≥75 years	• Previous stroke, TIA or embolism
• Age 65-74 years	• Hypertension	• Mitral stenosis
• Coronary artery disease	• Heart failure	• Prosthetic heart valve*
• Thyrotoxicosis	• LV ejection fraction ≤35% • Diabetes mellitus	

* indicates if mechanical valve, target INR greater than 2.5. INR = international normalized ratio; LV = left ventricular; TIA = transient ischaemic attack.

associated with stroke in all six studies in which it was evaluated, with incremental relative risk between 1.9 and 3.7 (averaging approximately 3.0). All patients with prior stroke or TIA require anticoagulation unless contra-indications exist in a given patient. Patient age is a consistent independent predictor of stroke, but older people are also at increased risk for anticoagulant-related bleeding. Special consideration of these older patients is therefore a critical aspect of effective stroke prophylaxis.

5.6 Risk stratification

Although these schemes for stratification of stroke risk identify patients who benefit most and least from anticoagulation, the threshold for use of anticoagulation is still controversial. Our recommendations for anti-thrombotic therapy are summarized in Table 9.

Anticoagulation is recommended for 3 weeks prior to and 4 weeks after cardioversion for patients with AF of unknown duration or with AF for longer than 48 h. Although left atrial thrombus and systemic embolism have been documented in patients with AF of shorter duration, the need for anticoagulation is less clear. When acute AF produces haemodynamic instability in the form of angina pectoris, MI, shock, or pulmonary oedema, immediate cardioversion should not be delayed to deliver therapeutic anticoagulation, but intravenous unfractionated heparin or subcutaneous injection of a low molecular weight heparin should be initiated before cardioversion by direct-current countershock or intravenous antiarrhythmic medication.

5.7. Catheter ablation

Catheter-directed ablation of AF represents a substantial achievement that promises better therapy for a large number of patients presently resistant to pharmacological or electrical conversion to sinus rhythm. The limited available studies suggest that catheter-based ablation offers benefit to selected patients with AF, but these studies do not provide convincing evidence of optimum catheter positioning or absolute rates of treatment success. Identification of patients who might benefit from ablation must take into account both potential benefits and short- and long-term risks. Rates of success and complications vary, sometimes considerably, from one study to another because of patient factors, patterns of AF, criteria for definition of success, duration of follow-up, and technical aspects.

6. Recommendations

6.1 Pharmacological rate control during atrial fibrillation

Class I

1. Measurement of the heart rate at rest and control of the rate using pharmacological agents are recommended for patients with persistent or permanent AF. (Level of Evidence: B)

2. In the absence of pre-excitation, intravenous administration of a beta-blockers (esmolol, metropolol, or propanolol) or diltiazem or verapamil is recommended to slow the ventricular response to AF in the acute setting, exercising caution in patients with hypotension or HF. (Level of Evidence: B)

3. Intravenous administration of digoxin or amiodarone is recommended to control the heart rate in patients with AF and HF who do not have an accessory pathway. (Level of Evidence: B)

4. In patients who experience symptoms related to AF during activity, the adequacy of heart rate control should be assessed during exercise, adjusting pharmacological treatment as necessary to keep the rate in the physiological range. (Level of Evidence: C)

5. Digoxin is effective following oral administration to control the heart rate at rest in patients with AF and is indicated for patients with HF or LV dysfunction or for sedentary individuals. (Level of Evidence: C)

Class IIa

1. A combination of digoxin and either a beta-blocker or diltiazem or verapamil is reasonable to control the heart rate both at rest and during exercise in patients with AF. (Level of Evidence: B)

2. It is reasonable to use ablation of the arterioventricular (AV) node or accessory pathway to control heart rate when pharmacological therapy is insufficient or associated with side effects. (Level of Evidence: B)

3. Intravenous amiodarone can be useful to control the heart rate in patients with AF when other measures are unsuccessful or contraindicated. (Level of Evidence: C)

4. When electrical cardioversion is not necessary in patients with AF and an accessory pathway, intravenous procainamide or ibutilide are reasonable alternatives. (Level of Evidence: C)

Class IIb

1. When the rate of ventricular response to AF cannot be adequately controlled using a beta-blocker, diltiazem, verapamil or digoxin, alone or in combination, oral amiodarone may be administered to slow the heart rate. (Level of Evidence: C)

2. Intravenous procainamide, disopyramide, ibutilide, or amiodarone may be considered for haemodynamically stable patients with AF involving conduction over an accessory pathway. (Level of Evidence: B)

3. When the rate of ventricular response to AF cannot be controlled with pharmacological agents or tachycardia-mediated cardiomyopathy is suspected, catheter-directed ablation of the AV node may be considered. (Level of Evidence: C)

Class III

1. Digitalis should not be used as the sole agent to control the rate of ventricular response in patients with paroxysmal AF. (Level of Evidence: B)

2. Catheter ablation of the AV node should not be attempted without a prior trial of medication to control the ventricular rate in patients with AF. (Level of Evidence: C)

3. In patients with decompensated HF and AF, intravenous administration of a nondihydropyridine calcium channel antagonist may exacerbate haemodynamic compromise and is not recommended. (Level of Evidence: C)

4. Intravenous administration of digitalis glyosides or nondihydropyridine calcium channel antagonists to patients with AF and pre-excitation may accelerate the ventricular response and is not recommended. (Level of Evidence: C)

6.2 Preventing thromboembolism

Class I

1. Antithrombotic therapy to prevent thromboembolism is recommended for all patients with AF, except those with lone AF or contraindications. (Level of Evidence: A)

2. The antithrombotic agent should be chosen based upon the absolute risks of stroke and bleeding and the relative risk and benefit for a given patient. (Level of Evidence: A)

3. For patients at high risk of stroke, chronic oral anticoagulant therapy with a vitamin K antagonist (INR 2.0 to 3.0) is recommended, unless contra-indicated. Factors associated with highest risk for stroke in patients with AF are prior stroke, TIA, or systemic embolism, rheumatic mitral stenosis and a mechanical prosthetic heart valve. (Level of Evidence: A)

4. Anticoagulation with a vitamin K antagonist is recommended for patients with more than 1 moderate risk factor (age greater than 75 years, hypertension, diabetes mellitus, HF, or impaired LV systolic function [ejection fraction less than or equal to 35% or less or fractional shortening less than 25%]). (Level of Evidence: A)

5. INR should be determined at least weekly during initiation of therapy and monthly when stable (Level of Evidence: A)

6. Aspirin, 81-325 mg daily, is recommended in low-risk patients or in those with contraindications to oral anticoagulation. (Level of Evidence: A)

7. For patients with AF who have mechanical heart valves, the target intensity of anticoagulation should be based on the type of prosthesis, maintaining an INR of at least 2.5. (Level of Evidence: B)

8. Antithrombotic therapy is recommended for patients with atrial flutter as for AF. (Level of Evidence: C)

Class IIa

1. For primary prevention of thromboembolism in patients with nonvalvular AF who have just one of the validated risk factors (age greater than 75 years (especially in female), hypertension, diabetes mellitus, HF, or impaired LV function), antithrombotic therapy with either aspirin or a vitamin K antagonist is reasonable, based upon an assessment of the risk of bleeding complications, ability to safely sustain anticoagulation, and patient preferences. (Level of Evidence: A)

2. For patients with nonvalvular AF who have one or more of the less well-validated risk factors (age 65-74 years, female gender, or CAD), treatment with either aspirin or a vitamin K antagonist is reasonable. (Level of Evidence: B)

3. It is reasonable to select antithrombotic therapy using the same criteria irrespective of the pattern (paroxysmal, persistent, or permanent) of AF. (Level of Evidence: B)

4. In patients with AF without a mechanical prosthetic heart valve, it is reasonable to interrupt anticoagulation for up to one week for procedures that carry a risk of bleeding. (Level of Evidence: C)

5. It is reasonable to re-evaluate the need for anti-coagulation at regular intervals. (Level of Evidence: C)

Class IIb

1. In patients 75 years of age and older at risk of bleeding but without contraindications to anticoagulant therapy, and in patients who unable to safely tolerate standard anticoagulation (INR 2.0 to 3.0), a lower INR target (2.0; range 1.6 to 2.5) may be considered for primary prevention of stroke and systemic embolism. (Level of Evidence: C)

2. When interruption of oral anticoagulant therapy for longer than 1 week is necessary in high-risk patients, unfractionated or low molecular weight heparin may be given by injection, although efficacy is uncertain. (Level of Evidence: C)

3. Following coronary revascularization in patients with AF, low-dose aspirin (less than 100 mg daily) and/or clopidogrel (75mg daily) may be given concurrently with anticoagulation, but these strategies are associated with an increased risk of bleeding. (Level of Evidence: C)

4. In patients undergoing coronary revascularization, anticoagulation may be interrupted to prevent bleeding, but should be resumed as soon as possible after the procedure and the dose adjusted to achieve a therapeutic INR. Aspirin may be given during the hiatus. For patients undergoing percutaneous intervention, the maintenance regimen should consist of clopidogrel, 75 mg daily, plus warfarin (INR 2.0 to 3.0). Clopidogrel should be given for a minimum of one month after a bare metal stent, at least three months for a sirolimus-eluting stent, at least six months for a paclitaxel-eluting stent, and twelve months or longer in selected patients, followed by warfarin alone. (Level of Evidence: C)

5. In patients with AF who sustain ischaemic stroke or systemic embolism during treatment with anticoagulation (INR 2.0 to 3.0), it may be reasonable to raise the intensity of anticoagulation up to a target INR of 3.0 to 3.5. (Level of Evidence: C)

Class III

1. Long-term anticoagulation is not recommended for primary stroke prevention in patients below age 60 years without heart disease (lone AF). (Level of Evidence: C)

6.3 Cardioversion of atrial fibrillation

Pharmacological cardioversion

Class I

1. Administration of flecainide, dofetilide, propafenone, or ibutilide is recommended for pharmacological cardioversion of AF. (Level of Evidence: A)

Class IIa

1. Administration of amiodarone is reasonable for pharmacological cardioversion of AF. (Level of Evidence: A)

2. A single oral dose of propafenone or flecainide ("pill-in-the-pocket") can be used to terminate persistent AF out of hospital for selected patients once treatment has proved safe in hospital. Before antiarrhythmic medication is initiated, a beta-blocker, diltiazem or verapamil should be given to prevent rapid AV conduction. (Level of Evidence: C)

3. Amiodarone can be beneficial on an outpatient basis in patients with paroxysmal or persistent AF when rapid restoration of sinus rhythm is unnecessary. (Level of Evidence: C)

Class IIb

1. Quinidine or procainamide might be considered for cardioversion of AF, but their usefulness is not well established. (Level of Evidence: C)

Class III

1. Digoxin and sotalol are not recommended for pharmacological cardioversion of AF. (Level of Evidence: A)

2. Quinidine, procainamide, disopyramide, and dofetilide should not be started out of hospital for conversion of AF. (Level of Evidence: B)

Direct-current cardioversion

Class I

1. When a rapid ventricular response to AF does not respond promptly to pharmacological measures, immediate direct-current cardioversion is recommended for patients with myocardial ischaemia, symptomatic hypotension, angina, or HF. (Level of Evidence: C)

2. Immediate direct-current cardioversion is recommended for patients with pre-excitation when AF occurs with extreme tachycardia or haemodynamic instability. (Level of Evidence: B)

3. Cardioversion is recommended when symptoms of AF are unacceptable to the patient. In case of relapse, direct-current cardioversion may be repeated following administration of antiarrhythmic medication. (Level of Evidence: C)

Class IIa

1. Direct-current cardioversion can be useful to restore sinus rhythm as part of a long-term management strategy for patients with AF. (Level of Evidence: B)

2. Patient preference is a reasonable consideration in the selection of infrequently repeated cardioversions for the management of symptomatic or recurrent AF. (Level of Evidence: C)

Class III

1. Frequent direct-current cardioversion is not recommended for patients with relatively short periods of sinus rhythm after multiple cardioversion procedures despite prophylactic antiarrhythmic drug therapy. (Level of Evidence: C)

2. Electrical cardioversion is contraindicated in patients with digitalis toxicity or hypokalemia. (Level of Evidence: C)

Pharmacological enhancement of direct-current cardioversion

Class IIa

1. Pretreatment with amiodarone, flecainide, ibutilide, propafenone, or sotalol can be useful to enhance direct-current cardioversion and prevent recurrent AF. (Level of Evidence: B)

2. In patients who relapse to AF after successful cardioversion, it can be useful to repeat the procedure

following administration of antiarrhythmic medication. (Level of Evidence: C)

Class IIb

1. For patients with persistent AF, administration of beta-blockers, disopyramide, diltiazem, dofetilide, procainamide, or verapamil may be considered, although the efficacy of these agents to enhance the success of direct-current cardioversion or to prevent early recurrence of AF is uncertain. (Level of Evidence: C)

2. Out-of-hospital initiation of antiarrhythmic medications may be considered in patients without heart disease to enhance the success of cardioversion of AF. (Level of Evidence: C)

3. Out-of-hospital administration of antiarrhythmic medications may be considered to enhance the success of cardioversion of AF in patients with certain forms of heart disease, once the safety of the drug has been verified for the patient. (Level of Evidence: C)

Prevention of Thromboembolism in Patients With Atrial Fibrillation Undergoing Cardioversion

Class I

1. For patients with AF of 48h duration or longer, or when the duration of AF is unknown, anticoagulation (INR 2.0 to 3.0) is recommended for at least 3 weeks prior to and 4 weeks after cardioversion, regardless of the method used to restore sinus rhythm. (Level of Evidence: B)

2. For patients with AF of more than 48h duration requiring immediate cardioversion because of haemodynamic instability, heparin should be administered concurrently by an initial intravenous injection followed by a continuous infusion (activated partial thromboplastin time [aPTT] 1.5 to 2 times control). Thereafter oral anticoagulation (INR 2.0 to 3.0) should be provided for at least 4 weeks, as for elective cardioversion. Limited data support subcutaneous low molecular weight heparin. (Level of Evidence: C)

3. For patients with AF of less than 48h duration associated with haemodynamic instability, cardioversion should be performed immediately without anticoagulation. (Level of Evidence: C)

Class IIa

1. During the 48 h after onset of AF, the need for anticoagulation before and after cardioversion may be based on the patient's risk of thromboembolism. (Level of Evidence: C)

2. As an alternative to anticoagulation prior to cardioversion of AF, it is reasonable to perform transoesophageal echocardiography in search of thrombus. (Level of Evidence: B)

2a. For patients with no identifiable thrombus, cardioversion is reasonable immediately after anticoagulation. (Level of Evidence: B) Thereafter, continuation of oral anticoagulation (INR 2.0 to 3.0) is reasonable for at least 4 weeks, as for elective cardioversion. (Level of Evidence: B) Limited data are available to support subcutaneous low molecular weight heparin in this indication. (Level of Evidence: C)

2b. For patients in whom thrombus is identified, oral anticoagulation (INR 2.0 to 3.0) is reasonable for at least 3 weeks before and 4 weeks after restoration of sinus rhythm, and longer anticoagulation may be appropriate after apparently successful cardioversion, because the risk of thromboembolism often remains elevated in such cases. (Level of Evidence: C)

3. For patients with atrial flutter undergoing cardioversion, anticoagulation can be beneficial according to the recommendations as for patients with AF. (Level of Evidence: C)

6.4 Maintenance of Sinus Rhythm

Class I

1. Before initiating antiarrhythmic drug therapy, treatment of precipitating or reversible causes of AF is recommended. (Level of Evidence: C)

Class IIa

1. Pharmacological therapy can be useful in patients with AF to maintain sinus rhythm and prevent tachycardia-induced cardiomyopathy. (Level of Evidence: C)

2. Infrequent, well-tolerated recurrence of AF is reasonable as a successful outcome of antiarrhythmic drug therapy. (Level of Evidence: C)

3. Outpatient initiation of antiarrhythmic drug therapy is reasonable in patients with AF who have no associated heart disease when the agent is well tolerated. (Level of Evidence: C)

4. In patients with lone AF without structural heart disease, propafenone or flecainide can be beneficial on an outpatient basis in patients with paroxysmal AF

who are in sinus rhythm at the time of drug initiation. (Level of Evidence: B)

5. Sotalol can be beneficial in outpatients in sinus rhythm with little or no heart disease prone to paroxysmal AF if the baseline uncorrected QT interval is less than 460 ms, electrolytes are normal, and risk factors associated with proarrhythmia are absent. (Level of Evidence: C)

6. Catheter ablation is a reasonable alternative to pharmacological therapy to prevent recurrent AF in symptomatic patients with little or no left atrial enlargement. (Level of Evidence: C)

Class III

1. Antiarrhythmic therapy with a particular drug is not recommended for maintenance of sinus rhythm in patients with AF who have risk factors for proarrhythmia with that agent. (Level of Evidence: A)

2. Pharmacological therapy is not recommended for maintenance of sinus rhythm in patients with advanced sinus node disease or AV node dysfunction unless they have a functioning pacemaker. (Level of Evidence: C)

6.5 Postoperative atrial fibrillation

Class I

1. Unless contraindicated, an oral beta-blocker is recommended to prevent postoperative AF for patients undergoing cardiac surgery. (Level of Evidence: A)

2. AV nodal blocking agents are recommended for rate control in patients who develop postoperative AF. (Level of Evidence: B)

Class IIa

1. Preoperative amiodarone reduces the incidence of AF in patients undergoing cardiac surgery and represents appropriate prophylactic therapy for patients at high risk for postoperative AF. (Level of Evidence: A)

2. It is reasonable to restore sinus rhythm by pharmacological cardioversion with ibutilide or direct current cardioversion in patients who develop postoperative AF. (Level of Evidence: B)

3. Antiarrhythmic medication is reasonable to maintain sinus rhythm in patients with recurrent or refractory postoperative AF. (Level of Evidence: B)

4. Antithrombotic medication is reasonable in patients who develop postoperative AF. (Level of Evidence: B)

Class IIb

1. Prophylactic sotalol may be considered for patients at risk of developing AF following cardiac surgery. (Level of Evidence: B)

6.6 Acute myocardial infarction

Class I

1. Direct-current cardioversion is recommended for patients with severe haemodynamic compromise, intractable ischaemia, or when adequate rate control cannot be achieved with pharmacological agents in patients with acute MI and AF. (Level of Evidence: C)

2. Intravenous amiodarone is recommended to slow a rapid ventricular response to AF and improve LV function in patients with acute MI. (Level of Evidence: C)

3. Intravenous beta-blockers and nondihydropyridine calcium antagonists are recommended to slow a rapid ventricular response to AF in patients with acute MI who do not have LV dysfunction, bronchospasm, or AV block. (Level of Evidence: C)

4. For patients with AF and acute MI, unfractionated heparin is recommended (aPTT 1.5 to 2.0 times control), unless contraindicated. (Level of Evidence: C)

Class IIa

1. Intravenous digitalis is reasonable to slow a rapid ventricular response and improve LV function in patients with acute MI and AF associated with severe LV dysfunction and HF. (Level of Evidence: C)

Class III

1. Class IC antiarrhythmic drugs are not recommended in patients with AF and acute MI. (Level of Evidence: C)

6.7 Management of atrial fibrillation associated with the Wolff-Parkinson White pre-excitation syndrome

Class I

1. Catheter ablation of the accessory pathway is recommended in symptomatic patients with AF who have WPW syndrome, particularly those with syncope due to rapid rate or short bypass tract refractory period. (Level of Evidence: B)

2. Immediate direct-current cardioversion is recommended to prevent ventricular fibrillation in patients with a short anterograde bypass tract refractory period in whom AF occurs with a rapid ventricular response associated with haemodynamic instability. (Level of Evidence: B)

3. Intravenous procainamide or ibutilide is recommended to restore sinus rhythm in patients with WPW in whom AF occurs without haemodynamic instability in association with a wide QRS complex on the ECG (.120ms duration) or rapid pre-excited ventricular response. (Level of Evidence: C)

Class IIa

1. Intravenous flecainide or direct current cardioversion are reasonable when very rapid ventricular rates occur in patients with AF involving an accessory pathway. (Level of Evidence: B)

Class IIb

1. It may be reasonable to administer intravenous quinidine, procainamide, disopyramide, ibutilide, or amiodarone to haemodynamically stable patients with AF involving an accessory pathway. (Level of Evidence: B)

Class III

1. Intravenous administration of digitalis glycosides or non-dihydropyridine calcium chanel antagonist is not recommended in patients with WPW syndrome who have pre-excited ventricular activation during AF. (Level of Evidence: B)

6.8 Hyperthyroidism

Class I

1. A beta-blocker is recommended to control the heart rate in patients with AF complicating thyrotoxicosis, unless contraindicated. (Level of Evidence: B)

2. When a beta-blocker cannot be used, a non-dihydropyridine calcium channel antagonist is recommended to control the ventricular rate in patients with AF and thyrotoxicosis.(Level of Evidence: B)

3. In patients with AF and thyrotoxicosis, oral anticoagulation (INR 2.0 to 3.0) is recommended. (Level of Evidence: C)

4. Once euthyroid state is achieved, antithrombotic prophylaxis is the same as for patients without hyperthyroidism. (Level of Evidence: C)

6.9 Management of atrial fibrillation during pregnancy

Class I

1. Digoxin, a beta-blocker, or nondihydropyridine calcium channel antagonists are recommended to control the ventricular rate in pregnant patients with AF. (Level of Evidence: C)

2. Direct-current cardioversion is recommended in pregnant patients who become haemodynamically unstable due to AF. (Level of Evidence: C)

3. Protection against thromboembolism is recommended throughout pregnancy for patients with AF except those at low thromboembolic risk. Anticoagulant or aspirin should be chosen according to the stage of pregnancy. (Level of Evidence: C)

Class IIb

1. During the first trimester and last month of pregnancy for patients with AF and risk factors for thromboembolism, consider administering unfractionated heparin by continuous intravenous infusion (apTT 1.5 to 2 times control) or by subcutaneous injection (10 000 to 20 000 units every 12h, adjusted to prolong the aPTT 6h after injection to 1.5 times control. (Level of Evidence: B)

2. During the first trimester and last month of pregnancy subcutaneous low molecular weight heparin may be considered for patients with AF and risk factors for thromboembolism despite limited data. (Level of Evidence: C)

3. During the second trimester, consider oral anticoagulation for pregnant women with AF at high thromboembolic risk. (Level of Evidence: C)

4. Quinidine or procainamide may be considered for pharmacological cardioversion in haemodynamically stable patients who develop AF during pregnancy. (Level of Evidence: C)

6.10 Management of atrial fibrillation in patients with hypertrophic cardiomyopathy

Class I

1. Oral anticoagulation (INR 2.0 to 3.0) is recommended in patients with HCM who develop AF. (Level of Evidence: B)

Class IIa

1. Antiarrhythmic medications can be useful to prevent recurrent AF in patients with HCM. Either disopyramide combined with a beta-blocker or nondihydropyridine calcium channel antagonist or amiodarone alone is generally preferred. (Level of Evidence: C)

6.11 Management of atrial fibrillation in patients with pulmonary disease

Class I

1. Correction of hypoxaemia and acidosis is the recommended primary therapeutic measure for patients who develop AF during an acute pulmonary illness or exacerbation or chronic pulmonary disease. (Level of Evidence C)

2. Diltiazem or verapamil is recommended to control the ventricular rate in patients with obstructive pulmonary disease who develop AF. (Level of Evidence: C)

3. Direct-current cardioversion should be attempted in patients with pulmonary disease who become haemodynamically unstable as a consequence of AF. (Level of Evidence: C)

Class III

1. Theophylline and beta-adrenergic agonist agents are not recommended in patients with bronchospastic lung disease who develop AF. (Level of Evidence: C)

2. Beta-blockers, sotalol, propafenone, and adenosine are not recommended in patients with obstructive lung disease who develop AF. (Level of Evidence: C)

Chapter 3

Management of Syncope*
2004

Chairperson:
Michele Brignole, MD, FESC
Dept. of Cardiology and Arrhythmologic Centre
Ospedali del Tigullio - Via Don Bobbio 25
16033 Lavagna - Italy
Phone : +39 0185 329569
Fax : +39 0185 306506
E-mail : mbrignole@ASL4.liguria.it

Task Force Members:
1. Alboni Paolo, Cento, Italy
2. Benditt David, Minneapolis, USA
3. Bergfeldt Lennart, Stockholm, Sweden
4. Blanc Jean-Jacques, Brest, France
5. Bloch Thomsen Poul Erik, Hellerup, Denmark
6. van Dijk J. Gert, Leiden, The Netherlands
7. Fitzpatrick Adam, Manchester, UK
8. Hohnloser Stefan, Frankfurt, Germany
9. Janousek Jan, Prague, Czech Republic
10. Kapoor Wishwa, Pittsburgh, USA
11. Kenny Rose-Anne, Newcastle, UK
12. Kulakowski Piotr, Warsaw, Poland
13. Masotti Giulio, Firenze, Italy[1]
14. Moya Angel, Barcelona, Spain
15. Raviele Antonio, Mestre-Venice, Italy
16. Sutton Richard, London, UK
17. Theodorakis George, Athens, Greece
18. Ungar Andrea, Firenze, Italy[1]
19. Wieling Wouter, Amsterdam, The Netherlands

ESC Staff:
1. Keith McGregor, Sophia Antipolis, France
2. Veronica Dean, Sophia Antipolis, France
3. Catherine Després, Sophia Antipolis, France
4. Xue Li, Sophia Antipolis, France

1. Evaluation of patients with syncope

The "Initial evaluation"

- Careful history from patient and witnesses about circumstances, attack onset and termination.
- Physical examination including orthostatic blood pressure measurements.
- Standard electrocardiogram (ECG).

The "3 key questions"

- Is loss of consciousness attributable to syncope or not?
- Are there important clinical features in the history that suggest the diagnosis?
- Is heart disease present or absent?

Definition of syncope

Syncope is a symptom, the defining clinical characteristics of which are a transient, self-limited loss of consciousness, usually leading to falling. The onset of syncope is relatively rapid, the subsequent recovery is spontaneous, complete and usually prompt. The underlying mechanism is a relatively abrupt cerebral hypoperfusion.

Classification of syncope

- Neurally-mediated (reflex) e.g. vasovagal, carotid sinus, situational, etc.
- Orthostatic hypotension.
- Cardiac arrhythmias as primary cause e.g. bradycardia, tachycardia, etc.

* Adapted from the ESC Guidelines on Management (Diagnosis and Treatment) of Syncope update 2004, executive summary (European Heart Journal 2004; 25: 2054-2072) and full text (Europace 2004; 6: 467-537). [1] Representative of the European Union Geriatric Medicine Society

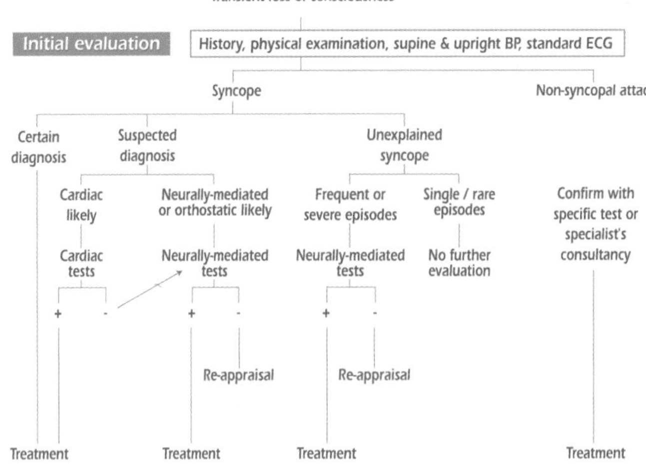

- Structural cardiac or cardiopulmonary disease e.g. acute myocardial infarction/ischaemia, aortic dissection, pulmonary embolus, etc.

Note: In syncopal conditions (and in the absence of head injury), EEG, CT scan and MRI are not helpful.

Classification of non-syncopal attack

- Disorders resembling syncope with impairment or loss of consciousness, e.g. seizure, transient ischaemic attacks, etc.

- Disorders resembling syncope with intact consciousness, e.g. psychogenic pseudo-syncope (somatisation disorders), etc.

Features that suggest a non-syncopal attack

- Confusion after attack for more than 5 minutes (seizure).

- Prolonged (>15 seconds) tonic-clonic movements starting at the onset of the attack (seizure).

- Frequent attacks with somatic complaints, no organic heart disease (psychiatric).

- Associated with vertigo, dysarthria, diplopia (transient ischaemic attack).

Diagnostic Criteria - certain

Initial evaluation may lead to a certain diagnosis based on symptoms, signs or ECG findings. This applies to the following cases:

- **Classical vasovagal syncope** is diagnosed if precipitating events such as fear, severe pain, emotional distress, instrumentation or prolonged standing are associated with typical prodromal symptoms.

- **Situational syncope** is diagnosed if syncope occurs during or immediately after urination, defaecation, cough or swallowing.

- **Orthostatic syncope** is diagnosed when there is a documentation of orthostatic hypotension (decrease of SBP ≥ 20 mmHg or to < 90 mmHg) associated with syncope or pre-syncope.

- **Syncope due to cardiac ischaemia** is diagnosed when symptoms are present with ECG evidence of acute ischaemia with or without myocardial infarction.

- **Syncope due to cardiac arrhythmia** is diagnosed by ECG when there is:
    - Sinus bradycardia < 40 bpm or repetitive sinoatrial blocks or sinus pauses > 3 seconds.
    - Atrioventricular block (2nd degree Mobitz II or 3rd degree atrioventricular block).
    - Alternating left and right bundle branch block.
    - Rapid paroxysmal supraventricular tachycardia or ventricular tachycardia.
    - Pacemaker malfunction with cardiac pauses.

Diagnostic criteria - suspected

Features that suggest a cardiac cause:

- Supine
- During exertion
- Preceded by palpitation
- Presence of severe heart disease
- ECG abnormalities summarised as:
  - wide QRS complex (≥ 0.12 seconds)
  - AV conduction abnormalities
  - sinus bradycardia (< 50 beats per minute (bpm)) or pauses
  - long QT interval

Features that suggest a neurally-mediated cause:

- Absence of cardiac disease
- Long history of syncope
- After sudden unexpected unpleasant sight, sound or smell
- Prolonged standing at attention or crowded, warm places
- Nausea, vomiting associated with syncope
- Within one hour of a meal
- After exertion
- Temporal relationship with start of medication or changes of dosage

When to hospitalise a patient with syncope:

- Features that suggest a cardiac cause
- Syncope causing severe injury
- Frequent recurrent syncopes

2. Diagnostic tests

Carotid sinus massage

Indications:

Patients > 40 years with syncope of unknown aetiology after the initial evaluation. In case of risk of stroke due to carotid artery disease, massage should be avoided.

Methodology:

Massage is performed with the patient both supine and erect, on the right and left side, during ECG and BP monitoring. Duration of massage of a minimum of 5 and a maximum of 10 seconds.

Diagnosis:

The procedure is considered positive if symptoms are reproduced during or immediately after the massage in presence of asystole ≥ 3 seconds and/or a fall in systolic blood pressure ≥ 50 mmHg. A positive response is diagnostic of the cause of syncope in the absence of any other competing diagnosis.

Classification of positive responses to tilt testing

- **Type 1 Mixed.** Heart rate falls at the time of syncope but the ventricular rate does not fall to < 40 bpm or falls to < 40 bpm for < 10 seconds with or without asystole of < 3 seconds. Blood pressure falls before the heart rate falls.
- **Type 2A Cardioinhibition without asystole.** Heart rate falls to a ventricular rate < 40 bpm for > 10 seconds but asystole of > 3 seconds does not occur. Blood pressure falls before the heart rate falls.
- **Type 2B Cardioinhibition with asystole.** Asystole occurs for > 3 seconds. Blood pressure fall coincides with or occurs before the heart rate fall.
- **Type 3 Vasodepressor**. Heart rate does not fall > 10% at the time of syncope from its peak during the tilt.
- **Exception 1. Chronotropic Incompetence.** No heart rate rise during tilt testing (i.e. < 10% from the pre-tilt rate).
- **Exception 2. Excessive heart rate rise (Postural Orthostatic Tachycardia Syndrome).** An excessive heart rate rises both at the onset of the upright position and throughout its duration before syncope (i.e. peak rate > 130 bpm).

Tilt testing

Indications:

- Unexplained single syncopal episode in high risk settings (e.g. occurrence or potential risk of physical injury or with occupational implications), or recurrent episodes in the absence of organic heart disease, or, in the presence of organic heart disease, after cardiac causes of syncope have been excluded.
- When it will be of clinical value to demonstrate susceptibility to neurally-mediated syncope to the patient.
- When an understanding of the haemodynamic pattern of syncope may alter the therapeutic approach.
- For differentiating syncope with jerking movements from epilepsy.
- For evaluating patients with recurrent unexplained falls.
- For assessing recurrent pre-syncope or dizziness.

Methodology:

Class I

- Supine pre-tilt phase of at least 5 min when no venous cannulation is performed, and at least 20 min when cannulation is undertaken.
- Tilt angle is 60 to 70 degrees.
- Passive phase of a minimum of 20 min and a maximum of 45 min.
- Use of either intravenous isoprenaline/isoproterenol or sublingual nitroglycerin for drug provocation if passive phase has been negative. Drug challenge phase duration of 15-20 min.
- For isoproterenol, an incremental infusion rate from 1 up to 3 μg/min in order to increase average heart rate by about 20-25% over baseline, administered without returning the patient to the supine position.
- For nitroglycerin, a fixed dose of 400 μg nitroglycerin spray sublingually administered in the upright position.
- The test is considered positive if syncope occurs.

Class II

Divergence of opinion exists in the case of induction of pre-syncope.

Diagnosis:

Class I

- In patients without structural heart disease, tilt testing is diagnostic, and no further tests need to be performed when spontaneous syncope is reproduced.
- In patients with structural heart disease, cardiac causes should be excluded prior to considering positive tilt test results as evidence suggesting neurally mediated syncope.

Class II

- The clinical meaning of abnormal responses other than induction of syncope is unclear.

Electrocardiographic monitoring

Indications:

Class I

- In-hospital monitoring (in bed or telemetric) is warranted when the patient has an important structural heart disease and is at high risk of life-threatening arrhythmias (see page 6).
- Holter monitoring is indicated in patients who have the clinical or ECG features suggesting an arrhythmic syncope such as those listed on page 6 and very frequent syncopes or pre-syncopes (e.g. ≥ 1 per week).
- When the mechanism of syncope remains unclear after full evaluation, Implantable Loop Recorder is indicated in patients who have the clinical or ECG features suggesting an arrhythmic syncope such as those listed on page 6 or a history of recurrent syncopes with injury.

Class II

- Holter monitoring may be useful in patients who have clinical or ECG features suggesting an arrhythmic syncope such as those listed on page 6 in order to guide subsequent examinations (i.e. electrophysiological study).

- External Loop Recorder may be indicated in patients who have the clinical or ECG features suggesting an arrhythmic syncope such as those listed on page 6 and inter-symptom interval ≤ 4 weeks.

- Implantable Loop Recorder may be indicated:
  - In an initial phase of the work-up instead of completion of conventional investigations in patients with preserved cardiac function who have the clinical or ECG features suggesting an arrhythmic syncope as those listed on page 6.
  - To assess the contribution of bradycardia before embarking on cardiac pacing in patients with suspected or certain neurally-mediated syncope presenting with frequent or traumatic syncopal episodes.

Class III

- ECG monitoring is unlikely to be useful in patients who do not have the clinical or ECG features suggesting an arrhythmic syncope as those listed on page 6 and therefore it should not be performed.

Diagnosis:

Class I

- ECG monitoring is diagnostic when a correlation between syncope and an electrocardiographic abnormality (brady- or tachyarrhythmia) is detected.

- ECG monitoring excludes an arrhythmic cause when there is a correlation between syncope and no rhythm variation.

- In the absence of such correlations, additional testing is recommended with possible exception of:
  - ventricular pauses longer than 3 sec when awake
  - periods of Mobitz 2nd or 3rd degree atrioventricular block when awake
  - rapid paroxysmal ventricular tachycardia.

Class II

- Pre-syncope may not be an accurate surrogate for syncope in establishing a diagnosis and, therefore, therapy should not be guided by pre-syncopal findings.

Electrophysiological testing

Indications:

When the initial evaluation suggests an arrhythmic cause of syncope (see initial evaluation, diagnostic criteria).

Diagnosis:

Class I

- Normal electrophysiological findings cannot completely exclude an arrhythmic cause of syncope; when an arrhythmia is likely, further evaluations (for example loop recording) are recommended.

- Depending on the clinical context, abnormal electrophysiological findings may not be diagnostic of the cause of syncope.

- An electrophysiological study is diagnostic, and usually no additional tests are required, in the following cases:
  - sinus bradycardia and a very prolonged sinus node recovery time
  - bifascicular block and:
    - a baseline His-Ventricular interval of ≥ 100ms, or
    - 2nd or 3rd degree His-Purkinje block is demonstrated during incremental atrial pacing, or
    - if the baseline electrophysiological study is inconclusive, high-degree His-Purkinje block is provoked by intravenous administration of ajmaline, procainamide, or disopyramide
  - induction of sustained monomorphic ventricular tachycardia
  - induction of rapid supraventricular arrhythmia which reproduces hypotensive or spontaneous symptoms

Class II

Divergence of opinion exists on the diagnostic value of electrophysiological study in case of:
  - His-Ventricular interval of > 70 ms but < 100 ms
  - Induction of polymorphic ventricular tachycardia or ventricular fibrillation in patients with ischaemic or dilated cardiomyopathy
  - Brugada syndrome

Echocardiogram

Indications:

When cardiac disease is suspected.

Diagnosis:

Even if echocardiography alone is only seldom diagnostic, this test provides information about the type and severity of underlying heart disease which may be useful for risk stratification. Echocardiography only makes a diagnosis in severe aortic stenosis and atrial myxoma.

ATP test

Indications:

In the absence of sufficient hard data, the test may be indicated at the end of the diagnostic work-up.

Methodology:

Rapid injection of a 20 mg bolus of ATP during ECG monitoring. Asystole lasting > 6 seconds, or Atrio Ventricular block lasting > 10 seconds, is considered abnormal.

Diagnosis:

ATP testing produces an abnormal response in some patients with syncope of unknown origin, but not in controls. ATP testing identifies a group of patients with otherwise unexplained syncope with definite clinical features and benign prognosis but possibly heterogeneous mechanism of syncope. Thus specific treatment should be postponed until a definite mechanism of syncope can be obtained (Class II).

Ventricular signal averaged electrocardiogram, T wave alternans

There is general agreement that ventricular signal-averaged electrocardiogram and T wave alternans are not diagnostic of the cause of syncope. In patients with syncope and no evidence of structural heart disease, the technique may be useful for guiding the use of electrophysiological studies. Its systematic use is not recommended.

Exercise testing

Indications:

Syncope during or shortly after exertion.

Diagnosis:

Class I

- When ECG and haemodynamic abnormalities are present and syncope is reproduced during or immediately after exercise.
- If Mobitz 2nd degree or 3rd degree AV block develop during exercise even without syncope.

Cardiac catheterisation and angiography

Indications:

In patients with syncope suspected to be due, directly or indirectly, to myocardial ischaemia, coronary angiography is recommended in order to confirm the diagnosis and to establish optimal therapy (Class I). Angiography alone is rarely diagnostic of the cause of syncope (Class III).

Neurological and psychiatric evaluation

Indications:

- Neurological referral is indicated in patients in whom loss of consciousness cannot be attributed to syncope.
- In case of unequivocal syncope, neurological referral is warranted when syncope may be due to autonomic failure or to a cerebrovascular steal syndrome.

Distinguishing seizure from syncope

	Seizure likely	Syncope likely
Findings during loss of consciousness (as observed by an eyewitness)	• Tonic-clonic movements prolonged and their onset coincides with loss of consciousness • Hemilateral clonic movement • Clear automatisms • Tongue biting	• Tonic-clonic movements always of short duration (< 15 seconds) and they start after the loss of consciousness
Symptoms before the event	• Aura (such as funny smell)	• Nausea, vomiting, abdominal discomfort, feeling of cold, sweating
Symptoms after the event	• Prolonged confusion • Aching muscles	• Usually short duration • Nausea, vomiting, pallor

- Psychiatric evaluation is recommended when symptoms suggest psychogenic pseudo-syncope or if true syncope is due to psychiatric medication, which may need to be altered.

- In all other patients with syncope, neurological and psychiatric investigations are not recommended.

3. Treatment

Neurally-mediated (reflex) syncope

In general, initial treatment, e.g. education and reassurance, is sufficient. Additional treatment may be necessary in high risk or high frequency settings when:

- Syncope is very frequent, e.g. alters the quality of life.

- Syncope is recurrent and unpredictable (absence of premonitory symptoms) and exposes patients at "high risk" of trauma.

- Syncope occurs during the prosecution of a 'high risk' activity (e.g., driving, machine operator, flying, competitive athletics, etc).

Treatment is not necessary in patients who have sustained a single syncope and are not having syncope in a high risk setting. It is valuable to assess the relative contribution of cardioinhibition and vasodepression before embarking on treatment as there are different therapeutic strategies for the two aspects. Even if evidence of utility of such an assessment exists only for the carotid sinus massage, it is recommended to extend this assessment also by means of tilt testing or implantable loop recorder.

Class I

- Explanation of the risk, and reassurance about the prognosis in vasovagal syncope.

- Avoidance of trigger events as much as possible and reducing magnitude of potential triggers when feasible (e.g. emotional upset) and causal situation in situational syncope.

- Modification or discontinuation of hypotensive drug treatment for concomitant conditions.

- Cardiac pacing in patients with cardioinhibitory or mixed carotid sinus syndrome.

Class II

- Volume expansion by salt supplements, an exercise programme or head-up tilt sleeping (> 10°) in posture-related syncope.

- Tilt training in patients with vasovagal syncope.

- Isometric leg and arm counter-pressure manoeuvres in patients with vasovagal syncope.

- Cardiac pacing in patients with cardioinhibitory vasovagal syncope with a frequency > 5 attacks per year or severe physical injury or accident and age > 40.

Class III

- The evidence fails to support the efficacy of beta-adrenergic blocking drugs. Beta-adrenergic blocking drugs may aggravate bradycardia in some cardioinhibitory cases.

Orthostatic hypotension

Class I

- Syncope due to orthostatic hypotension should be treated in all patients. In many instances, treatment entails only modification of drug treatment for concomitant conditions.

Cardiac arrhythmias as primary cause

Class I

- Patients who suffer from syncope due to cardiac arrhythmias and whose condition is life-threatening, or where there is a serious risk of injury, must receive the appropriate treatment.

Class II

- Treatment may be employed when the culprit arrhythmia has not been demonstrated and a diagnosis of life-threatening arrhythmia is presumed from surrogate data.

- Treatment may be employed when a culprit arrhythmia has been identified but is not life-threatening or presenting a high risk of injury.

4. Situations in which ICD therapy is likely to be useful

- **Documented** syncopal ventricular tachycardia or fibrillation without correctable causes (e.g., drug-induced) (Class I, Level A).

- **Undocumented** syncope likely to be due to ventricular tachycardia or fibrillation:
  - Inducible sustained monomorphic ventricular tachycardia with severe haemodynamic compromise, in the absence of another competing diagnosis as a cause of syncope (Class I, Level B).
  - Very depressed left ventricular systolic function in the absence of another competing diagnosis as a cause of syncope (Class II, Level B).
  - Established long QT syndrome, Brugada syndrome, arrhythmogenic right ventricular dysplasia, or hypertrophic obstructive cardiomyopathy, with a family history of sudden death, in the absence of another competing diagnosis for the cause of syncope (Class II).
  - Brugada syndrome or arrhythmogenic right ventricular dysplasia and inducible ventricular tachyarrhythmias with severe haemodynamic compromise in the absence of another competing diagnosis for the cause of syncope (Class II).

5. Syncope facility ("syncope unit")

- A cohesive, structured care pathway (either delivered within a single syncope facility or as a more multi-faceted service) is recommended for the global assessment of the patient with syncope.

- Experience and training in key components of cardiology, neurology, emergency and geriatric medicine are pertinent.

- Core equipment for the facility include: surface ECG recording, phasic blood pressure monitoring, tilt table testing equipment, external and internal (implantable) ECG loop recorder systems, 24 hour ambulatory blood pressure monitoring, 24 hour ambulatory ECG monitoring and autonomic function testing.

- Preferential access to other tests or therapy for syncope should be guaranteed and standardised.

- The majority of syncope patients should be investigated as out-patients or day cases.

Figure 2. A proposed model of organisation for the evaluation of the syncope patient in a community

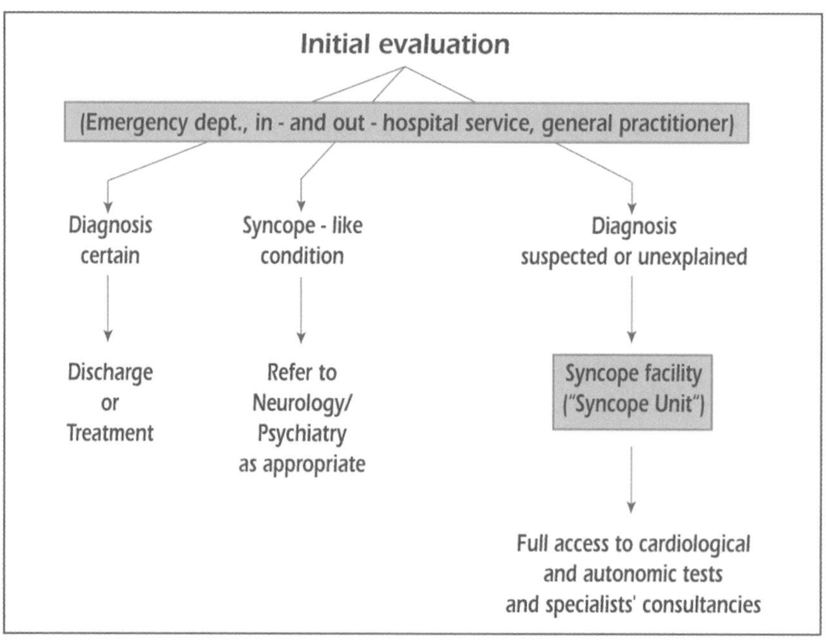

Chapter 4

Ventricular Arrhythmias and the Prevention of Sudden Cardiac Death*

2006

Co-chairperson:
Douglas P. Zipes
MD, MACC, FAHA, FESC
Division of Cardiology
Indiana University, School of Medicine
Krannert Institute of Cardiology
1801 N. Capitol Ave.
Indianapolis 46202-4800-USA
Phone: (+1) 317 962 0555
Fax: (+1) 317 962 0568
E-mail: dzipes@iupui.edu

Co-chairperson:
A. John Camm
MD, FACC, FAHA, FESC
Division of Cardiac And Vascular Sciences
St. George's University of London
Cranmer Terrace
London SW17 0RE
United Kingdom
Phone: (+44) 20 8725 3554
Fax: (+44) 20 8767 7141
E-mail: jcamm@sgul.ac.uk

Task Force Members:
1. Martin Borggrefe, MD, FESC
2. Alfred E. Buxton, MD, FACC, FAHA
3. Bernard Chaitman, MD, FACC, FAHA
4. Martin Fromer, MD
5. Gabriel Gregoratos, MD, FACC, FAHA
6. George Klein, MD, FACC
7. Arthur J. Moss, MD, FACC, FAHA
8. Robert J Myerburg, MD, FACC, FAHA
9. Silvia G. Priori, MD, PhD, FESC**
10. Miguel A. Quinones, MD, FACC
11. Dan M. Roden, MD, CM, FACC, FAHA
12. Michael J. Silka, MD, FACC, FAHA
13. Cynthia Tracy, MD, FACC, FAHA

ESC Staff:
1. Keith McGregor, Sophia Antipolis, France
2. Veronica Dean, Sophia Antipolis, France
3. Catherine Després, Sophia Antipolis, France
4. Karine Piellard, Sophia Antipolis, France

1. Introduction

The reader should note that the recommendations, text, figures, and tables included in these pocket guidelines represent a succinct summary of the more extensive evidence base, critical evaluation, supporting text, tables, figures, and references that are included in the full text guidelines. Readers are strongly encouraged to refer to the full text guidelines.

Classification of Recommendations and Level of Evidence are expressed in the American College of Cardiology (ACC)/American Heart Association (AHA)/European Society of Cardiology (ESC) format as follows:

*Adapted from the ACC/AHA/ESC Guidelines for the Management of Patients with Ventricular Arrhythmias and the Prevention of Sudden Cardiac Death - Executive Summary (European Heart Journal 2006;27:2099-2140) and Full Text (Europace 2006;8:746-837)

Class I:	Conditions for which there is evidence and/or general agreement that a given procedure or treatment is beneficial, useful and effective.
Class II:	Conditions for which there is conflicting evidence and/or divergence of opinion about the usefulness/efficacy of a procedure or treatment.
Class IIa:	Weight of evidence or opinion is in favor of usefulness/efficacy.
Class IIb:	Usefulness/efficacy is less well established by evidence/opinion.
Class III:	Conditions for which there is evidence and/or general agreement that a procedure/treatment is not useful/effective and in some cases may be harmful.

Level of Evidence A	Data derived from multiple randomized clinical trials or meta-analyses
Level of Evidence B	Data derived from a single randomized trial or large non-randomized studies
Level of Evidence C	Only consensus opinion of experts, case studies, or standard-of-care

The schema for classification of recommendations and level of evidence is summarized in Figure 1.

Figure 1. Applying Classification of Recommendations and Level of Evidence

Size of Treatment Effect →

Estimate of Certainty (Precision) of Treatment Effect

	CLASS I Benefit >>> Risk Procedure/Treatment should be performed/ administered	**CLASS IIa** Benefit >> Risk Additional studies with focused objectives needed It is reasonable to perform procedure/administer treatment	**CLASS IIb** Benefit ≥ Risk Additional studies with broad objectives needed; additional registry data would be helpful Procedure/Treatment may be considered	**CLASS III** Risk ≥ Benefit No additional studies needed Procedure/Treatment should not be performed/ administered since it is not helpful and may be harmful
LEVEL A Multiple (3-5) population risk strata evaluated* General consistency of direction and magnitude of effect	- Recommendation that procedure or treatment is useful/effective - Sufficient evidence from multiple randomized trials or meta-analyses	- Recommendation in favour of treatment or procedure being useful/effective - Some conflicting evidence from multiple randomized trials or meta-analyses	- Recommendation's usefulness/efficacy less well established - Greater conflicting evidence from multiple randomized trials or meta-analyses	- Recommendation that procedure or treatment is not useful/effective and may be harmful - Sufficient evidence from multiple randomized trials or meta-analyses
LEVEL B Limited (2-3) population risk strata evaluated*	- Recommendation that procedure or treatment is useful/effective - Limited evidence from single randomized trial or non-randomized studies	– Recommendation in favour of treatment or procedure being useful/effective - Some conflicting evidence from single randomized trial or non-randomized studies	- Recommendation's usefulness/efficacy less well established - Greater conflicting evidence from single randomized trial or non-randomized studies	- Recommendation that procedure or treatment is not useful/effective and may be harmful - Limited evidence from single randomized trial or non-randomized studies
LEVEL C Very limited (1-2) population risk strata evaluated*	- Recommendation that procedure or treatment is useful/effective - Only expert opinion, case studies, or standard-of-care	- Recommendation in favour of treatment or procedure being useful/effective - Only diverging expert opinion, case studies, or standard-of-care	- Recommendation's usefulness/efficacy less well established - Only diverging expert opinion, case studies, or standard-of-care	- Recommendation that procedure or treatment is not useful/effective and may be harmful - Only expert opinion, case studies, or standard-of-care

* Data available from clinical trials or registries about the usefulness/efficacy in different subpopulations, such as gender, age, history of diabetes, history of prior myocardial infarction, history of heart failure, and prior aspirin use. A recommendation with Level of Evidence B or C does not imply that the recommendation is weak. Many important clinical questions addressed in the guidelines do not lend themselves to clinical trials. Even though randomized trials are not available, there may be a very clear clinical consensus that a particular test or therapy is useful or effective.

Table 1. Inconsistencies Between ACC/AHA/ESC Guidelines for the Management of Patients With ventricular Arrhythmias and the Prevention of SCD and Other Published ACC/AHA and ESC Guidelines With Respect to ICD Therapy for Primary Prevention to Reduce Total Mortality by a Reduction in SCD

Group addressed in ecommendation	Guideline and Class of Recommendation with Level of Evidence* for Each Group				
	2005 ACC/AHA HF	2005 ESC HF	2004 ACC/AHA STEMI	2002 ACC/AHA/NASPE PM and ICD	Comment from the ACC/AHA/ESC VA & SCD Guidelines
LVD d/t MI, LVEF ≤30%, NYHA II, III	Class I; LOE: B	Class I; LOE: A	Class IIa; LOE: B	Class IIa; LOE: B	VA & SCD has combined all trials that enrolled patients with LVD d/t MI into one recommendation, Class I; LOE: A
LVD d/t MI, LVEF 30% to 35%, NYHA II, III	Class IIa; LOE: B	Class I; LOE: A	N/A	N/A	
LVD d/t MI, LVEF 30% to 40%, NSVT, positive EP study	N/A	N/A	Class I; LOE: B	Class IIb; LOE:B	
LVD d/t MI, LVEF ≤30%, NYHA I	Class IIa; LOE: B	N/A	N/A	N/A	VA & SCD has expanded the range of LVEF to ≤30% to 35% for patients with LVD d/t MI and NYHA functional class I into one recommendation, Class IIa; LOE: B.
LVD d/t MI, LVEF ≤31% to 35%, NYHA I	N/A	N/A	N/A	N/A	
NICM, L VEF ≤30%, NYHA II, III	Class I; LOE: B	Class I; LOE: A	N/A	N/A	VA & SCD has combined all trials of NICM, NYHA II, III into one recommendation, Class I; LOE: B
NICM, LVEF 30% to35%, NYHA II, III	Class IIa; LOE: B	Class I; LOE: A	N/A	N/A	
NICM, LVEF ≤30%, NYHA I	Class IIb; LOE: C	N/A	N/A	N/A	VA & SCD has expanded the range of LVEF to ≤30% to 35% for patients with NICM and NYHA functional class I into one recommendation, Class IIb; LOE: B.
NICM, LVEF ≤31% to35%, NYHA I	N/A	N/A	N/A	N/A	

*For an explanation of class of recommendation and level of evidence (LOE), see Figure 1.

ACC/AHA HF = ACC/AHA 2005 Guidelines Update for the Diagnosis and Management of Chronic Heart Failure in the Adult; ACC/AHA/NASPE PM and ICD = ACC/AHA/NASPE 2002 Guidelines Update for Implantation of Cardiac Pacemakers and Antiarrhythmia Devices; ACC/AHA STEMI = ACC/AHA 2004 Guidelines for the Management of Patients with ST-Elevation Myocardial Infarction; EP = electrophysiological; ESC HF = ESC 2005 Guidelines for the Diagnosis and Treatment of Chronic Heart Failure; LOE = level of evidence; LVD d/t MI = left ventricular dysfunction due to prior myocardial infarction; LVEF = left ventricular ejection fraction; N/A = not addressed; NICM = non-ischaemic cardiomyopathy; NSVT = nonsustained ventricular tachycardia; NYHA = New York Heart Association functional class; SCD = sudden cardiac death; VA = ventricular arrhythmias.

1.1 Prophylactic implantable cardioverter device recommendations across published guidelines

Please see Table 1 for prophylactic implantable cardioverter defibrillator (ICD) therapy recommendations across published guidelines. A detailed explanation of the rationale used in formulating these recommendations can be found in the full text guidelines.

1.2 Classification of ventricular arrhythmias and sudden cardiac death

This classification table is provided for direction and introduction to these pocket guidelines (Table 2).

Table 2. Classification of ventricular Arrhythmias

Classification by Electrocardiography	
Nonsustained VT	Three or more beats in duration, terminating spontaneously in less than 30 seconds.VT is a cardiac arrhythmia of 3 or more consecutive complexes in duration emanating from the ventricles at a rate of greater than 100 bpm (cycle length less than 600 msec).
Monomorphic	Nonsustained VT with a single QRS morphology.
Polymorphic	Nonsustained VT with a changing QRS morphology at cycle length between 600 and 180 msec.
Sustained VT	VT greater than 30 seconds in duration and/or requiring termination due to haemodynamic compromise in less than 30 seconds.
Monomorphic	Sustained VT with a stable single QRS morphology.
Polymorphic	Sustained VT with a changing or multiform QRS morphology at cycle length between 600 and 180 msec.
Bundle branch reentrant tachycardia	VT due to reentry involving the His-Purkinje system,usually with LBBB morphology; this usually occurs in the setting of cardiomyopathy.
Bidirectional VT	VT with a beat-to-beat alternans in the QRS frontal plane axis, often associated with digitalis toxicity.
Torsades de pointes	Characterized by VT associated with a long QT or QTc, and electrocardiographically characterized by twisting of the peaks of the QRS complexes around the isoelectric line during the arrhythmia: - "Typical" initiated following "short long short" coupling intervals. - Short coupled variant initiated by normal short coupling.
Ventricular flutter	A regular (cycle length variability 30 msec or less) ventricular arrhythmia approximately 300 bpm (cycle length 200 msec) with a monomorphic appearance; no isoelectric interval between successive QRS complexes.
Ventricular fibrillation	Rapid, usually more than 300 bpm/200 msec (cycle length 180 msec or less), grossly irregular ventricular rhythm with marked variability in QRS cycle length, morphology, and amplitude.

LBBB = left bundle-branch block; VT = ventricular tachycardia.

2. Incidence of sudden cardiac death

The geographic incidence of sudden cardiac death (SCD) varies as a function of coronary heart disease (CHD) prevalence in different regions. Estimates for the U.S. range from less than 200,000 to more than 450,000 SCDs annually, with the most widely used estimates in the range of 300,000 to 350,000 SCDs annually. The variation is based, in part, on the inclusion criteria used in individual studies. Overall, event rates in Europe are similar to those in the United States, with significant geographic variations reported.

Approximately 50% of all CHD deaths are sudden and unexpected, occurring shortly (within 1 hr) after the onset of a change in clinical status, with some geographical variation in the fraction of coronary deaths that are sudden.

3. Clinical presentations of patients with ventricular arrhythmias and sudden cardiac death

Ventricular arrhythmias can occur in individuals with or without cardiac disorders. There is a great deal of overlap

Table 3. Clinical Presentations of Patients With ventricular Arrhythmias and Sudden Cardiac Death

Clinical Presentations
Asymptomatic individuals with or without electrocardiographic abnormalities
Persons with symptoms potentially attributable to ventricular arrhythmias • Palpitations • Dyspnoea • Chest pain • Syncope and presyncope
Ventricular tachycardia that is haemodynamically stable
Ventricular tachycardia that is not haemodynamically stable
Cardiac arrest • Asystolic (sinus arrest, atrioventricular block) • Ventricular tachycardia • Ventricular fibrillation • Pulseless electrical activity

between clinical presentations (Table 3) and severity and type of heart disease. The prognosis and management are individualized according to symptom burden and severity of underlying heart disease in addition to the clinical presentation.

4. General evaluation of patients with documented or suspected ventricular arrhythmias

4.1 Resting ECG

Recommendations

Class I

1. Resting 12-lead electrocardiogram (ECG) is indicated in all patients who are evaluated for ventricular arrhythmias (VA). (Level of Evidence: A)

4.2 Exercise Testing

Recommendations

Class I

1. Exercise testing (ET) is recommended in adult patients with VA who have an intermediate or greater probability of having CHD by age, gender and symptoms* to provoke ischaemic changes or VA. (Level of Evidence: B)

2. ET is useful in patients regardless of age with known or suspected exercise-induced VA, including catecholaminergic ventricular tachycardia (VT) to provoke the arrhythmia, achieve a diagnosis, and determine the patient's response to tachycardia. (Level of Evidence: B)

Class IIa

1. ET can be useful in evaluating response to medical or ablation therapy in patients with known exercise-induced VA. (Level of Evidence: B)

Class IIb

1. ET might be useful in patients with VA and a low probability of CHD by age, gender, and symptoms.* (Level of Evidence: C)

2. ET might be useful in the investigation of isolated premature ventricular complexes (PVCs) in middle-aged or older patients without other evidence of CHD. (Level of Evidence: C)

Class III

1. See Table 1 in the ACC/AHA 2002 Guideline Update for Exercise Testing for contraindications. (Level of Evidence: B) *See Table 4 in the ACC/AHA 2002 Guideline Update for Exercise Testing for further explanation of CHD probability.

4.3 Ambulatory electrocardiography

Recommendations

Class I

1. Ambulatory ECG is indicated when there is a need to clarify the diagnosis by detecting arrhythmias, QT interval changes, T-wave alternans or ST-changes, evaluate risk, or judge therapy. (Level of Evidence: A)

2. Event monitors are indicated when symptoms are sporadic, to establish whether they are caused by transient arrhythmias. (Level of Evidence: B)

3. Implantable recorders are useful in patients with sporadic symptoms suspected to be related to arrhythmias such as syncope, when a symptom-rhythm correlation cannot be established by conventional diagnostic techniques. (Level of Evidence: B)

4.4. ECG techniques and measurements

Recommendations

Class IIa

1. It is reasonable to use T-wave alternans for improving the diagnosis and risk stratification of patients with VA or at risk for developing life-threatening VA. (Level of Evidence: A)

Class IIb

2. ECG techniques such as signal-averaged ECG, heart rate variability, baroflex sensitivity and heart rate turbulence may be useful for improving the diagnosis and risk stratification of patients with ventricular arrhythmias or who are at risk of developing life-threatening ventricular arrhythmias. (Level of Evidence: B)

4.5 Left ventricular function and imaging

Recommendations

Class I

1. Echocardiography is recommended in patients with VA who are suspected of having structural heart disease. (Level of Evidence: B)

2. Echocardiography is recommended for the subset of patients at high-risk for development of serious VA or SCD, such as those with dilated, hypertrophic, or right ventricular cardiomyopathies, acute myocardial infarction (AMI) survivors, or relatives of patients with inherited disorders associated with SCD. (Level of Evidence: B)

3. ET with an imaging modality (echocardiography or nuclear perfusion [single-photon emission computed tomography (SPECT)]) is recommended to detect silent ischaemia in patients with VA who have an intermediate probability of having CHD by age, symptoms and gender, and in whom ECG assessment is less reliable because of digoxin use, left ventricular (LV) hypertrophy, greater than 1 mm ST-segment depression at rest, Wolff-Parkinson-White Syndrome or LBBB. (Level of Evidence: B)

4. Pharmacological stress testing with an imaging modality (echocardiography or myocardial perfusion SPECT) is recommended to detect silent ischaemia in patients with VA who have an intermediate probability of having CHD by age, symptoms, and gender and are physically unable to perform a symptom-limited exercise test. (Level of Evidence: B)

Class IIa

1. Magnetic resonance imaging (MRI), cardiac computed tomography (CT), or radionuclide angiography can be useful in patients with VA when echocardiography does not provide accurate assessment of LV and right ventricular (RV) function, and/or evaluation of structural changes. (Level of Evidence: B)

2. Coronary angiography can be useful in establishing or excluding the presence of significant obstructive CHD in patients with life-threatening VA or in survivors of SCD, who have an intermediate or greater probability of having CHD by age, symptoms, and gender. (Level of Evidence: C)

3. LV imaging can be useful in patients undergoing biventricular pacing. (Level of Evidence: C)

4.6 Electrophysiological testing

Electrophysiological (EP) testing with intracardiac recording and electrical stimulation at baseline and with drugs, has been used for arrhythmia assessment and risk stratification for SCD. EP testing is used to document inducibility of VT, guide ablation, evaluate drug effects, assess the risks of recurrent VT or SCD, evaluate loss of consciousness in selected patients with arrhythmias suspected as a cause and assess the indications for ICD therapy.

EP testing in patients with CHD

Recommendations

Class I

1. EP testing is recommended for diagnostic evaluation of patients with remote myocardial infarction (MI) with symptoms suggestive of ventricular tachyarrhythmias including palpitations, pre-syncope, and syncope. (Level of Evidence: B)

2. EP testing is recommended in patients with CHD to guide and assess efficacy of VT ablation. (Level of Evidence: B)

3. EP testing is useful in patients with CHD for the diagnostic evaluation of wide QRS-complex tachycardias of unclear mechanism. (Level of Evidence: C)

Class IIa

1. EP testing is reasonable for risk stratification in patients with remote MI, nonsustained (NSVT) and LV ejection fraction (LVEF) ≤40%. (Level of Evidence: B)

EP Testing in Patients with Syncope

Recommendations

Class I

1. EP testing is recommended in patients with syncope of unknown cause with impaired LV function or structural heart disease. (Level of Evidence: B)

2. EP testing can be useful in patients with syncope when brady-or tachyarrhythmias are suspected, and in whom non-invasive diagnostic studies are not conclusive. (Level of Evidence: B)

5. Therapies for ventricular arrhythmias

Therapies for VA include antiarrhythmic drugs (e.g., beta-blockers, amiodarone, sotalol), devices (e.g., ICDs), ablation, surgery, and revascularization. With the exception of ablation, recommendations for each of these modalities can be found within specific disease-based sections (e.g., Heart Failure) of these pocket guidelines. The recommendations for ablation therapy are described below.

5.1 Ablation

Recommendations

Class I

1. Ablation is indicated in patients who are otherwise at low risk for SCD and have sustained predominantly monomorphic VT that is drug resistant, or who are drug intolerant, or who do not wish long-term drug therapy. (Level of Evidence: C)

2. Ablation is indicated in patients with bundle-branch reentrant VT. (Level of Evidence: C)

3. Ablation is indicated as adjunctive therapy in patients with an ICD who are receiving multiple shocks as a result of sustained VT that is not manageable by reprogramming or changing drug therapy, or the patient does not wish long term drug-therapy. (Level of Evidence: C)

4. Ablation is indicated in patients with Wolff-Parkinson-White syndrome resuscitated from sudden cardiac arrest due to atrial fibrillation (AF) and rapid conduction over the accessory pathway causing ventricular fibrillation (VF). (Level of Evidence: B)

Class IIa

1. Ablation can be useful therapy in patients who are otherwise at low risk for SCD and have symptomatic nonsustained monomorphic VT that is drug resistant, or who are drug intolerant, or who do not wish long-term drug therapy. (Level of Evidence: C)

2. Ablation can be useful therapy in patients who are otherwise at low risk for SCD and have frequent symptomatic predominantly monomorphic PVCs that are drug resistant, or who are drug intolerant, or who do not wish long-term drug therapy. (Level of Evidence: C)

3. Ablation can be useful in symptomatic patients with Wolff-Parkinson-White syndrome who have accessory pathways with refractory periods less than 240 ms in duration. (Level of Evidence: B)

Class IIb

1. Ablation of Purkinje fiber potentials may be considered in patients with ventricular arrhythmia storm consistently provoked by PVCs of similar morphology.

2. Ablation of asymptomatic PVCs may be considered when the PVCs are very frequent to avoid or treat tachycardia-induced cardiomyopathy. (Level of Evidence: C)

Class III

1. Ablation of asymptomatic relatively infrequent PVCs is not indicated. (Level of Evidence: C)

6. Acute management of specific arrhythmias

6.1 Management of cardiac arrest

Recommendations

Class I

1. After establishing the presence of definite, suspected, or impending cardiac arrest, the first priority should be activation of a response team capable of identifying the specific mechanism and carrying out prompt intervention. (Level of Evidence: B)

2. Cardiopulmonary resuscitation (CPR) should be implemented immediately after contacting a response team. (Level of Evidence: A)

3. In an out of hospital setting, if an automated external defibrillator (AED) is available, it should be applied

immediately and shock therapy administered according to the algorithms contained in the documents on CPR developed by either the AHA in association with the International Liaison Committee on Resuscitation (ILCOR) and/or the European Resuscitation Council (ERC). (Level of Evidence: C)

4. For victims with ventricular tachyarrhythmic mechanisms of cardiac arrest, when recurrences occur after a maximally defibrillating shock (generally 360 Joules for monophasic defibrillators), intravenous amiodarone should be the preferred antiarrhythmic drug for attempting to achieve a stable rhythm after further defibrillations. (Level of Evidence: B)

5. For recurrent ventricular tachyarrhythmias or nontachyarrhythmic mechanisms of cardiac arrest, it is recommended to follow the algorithms contained in the documents on CPR developed by either the AHA in association with the ILCOR and/or the ERC. (Level of Evidence: C)

6. Reversible causes and factors contributing to cardiac arrest should be managed during advanced life support, including management of hypoxia, electrolyte disturbances, mechanical factors, and volume depletion. (Level of Evidence: C)

Class IIa

1. For response times ≥ 5 min, a brief (< 90 to 180 sec) period of CPR is reasonable prior to attempting defibrillation. (Level of Evidence: B)

Class IIb

1. A single precordial thump may be considered by healthcare professional providers when responding to a witnessed cardiac arrest. (Level of Evidence: C)

6.2 Ventricular tachycardia associated with low troponin MI

Recommendations

Class I

1. Patients presenting with sustained VT in whom low level elevations in cardiac biomarkers of myocyte injury/necrosis are documented, should be treated similarly to patients that have sustained VT and in whom no biomarker rise is documented. (Level of Evidence: C)

6.3 Sustained monomorphic VT

Recommendations

Class I

1. Wide-QRS tachycardia should be presumed to be VT if the diagnosis is unclear. (Level of Evidence: C)

2. Direct-current (DC) cardioversion with appropriate sedation is recommended at any point in the treatment cascade in patients with suspected sustained monomorphic VT with haemodynamic compromise. (Level of Evidence: C)

Class IIa

1. Intravenous (IV) procainamide (or ajmaline in some European countries) is reasonable for initial treatment of patients with stable sustained monomorphic VT. (Level of Evidence: B)

2. IV amiodarone is reasonable in patients with sustained monomorphic VT that is haemodynamically unstable, that is refractory to conversion with countershock, or recurrent despite procainamide or other agents. (Level of Evidence: C)

3. Transvenous catheter pace-termination can be useful to treat patients with sustained monomorphic VT that is refractory to cardioversion or is frequently recurrent despite antiarrhythmic medication. (Level of Evidence: C)

Class IIb

1. IV lidocaine might be reasonable for the initial treatment of patients with stable sustained monomorphic VT specifically associated with acute myocardial ischaemia or infarction. (Level of Evidence: C)

Class III

2. Calcium-channel blockers such as verapamil and diltiazem should not be used in patients to terminate wide QRS-complex tachycardia of unknown origin, especially in patients with a history of myocardial dysfunction. (Level of Evidence: C)

6.4 Repetitive monomorphic VT

Recommendations

Class IIa

1. IV amiodarone, beta-blockers, and IV procainamide (sotalol or ajmaline in Europe) can be useful for treating repetitive monomorphic VT in the context of CHD and idiopathic VT. (Level of Evidence: C)

6.5 Polymorphic VT

Recommendations

Class I

1. DC cardioversion with appropriate sedation as necessary is recommended for patients with sustained polymorphic VT with haemodynamic compromise and is reasonable at any point in the treatment cascade. (Level of Evidence: B)

2. IV beta-blockers are useful for patients with recurrent polymorphic VT, especially if ischaemia is suspected or cannot be excluded. (Level of Evidence: B)

3. IV loading with amiodarone is useful for patients with recurrent polymorphic VT in the absence of abnormal repolarization related to congenital or acquired QT syndrome. (Level of Evidence: C)

4. Urgent angiography with a view to revascularization should be considered for patients with polymorphic VT when myocardial ischaemia cannot be excluded. (Level of Evidence: C)

Class IIb

1. IV lidocaine may be reasonable for treatment of polymorphic VT specifically associated with acute myocardial ischaemia or infarction. (Level of Evidence: C)

6.6 Torsades de Pointes

Recommendations

Class I

1. Withdrawal of any offending drugs and correction of electrolyte abnormalities are recommended in patients presenting with torsades de pointes. (Level of Evidence: A)

2. Acute and long-term pacing is recommended for patients presenting with torsades de pointes due to heart block and symptomatic bradycardia. (Level of Evidence: A)

Class IIa

1. Management with IV magnesium sulfate is reasonable for patients who present with long QT syndrome (LQTS) and few episodes of torsades de pointes. Magnesium is not likely to be effective in patients with a normal QT interval. (Level of Evidence: B)

2. Acute and long-term pacing is reasonable for patients who present with recurrent pause-dependent torsades de pointes. (Level of Evidence: B)

3. Beta-blockade combined with pacing is reasonable acute therapy for patients who present with torsades de pointes and sinus bradycardia. (Level of Evidence: C)

4. Isoproterenol is reasonable as temporary treatment in acute patients who present with recurrent pause-dependent torsades de pointes who do not have congenital LQTS. (Level of Evidence: B)

Class IIb

1. Potassium repletion to 4.5 to 5 mM/L may be considered for patients who present with torsades de pointes. (Level of Evidence: B)

2. IV lidocaine or oral mexiletine may be considered in patients who present with LQT3 and torsades de pointes. (Level of Evidence: C)

6.7 Incessant VT

Recommendations

Class I

1. Revascularization and beta-blockade, followed by antiarrhythmic drugs such as IV procainamide or IV amiodarone are recommended for patients with recurrent or incessant polymorphic VT due to acute myocardial ischaemia. (Level of Evidence: C)

Class IIa

1. IV amiodarone or procainamide followed by VT ablation can be effective in the management of patients with frequently recurring or incessant monomorphic VT. (Level of Evidence: B)

Class IIb

1. IV amiodarone and IV beta-blockers separately or together may be reasonable in patients with VT storm. (Level of Evidence: C)

2. Overdrive pacing or general anesthesia may be considered for patients with frequently recurring or incessant VT. (Level of Evidence: C)

3. Spinal cord modulation may be considered for some patients with frequently recurring or incessant VT. (Level of Evidence: C)

7. Ventricular arrhythmia and sudden cardiac death related to specific pathology

7.1 Left ventricular dysfunction due to prior MI

Recommendations

Class I

1. Aggressive attempts should be made to treat heart failure (HF) that may be present in some patients with LV dysfunction (LVD) due to prior MI and ventricular tachyarrhythmias. (Level of Evidence: C)

2. Aggressive attempts should be made to treat myocardial ischaemia that may be present in some patients with ventricular tachyarrhythmias. (Level of Evidence: C)

3. Coronary revascularization is indicated to reduce the risk of SCD in patients with VF when direct, clear evidence of acute myocardial ischaemia is documented to immediately precede the onset of VF. (Level of Evidence: B)

4. If coronary revascularization cannot be carried out, and there is evidence of prior MI and significant LVD, the primary therapy of patients resuscitated from VF should be the ICD in patients who are receiving chronic optimal medical therapy, and who have reasonable expectation of survival with a good functional status for more than 1 year. (Level of Evidence: A)

5. ICD therapy is recommended for primary prevention to reduce total mortality by a reduction in SCD in patients with LVD due to prior MI who are at least 40 days post-MI, have an LVEF ≤30% to 40%, are New York Heart Association (NYHA) functional class II or III, are receiving chronic optimal medical therapy, and who have reasonable expectation of survival with a good functional status for more than 1 year. (Level of Evidence: A)

6. The ICD is effective therapy to reduce mortality by a reduction in SCD in patients with LVD due to prior MI who present with haemodynamically unstable sustained VT, who are receiving chronic optimal medical therapy, and who have reasonable expectation of survival with a good functional status for more than 1 year. (Level of Evidence: A)

Class IIa

1. Implantation of an ICD is reasonable in patients with LVD due to prior MI who are at least 40 days post-MI, have an LVEF of ≤30% to 35%, are NYHA functional class I on chronic optimal medical therapy, and who have reasonable expectation of survival with a good functional status for more than 1 year. (Level of Evidence: B)

2. Amiodarone, often in combination with beta-blockers, can be useful for patients with LVD due to prior MI and symptoms due to VT unresponsive to beta-adrenergic blocking agents. (Level of Evidence: B)

3. Sotalol is reasonable therapy to reduce symptoms resulting from VT for patients with LVD due to prior MI unresponsive to beta-blocking agents. (Level of Evidence: C)

4. Adjunctive therapies to the ICD, including catheter ablation or surgical resection, and pharmacological therapy with agents such as amiodarone or sotalol are reasonable to improve symptoms due to frequent episodes of sustained VT or VF in patients with LVD due to prior MI. (Level of Evidence: C)

5. Amiodarone is reasonable therapy to reduce symptoms due to recurrent haemodynamically stable VT for patients with LVD due to prior MI who cannot or refuse to have an ICD implanted. (Level of Evidence: C)

6. ICD implantation is reasonable for treatment of recurrent sustained VT in patients post-MI with normal or near normal ventricular function who are receiving chronic optimal medical therapy, and who have reasonable expectation of survival with a good functional status for more than 1 year. (Level of Evidence: C)

Class IIb

1. Curative catheter ablation or amiodarone may be considered in lieu of ICD therapy to improve symptoms in patients with LVD due to prior MI and recurrent haemodynamically stable VT whose LVEF is > 40%. (Level of Evidence: B)

2. Amiodarone may be reasonable therapy for patients with LVD due to prior MI with an ICD indication, as defined above, in patients who cannot, or refuse to have an ICD implanted. (Level of Evidence: C)

Class III

1. Prophylactic antiarrhythmic drug therapy is not indicated to reduce mortality in patients with asymptomatic nonsustained VA. (Level of Evidence: B)

2. Class IC antiarrhythmic drugs in patients with a past history of MI should not be used. (Level of Evidence: A)

7.2 Valvular Heart Disease

Recommendations

Class I

1. Patients with valvular heart disease and VA should be evaluated and treated following current recommendations for each disorder. (Level of Evidence: C)

Class IIb

1. The effectiveness of mitral valve repair or replacement to reduce the risk of SCD in patients with mitral valve prolapse, severe mitral regurgitation and serious VA is not well established. (Level of Evidence: C)

7.3 Congenital heart disease

Recommendations

Class I

1. ICD implantation is indicated in patients with congenital heart disease who are survivors of cardiac arrest after evaluation to define the cause of the event and exclude any reversible causes. ICD implantation is indicated in patients who are receiving chronic optimal medical therapy, and who have reasonable expectation of survival with a good functional status for more than 1 year. (Level of Evidence: B)

2. Patients with congenital heart disease and spontaneous sustained VT should undergo invasive haemodynamic and EP evaluation. Recommended therapy includes catheter ablation or surgical resection to eliminate the VT. If that is not successful, ICD implantation is recommended. (Level of Evidence: C)

Class IIa

1. Invasive haemodynamic and EP evaluation is reasonable in patients with congenital heart disease and unexplained syncope and impaired ventricular function. In the absence of a defined and reversible cause, ICD implantation is reasonable in patients who are receiving chronic optimal medical therapy, and who have reasonable expectation of survival with a good functional status for more than 1 year. (Level of Evidence: B)

Class IIb

1. EP testing may be considered for patients with congenital heart disease and ventricular couplets or NSVT to determine the risk of a sustained VA. (Level of Evidence: C)

Class III

1. Prophylactic antiarrhythmic therapy is not indicated for asymptomatic patients with congenital heart disease and isolated PVCs. (Level of Evidence: C)

7.4 Pericardial diseases

Recommendations

Class I

1. VA that develop in patients with pericardial disease should be treated in the same manner that such arrhythmias are treated in patients with other diseases, including ICD pacemaker implantation as required. Patients receiving ICD implantation should be receiving chronic optimal medical therapy, and have reasonable expectation of survival with a good functional status for more than 1 year. (Level of Evidence: C)

7.5 Pulmonary arterial hypertension

Recommendations

Class III

1. Prophylactic antiarrhythmic therapy generally is not indicated for primary prevention of SCD in patients with pulmonary arterial hypertension or other pulmonary conditions. (Level of Evidence: C)

7.6 Transient Arrhythmias of Reversible Cause

Recommendations

Class I

1. Myocardial revascularization should be performed, when appropriate, to reduce the risk of SCD in patients experiencing cardiac arrest due to VF or polymorphic VT in the setting of acute ischaemia or myocardial infarction. (Level of Evidence: C)

2. Unless electrolyte abnormalities are proven to be the cause, survivors of cardiac arrest due to VF or polymorphic VT in whom electrolyte abnormalities are discovered, in general should be evaluated and treated in a similar manner as survivors of cardiac arrest without electrolyte abnormalities. (Level of Evidence: C)

3. Patients who experience sustained monomorphic VT in the presence of antiarrhythmic drugs or electrolyte abnormalities should be evaluated and treated in a manner similar to that of patients with VT without electrolyte abnormalities or antiarrhythmic drugs present. Antiarrhythmic drugs or electrolyte abnormalities should not be assumed to be the sole cause of sustained monomorphic VT. (Level of Evidence: B)

4. Patients who experience polymorphic VT in association with prolonged QT interval due to antiarrhythmic medications or other drugs should be advised to avoid exposure to all agents associated with QT prolongation. A list of such drugs can be found on the web sites www.qtdrugs.org and www.torsades.org. (Level of Evidence: B)

8. Ventricular arrhythmias associated with cardiomyopathies

8.1 Dilated Cardiomyopathy (DCM) (Nonischaemic)

Recommendations

Class I

1. EP testing is useful to diagnose bundle branch-reentrant tachycardia, and to guide ablation in patients with nonischaemic DCM. (Level of Evidence: C)

2. EP testing is useful for diagnostic evaluation in patients with nonischaemic DCM with sustained palpitations, wide QRS-complex tachycardia, syncope or presyncope. (Level of Evidence: C)

3. An ICD should be implanted in patients with nonischaemic DCM and significant LVD who have sustained VT or VF, who are receiving chronic optimal medical therapy, and who have reasonable expectation of survival with a good functional status for more than 1 year. (Level of Evidence: A)

4. ICD therapy is recommended for primary prevention to reduce total mortality by a reduction in SCD in patients with nonischaemic DCM who have an LVEF ≤30% to 35%, are NYHA functional class II or III receiving chronic optimal medical therapy, and who have reasonable expectation of survival with a good functional status for more than 1 year. (Level of Evidence: B)

Class IIa

1. ICD implantation can be beneficial for patients with unexplained syncope, significant LVD, and nonischaemic DCM who are receiving chronic optimal medical therapy, and who have reasonable expectation of survival with a good functional status for more than 1 year. (Level of Evidence: C)

2. ICD implantation can be effective for termination of sustained VT in patients with normal or near normal ventricular function and nonischaemic DCM who are receiving chronic optimal medical therapy, and who have reasonable expectation of survival with a good functional status for more than 1 year. (Level of Evidence: C)

Class IIb

1. Amiodarone may be considered for sustained VT or VF in patients with nonischaemic DCM. (Level of Evidence: C)

2. Placement of an ICD might be considered in patients who have nonischaemic DCM, LVEF ≤30% to 35%, are NYHA functional class I receiving chronic optimal medical therapy, and who have reasonable expectation of survival with a good functional status for more than 1 year. (Level of Evidence: C)

8.2 Hypertrophic Cardiomyopathy (HCM)

Recommendations

Class I

1. ICD therapy should be used for treatment in patients with HCM who have sustained VT and/or VF and who are receiving chronic optimal medical therapy, and who have reasonable expectation of survival with a

Table 4. Risk Factors for SCD in Hypertrophic Cardiomyopathy

Major risk factors	Possible in individual patients
Cardiac arrest (VF)	AF
Spontaneous sustained VT	Myocardial ischaemia
Family history of premature sudden death	LV outflow obstruction
Unexplained syncope	High-risk mutation
LV thickness greater than or equal to 30 mm	Intense (competitive) physical exertion
Abnormal exercise BP	
Nonsustained spontaneous VT	

Modified with permission from Maron BJ, McKenna WJ, Danielson GK, et al. American College of Cardiology/European Society of Cardiology clinical expert consensus document on hypertrophic cardiomyopathy. A report of the American College of Cardiology Foundation Task Force on Clinical Expert Consensus Documents and the European Society of Cardiology Committee for Practice Guidelines. Eur Heart J 2003;24: 1965-1991.

AF = atrial fibrillation; BP = blood pressure; LV = left ventricular; SCD = sudden cardiac death; VF = ventricular fibrillation; VT = ventricular tachycardia.

good functional status for more than 1 year. (Level of Evidence: B)

Class IIa

1. ICD implantation can be effective for primary prophylaxis against SCD in patients with HCM who have one or more major risk factor (See Table 4) for SCD and who are receiving chronic optimal medical therapy, and who have reasonable expectation of survival with a good functional status for more than 1 year. (Level of Evidence: C)

2. Amiodarone therapy can be effective for treatment in patients with HCM with a history of sustained VT and/or VF when ICD is not feasible. (Level of Evidence: C)

Class IIb

1. EP testing may be considered for risk assessment for SCD in patients with HCM. (Level of Evidence: C)

2. Amiodarone may be considered for primary prophylaxis against SCD in patients with HCM who have one or more major risk factor for SCD (See Table 4), if ICD implantation is not feasible. (Level of Evidence: C)

8.3 Arrhythmogenic right ventricular cardiomyopathy

Recommendations

Class II

1. ICD implantation is recommended for prevention of SCD in patients with arrhythmogenic RV cardiomyopathy (ARVC) with documented sustained VT or VF who are receiving chronic optimal medical therapy, and who have reasonable expectation of survival with a good functional status for more than 1 year. (Level of Evidence: B)

Class IIa

1. ICD implantation can be effective for prevention of SCD in patients with ARVC with extensive disease, including those with LV involvement, one or more affected family member with SCD, or undiagnosed syncope when VT/VF has not been excluded as the cause of syncope, who are receiving chronic optimal medical therapy, and who have reasonable expectation of survival with a good functional status for more than 1 year. (Level of Evidence: C)

2. Amiodarone or sotalol can be effective for treatment of sustained VT/VF in patients with ARVC when ICD implantation is not feasible. (Level of Evidence: C)

3. Ablation can be useful as adjunctive therapy in management of patients with ARVC with recurrent VT, despite optimal anti-arrhythmic drug therapy. (Level of Evidence: C)

Class IIb

1. EP testing might be useful for risk assessment of SCD in patients with ARVC. (Level of Evidence: C)

9. Heart failure

Recommendations

Class I

1. ICD therapy is recommended for secondary prevention of SCD in patients who survived VF or haemodynamically unstable VT, or VT with syncope and have an LVEF ≤40%, who are receiving chronic optimal medical therapy and who have a reasonable expectation of survival with a good functional status for more than 1 year. (Level of Evidence: A)

2. ICD therapy is recommended for primary prevention to reduce total mortality by a reduction in SCD in patients with LVD due to prior MI who are at least 40 days post-MI, have an LVEF ≤30% to 40%, are NYHA functional class II or III receiving chronic optimal medical therapy, and who have reasonable expectation of survival with a good functional status for more than 1 year. (Level of Evidence: A)

3. ICD therapy is recommended for primary prevention to reduce total mortality by a reduction in SCD in patients with nonischaemic heart disease who have an LVEF ≤30% to 35%, are NYHA functional class II or III receiving chronic optimal medical therapy, and who have reasonable expectation of survival with a good functional status for more than 1 year. (Level of Evidence: B)

4. Amiodarone, sotalol and/or other beta-blockers are recommended pharmacological adjuncts to ICD therapy to suppress symptomatic ventricular tachyarrhythmias (both sustained and nonsustained) in otherwise optimally treated patients with heart failure (HF). (Level of Evidence: C)

5. Amiodarone is indicated for the suppression of acute haemodynamically compromising ventricular or supraventricular tachyarrhythmias when cardioversion and/or correction of reversible causes has failed to terminate the arrhythmia or prevent its early recurrence. (Level of Evidence: B)

Class IIa

1. ICD therapy combined with biventricular pacing can be effective for primary prevention to reduce total mortality by a reduction in SCD, in patients with NYHA functional class III or IV receiving optimal medical therapy, in sinus rhythm with a QRS complex of at least 120ms and who have reasonable expectation of survival with a good functional status for more than 1 year. (Level of Evidence: B)

2. ICD therapy is reasonable for primary prevention to reduce total mortality by a reduction in SCD in patients with LVD due to prior MI who are at least 40 days post-MI, have an LVEF of ≤30% to 35%, are NYHA functional class I receiving chronic optimal medical therapy, and have reasonable expectation of survival with a good functional status for more than 1 year. (Level of Evidence: B)

3. ICD therapy is reasonable in patients with recurrent stable VT, a normal or near normal LVEF and optimally treated HF, and who have a reasonable expectation of survival with a good functional status for more than 1 year. (Level of Evidence: C)

4. Biventricular pacing in the absence of ICD therapy is reasonable for the prevention of SCD in patients with NYHA functional class III or IV HF, an LVEF ≤35% and a QRS complex 3160ms (or at least 120ms in the presence of other evidence of ventricular dyssynchrony) who are receiving chronic optimal medical therapy and who have reasonable expectation of survival with a good functional status for more than 1 year. (Level of Evidence: B)

Class IIb

1. Amiodarone, sotalol and/or beta-blockers may be considered as pharmacological alternatives to ICD therapy to suppress symptomatic ventricular tachyarrhythmias (both sustained and nonsustained) in optimally treated patients with HF for whom ICD therapy is not feasible. (Level of Evidence: C)

2. ICD therapy may be considered for primary prevention to reduce total mortality by a reduction in SCD in patients with nonischaemic heart disease who have an LVEF of ≤30% to 35%, are NYHA functional class I receiving chronic optimal medical therapy, and who have a reasonable expectation of survival with a good functional status for more than 1 year. (Level of Evidence: B)

10. Genetic arrhythmia syndromes

10.1 Long QT syndrome

Recommendations

Class I

1. Life style modification (see full-text guidelines) is recommended for patients with an LQTS diagnosis (clinical and/or molecular). (Level of Evidence: B)

2. Beta-blockers are recommended for patients with an LQTS clinical diagnosis (i.e., in the presence of prolonged QT interval). (Level of Evidence: B)

3. Implantation of an ICD along with use of beta-blockers is recommended for LQTS patients with previous cardiac arrest and who have reasonable expectation of survival with a good functional status for more than 1 year. (Level of Evidence: A)

Class IIa

1. Beta-blockers can be effective to reduce SCD in patients with a molecular LQTS analysis and normal QT interval. (Level of Evidence: B)

2. Implantation of an ICD with continued use of beta-blockers can be effective to reduce SCD in LQTS patients who are experiencing syncope and/or VT while receiving beta-blockers and who have reasonable expectation of survival with a good functional status for more than 1 year. (Level of Evidence: B)

Class IIb

1. Left cardiac sympathetic neural denervation may be considered for LQTS patients with syncope, torsades de pointes, or cardiac arrest while receiving beta-blockers. (Level of Evidence: B)

2. Implantation of an ICD with use of beta-blockers may be considered for prophylaxis of SCD for patients who are in categories possibly associated with higher risk of cardiac arrest such as LQT2 and LQT3, and who have reasonable expectation of survival with a good functional status for more than 1 year. (Level of Evidence: B)

10.2 Brugada Syndrome

Recommendations

Class I

1. An ICD is indicated for Brugada syndrome patients with previous cardiac arrest receiving chronic optimal medical therapy and who have reasonable expectation of survival with a good functional status for more than 1 year. (Level of Evidence: C)

Class IIa

1. An ICD is reasonable for Brugada syndrome patients with spontaneous ST-segment elevation in V1, V2, or V3 who have had syncope with or without mutations demonstrated in the SCN5A gene and who have reasonable expectation of survival with a good functional status for more than 1 year. (Level of Evidence: C)

2. Clinical monitoring for the development of a spontaneous ST-segment elevation pattern is reasonable for the management of patients with ST-segment elevation induced only with provocative pharmacological challenge with or without symptoms. (Level of Evidence: C)

3. An ICD is reasonable for Brugada syndrome patients with documented VT that has not resulted in cardiac arrest and who have reasonable expectation of survival with a good functional status for more than 1 year. (Level of Evidence: C)

4. Isoproterenol can be useful to treat an electrical storm in the Brugada syndrome. (Level of Evidence: C)

Class IIb

1. EP testing may be considered for risk stratification in asymptomatic Brugada syndrome patients with spontaneous ST-segment elevation with or without a mutation in the SCN5A gene. (Level of Evidence: C)

2. Quinidine might be reasonable for the treatment of electrical storm in patients with Brugada syndrome. (Level of Evidence: C)

10.3 Catecholaminergic polymorphic ventricular tachycardia

Recommendations

Class I

1. Beta-blockers are indicated for patients who are clinically diagnosed with catecholaminergic polymorphic VT (CPVT) based on the presence of spontaneous or documented stress-induced VA. (Level of Evidence: C)

2. Implantation of an ICD with use of beta-blockers is indicated for patients with CPVT who are survivors of cardiac arrest and who have reasonable expectation of survival with a good functional status for more than 1 year. (Level of Evidence: C)

Class IIa

1. Beta-blockers can be effective in patients without clinical manifestations when the diagnosis of CPVT is established during childhood based on genetic analysis. (Level of Evidence: C)

2. Implantation of an ICD with use of beta-blockers can be effective for affected patients with CPVT with syncope and/or documented sustained VT who are receiving beta- blockers and who have reasonable expectation of survival with a good functional status for more than 1 year. (Level of Evidence: C)

Class IIb

1. Beta-blockers may be considered for patients with CPVT who were genetically diagnosed in adulthood and never manifested clinical symptoms of tachyarrhythmias. (Level of Evidence: C)

11. Ventricular arrhythmias and sudden cardiac death related to specific populations

11.1 Athletes

Recommendations

Class I

1. Pre-participation history and physical examination, including family history of premature or sudden death and specific evidence of cardiovascular diseases such as cardiomyopathies and ion channel abnormalities is recommended in athletes. (Level of Evidence: C)

2. Athletes presenting with rhythm disorders, structural heart disease, or other signs or symptoms suspicious for cardiovascular disorders, should be evaluated as any other patient but recognizing the potential uniqueness of their activity. (Level of Evidence: C)

3. Athletes presenting with syncope should be carefully evaluated to uncover underlying cardiovascular disease or rhythm disorder. (Level of Evidence: B)

4. Athletes with serious symptoms should cease competition while cardiovascular abnormalities are being fully evaluated. (Level of Evidence: C)

Class IIb

1. 12-lead ECG and possibly echocardiography may be considered as pre-participation screening for heart disorders in athletes. (Level of Evidence: B)

11.2 Gender and pregnancy

Recommendations

Class I

1. Pregnant women developing haemodynamically unstable VT or VF should be electrically cardioverted or defibrillated. (Level of Evidence: B)

2. In pregnant women with LQTS who have had symptoms, it is beneficial to continue beta-blocker medications throughout pregnancy and afterwards, unless there are definite contraindications. (Level of Evidence: C)

11.3 Elderly patients

Recommendations

Class I

1. Elderly patients with VA should generally be treated in the same manner as younger individuals. (Level of Evidence: A)

2. The dosing and titration schedule of antiarrhythmic drugs prescribed to elderly patients should be adjusted to the altered pharmacokinetics of such patients. (Level of Evidence: C)

Class III

1. Elderly patients with projected life expectancy less than 1 year due to major comorbidities should not receive ICD therapy. (Level of Evidence: C)

Despite the demonstrated efficacy in reducing all-cause mortality and SCD, beta-blockers are underused in the elderly. Several randomized prospective trials have demonstrated the efficacy of ICDs in primary and secondary prevention of SCD when compared with antiarrhythmic drug therapy, across all age groups.

11.4 Patients with ICDs

Recommendations

Class I

1. Patients with implanted ICDs should receive regular follow-up and analysis of the device status. (Level of Evidence: C)

2. Implanted ICDs should be programmed to obtain optimal sensitivity and specificity. (Level of Evidence: C)

3. Measures should be undertaken to minimize the risk of inappropriate ICD therapies. (Level of Evidence: C)

4. Patients with implanted ICDs who present with incessant VT should be hospitalized for management. (Level of Evidence: C)

Class IIa

1. Catheter ablation can be useful for patients with implanted ICDs who experience incessant or frequently recurring VT. (Level of Evidence: B)

2. In patients experiencing inappropriate ICD therapy, electrophysiologic evaluation can be useful for

diagnostic and therapeutic purposes. (Level of Evidence: C)

11.5 Drug-induced arrhythmias

Digitalis Toxicity

Recommendations

Class I

1. An anti-digitalis antibody is recommended for patients who present with sustained ventricular arrhythmias, advanced AV block, and/or asystole that are considered due to digitalis toxicity. (Level of Evidence: A)

Class IIa

1. Patients taking digitalis who present with mild cardiac toxicity (e.g., isolated ectopic beats only), can be managed effectively with recognition, continuous monitoring of cardiac rhythm, withdrawal of digitalis, restoration of normal electrolyte levels (including serum potassium > 4 mM/L) and oxygenation. (Level of Evidence: C)

2. Magnesium or pacing is reasonable for patients who take digitalis and present with severe toxicity.* (Level of Evidence: C)

Class IIb

1. Dialysis for the management of hyperkalemia may be considered for patients who take digitalis and present with severe toxicity (sustained VA, advanced AV block, and/or asystole). (Level of Evidence: C)

Class III

1. Management by lidocaine or phenytoin is not recommended for patients taking digitalis and who present with severe toxicity (sustained VA, advanced AV block, and/or asystole). (Level of Evidence: C)

Drug-induced LQTS

Recommendations

Class I

1. In patients with drug-induced LQTS, removal of the offending agent is indicated. (Level of Evidence: A)

Class IIa

1. Management with IV magnesium sulfate is reasonable for patients who take QT-prolonging drugs and present with few episodes of torsades de pointes in which the QT remains long. (Level of Evidence: B)

2. Atrial or ventricular pacing or isoproterenol is reasonable for patients taking QT-prolonging drugs who present with recurrent torsades de pointes. (Level of Evidence: B)

Class IIb

1. Potassium ion repletion to 4.5 to 5 mmol/L may be reasonable for patients who take QT-prolonging drugs and present with few episodes of torsades de pointes in whom the QT remains long. (Level of Evidence: C)

Sodium channel blocker-related toxicity

Recommendations

Class I

1. In patients with sodium channel blocker-related toxicity, removal of the offending agent is indicated. (Level of Evidence: A)

Class IIa

1. Stopping the drug, reprogramming the pacemaker or repositioning leads can be useful in patients taking sodium-channel blockers who present with elevated defibrillation thresholds or pacing requirement. (Level of Evidence: C)

2. In patients taking sodium-channel blockers who present with atrial flutter with 1:1 AV conduction, withdrawal of the offending agent is reasonable. If the drug needs to be continued, additional A-V nodal blockade with diltiazem, verapamil or beta-blocker or atrial flutter ablation can be effective. (Level of Evidence: C)

Class IIb

1. Administration of a beta-blocker and a sodium bolus may be considered for patients taking sodium-channel blockers if the tachycardia becomes more frequent or more difficult to cardiovert. (Level of Evidence: C)

Arrhythmias caused by sodium channel-blocking drugs and other drugs are included in Table 5.

Table 5. Syndromes of Drug-Induced Arrhythmia and their Management

Drugs	Clinical setting	Management*
Digitalis	Mild cardiac toxicity (isolated arrhythmias only)	
	Severe toxicity: Sustained ventricular arrhythmias; advanced AV block; asystole	Anti digitalis antibody Pacing Dialysis for hyperkalemia
QT prolonging drugs	Torsades de pointes: few episodes, QT remains long	IV magnesium sulfate ($MgSO_4$)
		Replete potassium (K^+) to 4.5 to 5 mEq/L
	Recurrent torsades de pointes	Ventricular pacing
		Isoproterenol
Sodium channel blockers	Elevated defibrillation or pacing requirement	Stop drug; reposition leads
	Atrial flutter with 1:1 AV conduction	Diltiazem, verapamil, beta blocker (IV)
	Ventricular tachycardia (more frequent; difficult to cardiovert)	Beta blocker; sodium
	Brugada syndrome	Stop drug; treat arrhythmia

*Always includes recognition, continuous monitoring of cardiac rhythm, withdrawal of offending agents, restoration of normal electrolytes (including serum potassium to greater than 4 mEq/L) and oxygenation. Order of management is not meant to represent the preferred sequence when more than one treatment is listed. AV = atrioventricular; IV = intravenous.

Chapter 5

Cardiac Pacing and Cardiac Resynchronization Therapy*

2007

Developed in collaboration with the European Heart Rhythm Association

Chairperson:
Panos E. Vardas
Department of Cardiology
Heraklion University Hospital
P.O. Box 1352 Stavrakia
GR-711 10 Heraklion
Crete, Greece
Phone: +30 2810 392706
Fax: +30 2810 542 055
Email: cardio@med.uoc.gr

Task Force Members:

1. Angelo Auricchio, Lugano, Switzerland
2. Jean-Jacques Blanc, Brest, France
3. Jean-Claude Daubert, Rennes, France
4. Helmut Drexler, Hannover, Germany
5. Hugo Ector, Leuven, Belgium
6. Maurizio Gasparini, Milano, Italy
7. Cecilia Linde, Stockholm, Sweden
8. Francisco Bello Morgado, Lisboa, Portugal
9. Ali Oto, Ankara, Turkey
10. Richard Sutton, London, UK
11. Maria Trusz-Gluza, Katowice, Poland

ESC Staff:
1. Keith McGregor, Sophia Antipolis, France
2. Veronica Dean, Sophia Antipolis, France
3. Catherine Després, Sophia Antipolis, France

Introduction

The guidelines for the appropriate use of pacemaker devices presented in this document, a joint ESC and EHRA initiative, aim to provide for the first time in Europe an up to date specialists' view of the field. The guidelines cover two main areas: the first includes permanent pacing in bradyarrhythmias, syncope, and other specific conditions, while the second refers to ventricular resynchronization as an adjunct therapy in patients with heart failure.

The reader should note that the recommendations, text, figures, and tables included in these pocket guidelines represent a succinct summary of the more extensive evidence base, critical evaluation, supporting text, tables, figures, and references that are included in the full-text guidelines. Readers are strongly encouraged to refer to the full-text guidelines.

Classification of Recommendations and Level of Evidence are expressed in the European Society of Cardiology (ESC) format as follows:

Class I	**Evidence and/or general agreement that a given treatment or procedure is beneficial, useful and effective**
Class II	**Conflicting evidence and/or a divergence of opinion about the usefulness/efficacy of a given treatment or procedure**
Class IIa	**Weight of evidence/opinion is in favour of usefulness/efficacy**
Class IIb	**Usefulness/efficacy is less well established by evidence/opinion**
Class III	**Evidence or general agreement that the given treatment or procedure is not useful/effective and in some cases may be harmful**

*Adapted from the 2007 Guidelines for Cardiac Pacing and Cardiac Resynchronization Therapy (European Heart Journal 2007;28:2256-2295).

Levels of evidence

Level of Evidence A	**Data derived from multiple randomized clinical trials or meta-analyses**
Level of Evidence B	**Data derived from a single randomized clinical trial or large non-randomized studies**
Level of Evidence C	**Consensus of opinion of the experts and/or small studies, retrospective studies, registries**

*Recommendations for ESC Guidelines Production at www.escardio.org.

1. Pacing in arrhythmias

1.1. Sinus node disease

Recommendations for cardiac pacing in sinus node disease

Class	Clinical Indication	Level of evidence
Class I	1. Sinus node disease manifests as symptomatic bradycardia with or without bradycardia-dependant tachycardia. Symptom-rhythm correlation must have been: ▪ spontaneously occurring ▪ drug-induced where alternative drug therapy is lacking. 2. Syncope with sinus node disease, either spontaneously occurring or induced at electrophysiological study. 3. Sinus node disease manifests as symptomatic chronotropic incompetence: ▪ spontaneously occurring ▪ drug-induced where alternative drug therapy is lacking.	**C**
Class IIa	1. Symptomatic sinus node disease, which is either spontaneous or induced by a drug for which there is no alternative but no symptom rhythm correlation has been documented. Heart rate at rest should be < 40 bpm. 2. Syncope for which no other explanation can be made but there are abnormal electrophysiological findings (CSNRT > 800 ms).	**C**
Class IIb	1. Minimally symptomatic patients with sinus node disease, resting heart rate < 40 bpm while awake and no evidence of chronotropic incompetence.	**C**
Class III	1. Sinus node disease without symptoms including use of bradycardia-provoking drugs. 2. ECG findings of sinus node dysfunction with symptoms not due directly or indirectly to bradycardia. 3. Symptomatic sinus node dysfunction where symptoms can reliably be attributed to non-essential medication.	**C**

Note: when sinus node disease is diagnosed atrial tachyarrhythmias are likely even if not yet recorded, implying that serious consideration should be given to anticoagulant therapy.

1.2. Atrioventricular and intraventricular conduction disturbances

Recommendations for cardiac pacing in acquired atrioventricular block

Class	Clinical Indication	Level of evidence
Class I	1. Chronic symptomatic third or second degree (Mobitz I or II) atrioventricular block. 2. Neuromuscular diseases (e.g. myotonic muscular dystrophy, Kearns-Sayre syndrome etc.) with third-degree or second-degree atrioventricular block. 3. Third or second degree (Mobitz I or II) atrioventricular block: a) after catheter ablation of the atrioventricular junction b) after valve surgery when the block is not expected to resolve	**C** **B** **C**
Class IIa	1. Asymptomatic third or second degree (Mobitz I or II) atrioventricular block. 2. Symptomatic prolonged first degree atrioventricular block.	**C** **C**
Class IIb	1. Neuromuscular diseases (e.g. myotonic muscular dystrophy, Kearns-Sayre syndrome, etc.) with first degree atrioventricular block.	**B**
Class III	1. Asymptomatic first degree atrioventricular block. 2. Asymptomatic second degree Mobitz I with supra-Hisianconduction block. 3. Atrioventricular block expected to resolve.	**C** **C** **C**

Figure 1. Pacemaker mode selection in sinus node disease

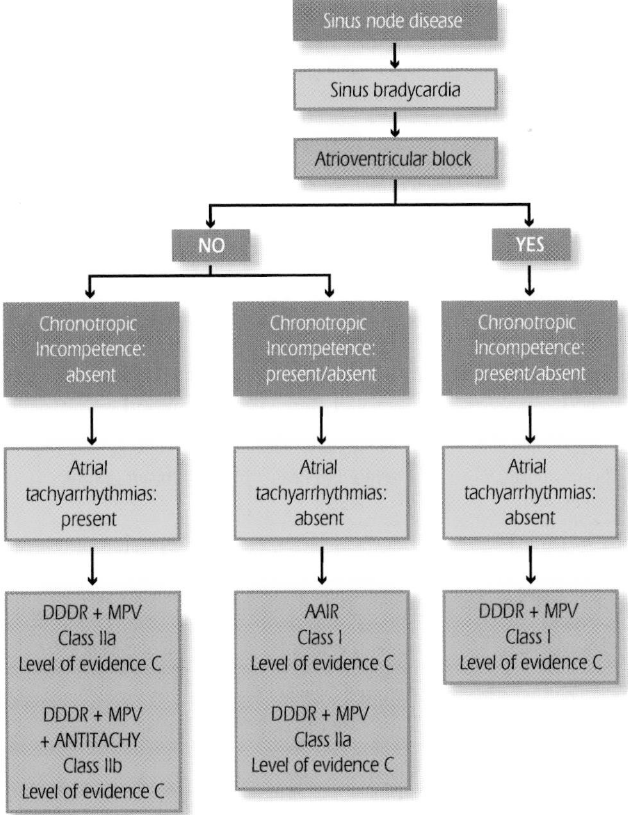

ANTITACHY = antitachycardia algorithms in pacemaker; MPV = minimisation of pacing in the ventricles.

Note: In sinus node disease VVIR and VDDR modes are considered unsuitable and are not recommended. Where Atrioventricular block exists AAIR is considered inappropriate.

Recommendations for cardiac pacing in chronic bifascicular and trifascicular block.

Class	Clinical Indication	Level of evidence
Class I	1. Intermittent third degree atrioventricular block. 2. Second degree Mobitz II atrioventricular block. 3. Alternating bundle-branch block. 4. Findings on electrophysiological study of markedly prolonged HV interval (≥ 100 ms) or pacing- induced infra-His block in patients with symptoms.	**C**
Class IIa	1. Syncope not demonstrated to be due to atrioventricular block when other likely causes have been excluded, specifically ventricular tachycardia. 2. Neuromuscular diseases (e.g. myotonic muscular dystrophy, Kearns-Sayre syndrome, etc.) with any degree of fascicular block. 3. Incidental findings on electrophysiological study of markedly prolonged HV interval (≥ 100 ms) or pacing- induced infra-His block in patients without symptoms.	**B** **C** **C**
Class IIb	None.	
Class III	1. Bundle branch block without atrioventricular block or symptoms. 2. Bundle branch block with first-degree atrioventricular block without symptoms.	**B**

Figure 2. Pacemaker mode selection in acquired atrioventricular block, chronic bifascicular and trifascicular block

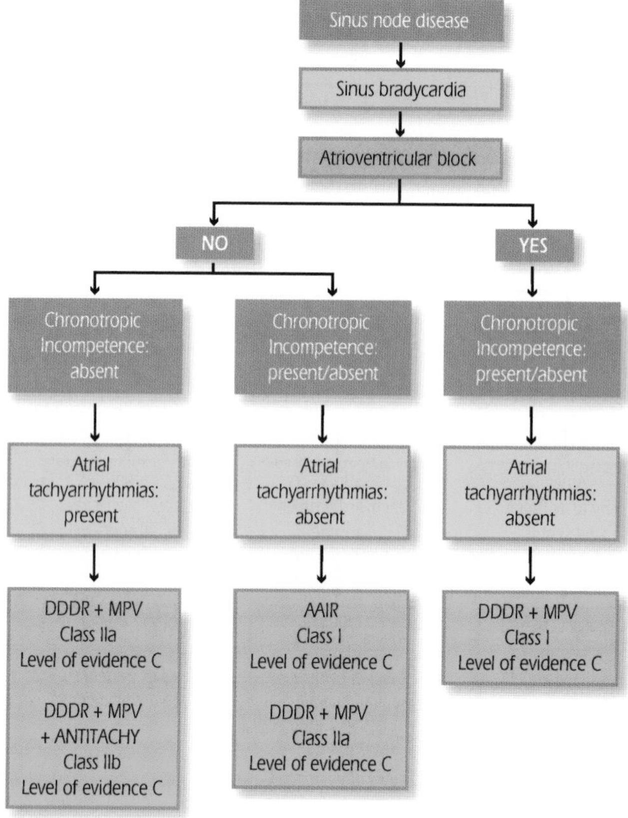

When atrioventricular block is not permanent, pacemakers with algorithms for preservation of native atrioventricular conduction should be selected.

* VVIR could be an alternative, especially in patients who have a low level of physical activity and in those with a short expected lifespan.

1.3. Recent myocardial infarction

Recommendations for permanent cardiac pacing in conduction disturbances related to acute myocardial infarction

Class	Clinical Indication	Level of evidence
Class I	1. Persistent third degree heart block preceded or not by intraventricular conduction disturbances. 2. Persistent Mobitz type II second degree heart block associated with bundle branch block, with or without PR prolongation. 3. Transient Mobitz type II second or third degree heart block associated with new onset bundle branch block.	**B**
Class IIa	None.	
Class IIb	None.	
Class III	1. Transient second or third degree heart block without bundle branch block. 2. Left anterior hemiblock newly developed or present on admission. 3. Persistent first degree atrioventricular block.	**B**

1.4. Reflex syncope

The main causes of reflex syncope

▪ Vasovagal syncope (common faint)
▪ Carotid sinus syncope
▪ Situational syncope: acute haemorrhage (or acute fluid depletion) cough, sneeze gastrointestinal stimulation (swallowing, defecation, visceral pain) micturition (post-micturition) post-exercise post-prandial others (e.g. brass instrument playing, weightlifting)
▪ Glossopharyngeal neuralgia

Recommendations for cardiac pacing in carotid sinus syndrome

Class	Clinical Indication	Level of evidence
Class I	1. Recurrent syncope caused by inadvertent carotid sinus pressure and reproduced by carotid sinus massage, associated with ventricular asystole of more than three seconds' duration (patient may be syncopal or presyncopal), in the absence of medication known to depress sinus node activity.	**C**
Class IIa	1. Recurrent unexplained syncope, without clear inadvertent carotid sinus pressure, but syncope is reproduced by carotid sinus massage, associated with a ventricular asystole of more than three seconds' duration (patient may be syncopal or presyncopal), in the absence of medication known to depress sinus node activity.	**B**
Class IIb	1. First syncope, with or without clear inadvertent carotid sinus pressure, but syncope (or pre-syncope) is reproduced by carotid sinus massage, associated with a ventricular asystole of more than three seconds' duration, in the absence of medicationknown to depress sinus node activity.	**C**
Class III	1. Hypersensitive carotid sinus reflex without symptoms.	**C**

Recommendations for cardiac pacing in vasovagal syncope

Class	Clinical Indication	Level of evidence
Class I	None.	
Class IIa	1. Patients over 40 years of age with recurrent severe vasovagal syncope who show prolonged asystole during ECG recording and/or tilt testing, after failure of other therapeutic options and being informed of the conflicting results of trials.	**C**
Class IIb	1. Patients under 40 years of age with recurrent severe vasovagal syncope who show prolonged asystole during ECG recording and/or tilt testing, after failure of other therapeutic options and being informed of the conflicting results of trials.	**C**
Class III	1. Patients without demonstrable bradycardia during reflex syncope.	**C**

1.5. Paediatrics and congenital heart diseases

Recommendations for cardiac pacing in paediatrics and congenital heart disease

Class	Clinical Indication	Level of evidence
Class I	1. Congenital third degree atrioventricular block with any of the following conditions: ▪ symptoms ▪ ventricular rate less than 50-55/min in infants ▪ ventricular rate less than 70/min in congenital heart disease ▪ ventricular dysfunction ▪ wide QRS escape rhythm ▪ complex ventricular ectopy ▪ abrupt ventricular pauses > 2-3x basic cycle length ▪ prolonged QTc, or ▪ presence of maternal antibodies-mediated block. 2. Second or third degree atrioventricular block with ▪ symptomatic bradycardia* ▪ ventricular dysfunction 3. Postoperative Mobitz type II second- or third-degree block which persists at least 7 days after cardiac surgery. 4. Sinus node dysfunction with correlation of symptoms.	**B** **C** **C** **C**
Class IIa	1. Asymptomatic sinus bradycardia in the child with complex congenital heart disease and ▪ resting heart rate less than 40/min, or ▪ pauses in ventricular rate more than 3 s. 2. Bradycardia-tachycardia syndrome with the need of antiarrhythmics when other therapeutical options, such as catheter ablation, are not possible. 3. Long-QT syndrome with ▪ 2:1 or third-degree atrioventricular block ▪ Symptomatic bradycardia* (spontaneous or due to beta-blocker) ▪ pause dependent ventricular tachycardia. 4. Congenital heart disease and impaired haemodynamics due to sinus bradycardia* or loss of atrioventricular synchrony	**C** **C** **B** **C**
Class IIb	1. Congenital third degree atrioventricular blocks without a Class I indication for pacing. 2. Transient postoperative third-degree atrioventricular block with residual bifascicular block. 3. Asymptomatic sinus bradycardia in the adolescent with congenital heart disease and ▪ resting heart rate less than 40/min or ▪ pauses in ventricular rate more than 3 s. 4. Neuromuscular diseases with any degree of atrioventricular block without symptoms.	**B** **C** **C** **C**
Class III	1. Transient postoperative atrioventricular block with return of atrioventricular conduction within 7 days. 2. Asymptomatic postoperative bifascicular block with and without first degree atrioventricular block. 3. Asymptomatic type I second-degree atrioventricular block. 4. Asymptomatic sinus bradycardia in the adolescent with minimum heart rate more than 40/min and maximum pause in ventricular rhythm less than 3 s.	**B** **C** **C** **C**

* Clinical significance of bradycardia is age dependent

1.6. Cardiac transplantation

Recommendations for cardiac pacing after cardiac transplantation

Class	Clinical Indication	Level of evidence
Class I	1. Symptomatic bradyarrhythmias due to sinus node dysfunction or atrioventricular block three weeks after transplantation.	**C**
Class IIa	1. Chronotropic incompetence impeding the quality of life late in the post-transplant period.	**C**
Class IIb	1. Symptomatic bradyarrhythmias between the first and third week after transplantation.	**C**
Class III	1. Asymptomatic bradyarrhythmias and tolerated chronotropic incompetence. 2. Monitoring of cardiac rejection alone. 3. Bradyarrhythmias during the first week of transplantation.	**C**

2. Pacing for specific conditions

2.1. Hypertrophic cardiomyopathy

Recommendations for cardiac pacing in hypertrophic cardiomyopathy

Class	Clinical Indication	Level of evidence
Class I	None.	
Class IIa	Symptomatic bradycardia due to beta blockade when alternative therapies are unacceptable.	**C**
Class IIb	Patients with drug refractory hypertrophic cardiomyopathy with significant resting or provoked LVOT gradient and contra-indications for septal ablation or myectomy.	**A**
Class III	1. Asymptomatic patients. 2. Symptomatic patients who do not have LVOT obstruction.	**C**

LVOT = left ventricular outflow tract

3. Cardiac resynchronization therapy in patients with heart failure

3.1. Introduction

Evidence-based clinical effects of cardiac resynchronization therapy

State-of-the-art management of congestive heart failure (CHF), besides alleviating symptoms, preventing major morbidity, and lowering mortality, increasingly strives to prevent disease progression, in particularly the transition between asymptomatic LV dysfunction and overt CHF. The clinical effects of long-term CRT were firstly evaluated in non-controlled studies, in which a sustained benefit conferred by biventricular pacing was measured. Randomised multi-centre trials with crossover or parallel treatment assignments were subsequently conducted to ascertain the clinical value of CRT in patients with advanced CHF and in sinus rhythm, with or without indications for an implantable cardioverter-defibrillator (ICD). Meta-analyses were also published. The usual study enrolment criteria were: 1) CHF in New York Heart Association (NYHA) functional Class III or IV despite optimal pharmacological treatment; 2) LV ejection fraction (EF) < 35%, LV end-diastolic diameter > 55 mm, and QRS duration ≥ 120 or 150 ms.

3.2. Recommendations

Pacing for heart failure can be applied either by biventricular pacing or, in selected cases, by left ventricular pacing alone. The following recommendations consider cardiac pacing for heart failure delivered through biventricular pacing, since this mode is supported by the greatest body of evidence. This, however, does not preclude other pacing modes, such as LV pacing, to correct ventricular dyssynchrony.

Ventricular conduction delay continues to be defined according to QRS duration (QRS ≥ 120 ms). It is recognised that ventricular conduction delay may not result in mechanical dyssynchrony. Dyssynchrony is defined as an uncoordinated regional contraction-relaxation pattern. Although from the theoretical point of view it may be more appropriate to target mechanical dyssynchrony, rather than electrical conduction delay, no large controlled study has prospectively assessed the value of mechanical dyssynchrony in heart failure patients undergoing pacing for heart failure.

Recommendations for the use of cardiac resynchronization therapy by biventricular pacemaker (CRT-P) or biventricular pacemaker combined with an ICD (CRT-D) in HF patients.

Heart failure patients who remain symptomatic in NYHA Class III-IV despite optimal pharmacological treatment, with low ejection fraction (LVEF ≤ 35%), left ventricular dilatation*, normal sinus rhythm and wide QRS complex (≥ 120 ms)

- Class I - Level of evidence A for CRT-P to reduce morbidity and mortality.
- CRT-D is an acceptable option for patients who have expectancy of survival with a good functional status for more than 1 year, Class I - Level of evidence B.

Recommendations for the use of biventricular pacing in HF patients with a concomitant indication for permanent pacing.

Heart failure patients with NYHA Class III-IV symptoms, low ejection fraction (LVEF ≤ 35%), left ventricular dilatation* and a concomitant indication for permanent pacing (first implant or upgrading of conventional pacemaker).

- Class IIa - Level of evidence C

Recommendations for the use of an ICD combined with biventricular pacemaker (CRT-D) in HF patients with an indication for an ICD.

Heart failure patients with a Class I indication for an ICD (first implant or upgrading at device change) who are symptomatic in NYHA Class III-IV despite optimal pharmacological treatment, with low ejection fraction (LVEF ≤ 35%), left ventricular dilatation*, wide QRS complex (≥ 120 ms).

- Class I - Level of evidence B.

Recommendations for the use of biventricular pacing in HF patients with permanent atrial fibrillation.
Heart failure patients who remain symptomatic in NYHA Class III-IV despite optimal pharmacological treatment, with low ejection fraction (LVEF ≤ 35%), LV dilatation*, permanent atrial fibrillation and indication for AV junction ablation. ▪ Class IIa - Level of evidence C.

* Left ventricular dilatation/Different criteria have been used to define LV dilatation in controlled studies on CRT: LV end diastolic diameter > 55 mm; LV end diastolic diameter > 30 mm/m^2, LV end diastolic diameter > 30 mm/m (height).

Section XIII: Myocardial Infarction

Universal Definition of Myocardial Infarction

Chapter 1

Universal Definition of Myocardial Infarction*

2007

The joint ESC-ACCF-AHA-WHF Task force for the Redefinition of Myocardial Infarction

Co-Chairpersons

Prof. Kristian Thygesen
Dept. of Medicine & Cardiology
Aarhus University Hospital
Tage Hansens Gade 2
DK-8000 Aarhus C
Denmark
Phone: +45 89 49 76 14
Fax: +45 89 49 76 19
Email: Kristian.Thygesen@as.aaa.dk

Prof. Joseph Alpert
Dept. of Medicine
Univ. of Arizona College of Medicine
1501 N. Campbell Ave.
P.O. Box 245017
Tucson AZ 85724-5017
USA
Phone: +1 520 626 6102
Fax: +1 520 626 2919
Email: jalpert@email.arizona.edu

Prof. Harvey White
Green Lane Cardiovascular Service
Auckland City Hospital
Private Bag 92024
1030 Auckland
New Zealand
Phone: +64 96309992
Fax: +64 96309915
Email: harveyw@adhb.govt.nz

Task Force Members:

Biomarker Group:
Allan S. Jaffe, Coordinator, USA
Fred S. Apple, USA
Marcello Galvani, Italy
Hugo A. Katus, Germany
L. Kristin Newby, USA
Jan Ravkilde, Denmark

ECG Group:
Bernard Chaitman, Coordinator, USA
Peter M. Clemmensen, Denmark
Mikael Dellborg, Sweden
Hanoch Hod, Israel
Pekka Porela, Finland

Imaging Group:
Richard Underwood, Coordinator, UK
Jeroen J. Bax, Netherlands
George A. Beller, USA
Robert Bonow, USA
Ernst E. Van Der Wall, Netherlands

Intervention Group:
Jean-Pierre Bassand, Co-coordinator, France
William Wijns, Co-coordinator, Belgium
T. Bruce Ferguson, USA
Philippe G. Steg, France
Barry F. Uretsky, USA
David O. Williams, USA

Clinical Investigation Group:
Paul W. Armstrong, Coordinator, Canada
Elliott M. Antman, USA
Keith A. Fox, UK
Christian W. Hamm, Germany
E. Magnus Ohman, USA
Maarten L. Simoons, Netherlands

Global Perspective Group:
Philip A. Poole-Wilson, Coordinator, UK
Enrique P. Gurfinkel, Argentina
José-Luis Lopez-Sendon, Spain
Prem Pais, India
Shanti Mendis*, Switzerland
Jun-Ren Zhu, China

Implementation Group:
Lars C. Wallentin, Coordinator, Sweden
Francisco Fernandez-Avilés, Spain
Kim M. Fox, UK
Alexander N. Parkhomenko, Ukraine
Silvia G. Priori, Italy
Michal Tendera, Poland
Liisa-Maria Voipio-Pulkki, Finland

ESC Staff:
1. Keith McGregor, Sophia Antipolis, France
2. Veronica Dean, Sophia Antipolis, France
3. Catherine Després, Sophia Antipolis, France

*Adapted from the ESC-ACCF-AHA-WHF Expert Consensus Document on the Universal Definition of Myocardial Infarction (European Heart Journal 2007;28:2525-2538).

*Dr. Shanti Mendis of the WHO participated in the task force in her personal capacity but this does not represent WHO approval of this document at the present time.

Definition of myocardial infarction

Criteria for acute myocardial infarction

The term myocardial infarction should be used when there is evidence of myocardial necrosis in a clinical setting consistent with myocardial ischaemia. Under these conditions any one of the following criteria meets the diagnosis for myocardial infarction:

- Detection of rise and/or fall of cardiac biomarkers (preferably troponin) with at least one value above the 99th percentile of the upper reference limit (URL) together with evidence of myocardial ischaemia with at least one of the following:
  - Symptoms of ischaemia;
  - ECG changes indicative of new ischaemia (new ST-T changes or new left bundle branch block (LBBB);
  - Development of pathological Q waves in the ECG;
  - Imaging evidence of new loss of viable myocardium or new regional wall motion abnormality.
- Sudden, unexpected cardiac death, involving cardiac arrest, often with symptoms suggestive of myocardial ischaemia, and accompanied by presumably new ST-elevation, or new LBBB, and/or evidence of fresh thrombus by coronary angiography and/or at autopsy, but death occurring before blood samples could be obtained, or at a time before the appearance of cardiac biomarkers in the blood.
- For percutaneous coronary interventions (PCI) in patients with normal baseline troponin values, elevations of cardiac biomarkers above the 99th percentile URL are indicative of peri-procedural myocardial necrosis. By convention, increases of biomarkers greater than 3 X 99th percentile URL have been designated as defining PCI-related myocardial infarction. A subtype related to a documented stent thrombosis is recognized.
- For coronary artery bypass grafting (CABG) in patients with normal baseline troponin values, elevations of cardiac biomarkers above the 99th percentile URL are indicative of peri-procedural myocardial necrosis. By convention, increases of biomarkers greater than 5 X 99th percentile URL plus either new pathological Q waves or new LBBB, or angiographically documented new graft or native coronary artery occlusion, or imaging evidence of new loss of viable myocardium have been designated as defining CABG-related myocardial infarction.
- Pathological findings of an acute myocardial infarction.

Criteria for prior myocardial infarction

Any one of the following criteria meets the diagnosis for prior myocardial infarction:

- Development of new pathological Q waves with or without symptoms.
- Imaging evidence of a region of loss of viable myocardium that is thinned and fails to contract, in the absence of a non-ischaemic cause.
- Pathological findings of a healed or healing myocardial infarction.

Pathology

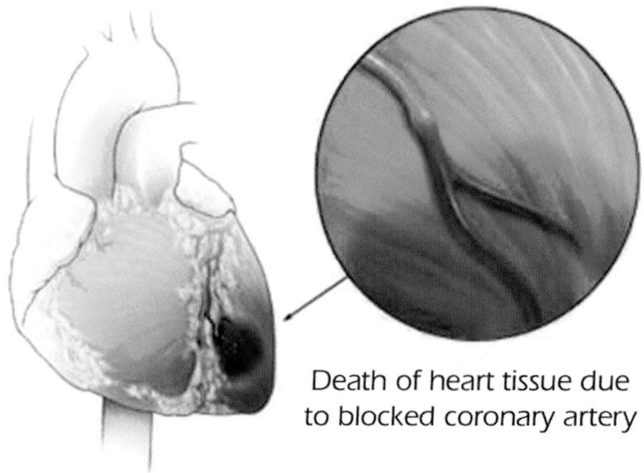

Myocardial Infarction is defined as myocardial cell death due to prolonged myocardial ischaemia.

Classification of myocardial infarction

Type 1	**Spontaneous myocardial infarction related to ischaemia due to a primary coronary event such as plaque erosion and/or rupture, fissuring, or dissection.**
Type 2	**Myocardial infarction secondary to ischaemia due to either increased oxygen demand or decreased supply e.g. coronary artery spasm, coronary embolism, anaemia, arrhythmias, hypertension, or hypotension.**
Type 3	**Sudden unexpected cardiac death, including cardiac arrest, often with symptoms suggestive of myocardial ischaemia, accompanied by presumably new ST-elevation, or new LBBB, or presumably new, major obstruction in a coronary artery by angiography and/or pathology, but death occurring before blood samples could be obtained, or at a time before the appearance of cardiac biomarkers in the blood.**
Type 4a	**Myocardial infarction associated with PCI.**
Type 4b	**Myocardial infarction associated with stent thrombosis as documented by angiography or autopsy**
Type 5	**Myocardial infarction associated with CABG.**

Cardiac biomarkers for detecting myocardial infarction

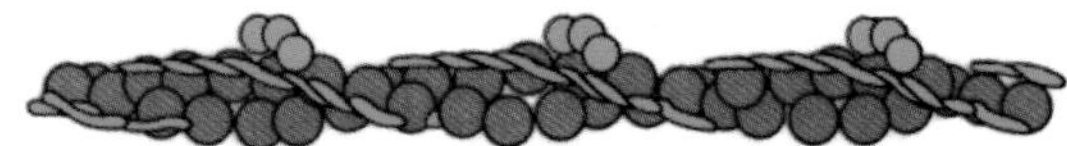

Preferably

Detection of rise and/or fall of Troponin (I or T) with at least one value above the 99th percentile of a control group measured with a coefficient of variation ≤ 10%.

When Troponin is not available

Detection of rise and/or fall of CKMB mass with at least one value above the 99th percentile of a control group measured with a coefficient of variation ≤ 10%.

Reinfarction

In patients where recurrent myocardial infarction is suspected from clinical signs or symptoms following the initial infarction, an immediate measurement of cardiac troponin is recommended. A second sample should be obtained 3-6 hrs later. Recurrent infarction is diagnosed if there is a 20% or more increase of the value in the second sample. This value should also exceed the 99th percentile for a control group.

Elevations of Troponin in the absence of overt ischaemic heart disease

- Cardiac contusion, or other trauma including surgery, ablation, pacing etc
- Congestive heart failure - acute and chronic
- Aortic dissection
- Aortic valve disease
- Hypertrophic cardiomyopathy
- Tachy- or bradyarrhythmias, or heart block
- Apical ballooning syndrome
- Rhabdomyolysis with cardiac injury
- Pulmonary embolism, severe pulmonary hypertension
- Renal failure
- Acute neurological disease, including stroke, or subarachnoid haemorrhage
- Infiltrative diseases, e.g., amyloidosis, haemochromatosis, sarcoidosis, and scleroderma
- Inflammatory diseases, e.g., myocarditis or myocardial extension of endo-/pericarditis
- Drug toxicity or toxins
- Critically ill patients, especially with respiratory failure, or sepsis
- Burns, especially if affecting > 30% of body surface area
- Extreme exertion

Electrocardiographic detection of myocardial infarction

ECG manifestations of acute myocardial ischaemia (in absence of LVH and LBBB)

ST-elevation

New ST-elevation at the J point in two contiguous leads with the cut-off points: ≥ 0.2 mV in men or ≥ 0.15 mV in women in leads V_2-V_3 and/or ≥ 0.1 mV in other leads

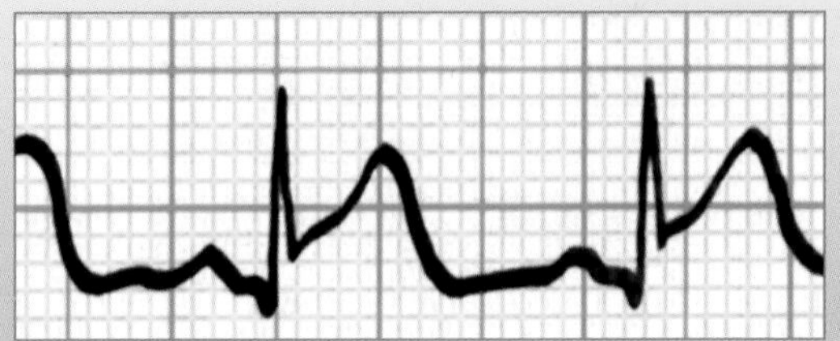

ST-depression and T wave changes

New horizontal or down-sloping ST-depression ≥ 0.05 mV in two contiguous leads; and/or T-inversion ≥ 0.1 mV in two contiguous leads with prominent R wave or R/S ratio > 1

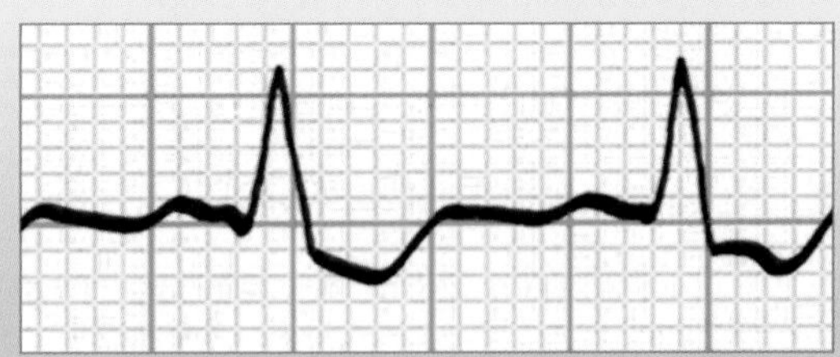

ECG changes associated with prior myocardial infarction

- Any Q wave in leads V_2-V_3 ≥ 0.02 sec or QS complex in leads V_2 and V_3.
- Q-wave ≥ 0.03 sec and ≥ 0.1 mV deep or QS complex in leads I, II, aVL, aVF or V_4-V_6 in any two leads of a contiguous lead grouping (I, aVL, V_6; V_4-V_6; II, III, aVF).
- R-wave ≥ 0.04 sec in V_1-V_2 and R/S ≥ 1 with a concordant positive T-wave in the absence of a conduction defect.

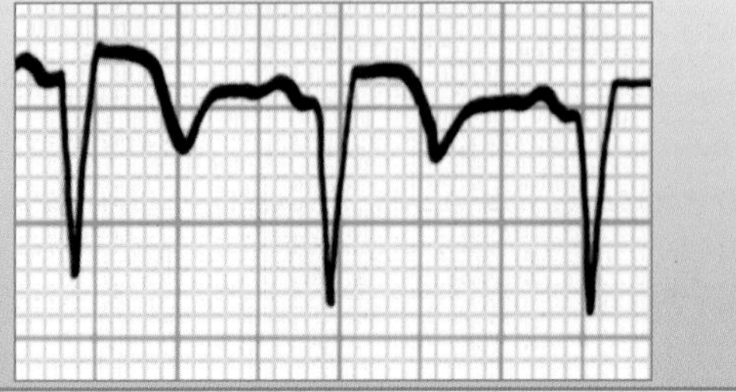

Common ECG pitfalls in diagnosing myocardial infarction

False positives:

- Benign early repolarization
- LBBB
- Pre-excitation
- Brugada syndrome
- Peri-/myocarditis
- Pulmonary embolism
- Subarachnoid haemorrhage
- Metabolic disturbances such as hyperkalemia
- Failure to recognize normal limits for J-point displacement
- Lead transposition or use of modified Mason-Likar configuration
- Cholecystitis

False Negatives:

- Prior myocardial infarction with Q waves and/or persistent ST-elevation
- Paced rhythm
- LBBB

Reinfarction

Reinfarction should be considered when ST-elevation ≥ 0.1 mV reoccurs in a patient having a lesser degree of ST-elevation or new pathognomonic Q waves, particularly when associated with ischaemic symptoms. ST-depression or LBBB on their own should not be considered valid criteria for myocardial infarction.

Imaging techniques for detection of myocardial infarction

Imaging techniques can be useful in the diagnosis of myocardial infarction because of the ability to detect wall motion abnormalities in the presence of elevated cardiac biomarkers. If for some reason biomarkers have not been measured or may have normalized, demonstration of new loss of myocardial viability alone in the absence of non-ischaemic causes meets the criteria for myocardial infarction. However, if biomarkers have been measured at appropriate times and are normal, the determinations of these take precedence over the imaging criteria.

Echocardiography and radionuclide techniques, in conjunction with exercise or pharmacologic stress can identify ischaemia and myocardial viability. Non-invasive imaging techniques can diagnose healing or healed infarction by demonstrating regional wall motion, thinning or scar in the absence of other causes.

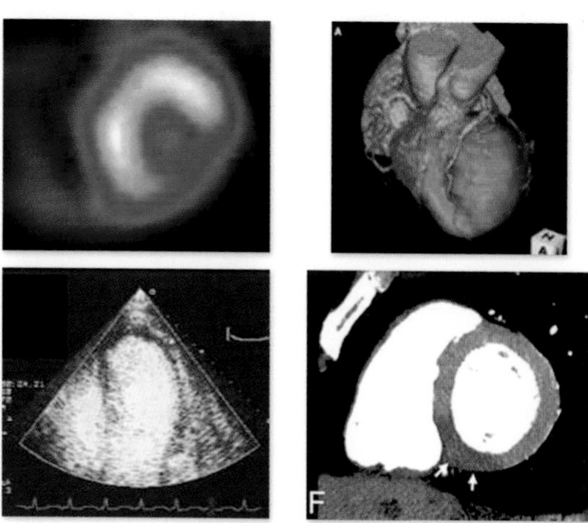

Myocardial infarction associated with interventions

Diagnostic criteria for myocardial infarction with PCI

In the setting of PCI, the occurrence of procedure-related cell necrosis can be detected by measurement of cardiac biomarkers before or immediately after the procedure, and again at 6-12 and 18-24 hours. Elevations of biomarkers above the 99th percentile after PCI, assuming a normal baseline troponin value, are indicative of post-procedural myocardial necrosis. There is currently no solid scientific basis for defining a biomarker threshold for the diagnosis of peri-procedural myocardial infarction.

By arbitrary convention, it is suggested to designate increases greater than 3 X 99th percentile for a control group as PCI-related myocardial infarction (type 4a). If cardiac troponin is elevated before the procedure and not stable for at least two samples 6 hours apart, there are insufficient data to recommend biomarker criteria for the diagnosis of peri-procedural myocardial infarction. If the values are stable, criteria for reinfarction by further measurement of biomarkers together with the features of the ECG or imaging can be applied.

A separate subcategory of myocardial infarction (type 4b) is related to stent thrombosis as documented by angiography and/or autopsy.

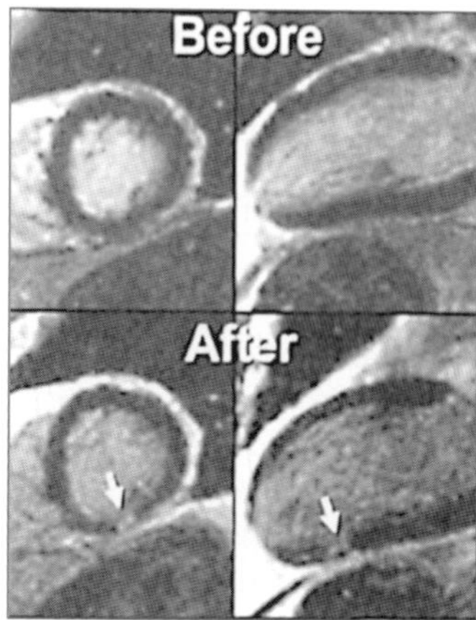

Diagnostic criteria for myocardial infarction with CABG

Any increase of cardiac biomarkers after CABG indicates myocyte necrosis, implying that an increasing magnitude of biomarker is likely to be related to an impaired outcome. However, scant literature exists concerning the use of biomarkers for defining myocardial infarction in the setting of CABG. Therefore, biomarkers cannot stand alone in diagnosing myocardial infarction.

In view of the adverse impact on survival observed in patients with significant biomarker elevations, it is suggested, by arbitrary convention, that biomarker values greater than the 5 x 99th percentile for a control group during the first 72 hrs following CABG when associated with the appearance of new pathological Q waves or new LBBB, or angiographically documented new graft or native coronary artery occlusion, or imaging evidence of new loss of viable myocardium should be considered as diagnostic of a CABG related myocardial infarction (type 5).

Clinical investigations involving myocardial infarction

Consistency among investigators and regulatory authorities with regard to the definition of myocardial infarction used in clinical investigations is essential. Furthermore, investigators should ensure that a trial provides comprehensive data for the classification of the different types of myocardial infarction according to multiples of the 99th percentile for a control group of the applied cardiac biomarker.

Classification of the different types of myocardial infarction according to multiples of the 99th percentile URL of the applied cardiac biomarker

Multiples X 99%	MI Type 1 (spontaneous)	MI Type 2 (secondary)	MI Type 3* (sudden death)	MI Type 4a** (PCI)	MI Type 4b (stent thrombosis)	MI Type 5** (CABG)	Total Number
1-2 X							
2-3 X							
3-5 X							
5-10 X							
> 10 X							
Total number							

*Biomarkers are not available for this type of myocardial infarction since the patients expired before biomarker determination could be performed.

**For the sake of completeness, the total distribution of biomarker values should be reported. The hatched areas represent biomarker elevations below the decision limit used for these types of myocardial infarction.

Sample clinical trial tabulation of randomized patients by types of myocardial infarction

Types of MI	Treatment A Number of patients	Treatment B Number of patients
MI Type 1		
MI Type 2		
MI Type 3		
MI Type 4a		
MI Type 4b		
MI Type 5		
Total number		

Section XIV: Pulmonary Embolism

1. Diagnosis and Management of Acute Pulmonary Embolism

Chapter 1

Diagnosis and Management of Acute Pulmonary Embolism* 2008

The Task Force on Acute Pulmonary Embolism of the European Society of Cardiology

Chairperson:
Adam Torbicki, MD, PhD, FESC
Dept. of Chest Medicine
Institute for Tuberculosis and Lung Diseases
ul. Plocka 26
01-138 Warsaw
Poland
Tel.: +48 22 431 2114
Fax: +48 22 431 2414
E-mail: a.torbicki@igichp.edu.pl

Task Force Members:
1. Arnaud Perrier, Geneva, Switzerland
2. Stavros Konstantinides, Goettingen, Germany
3. Giancarlo Agnelli, Perugia, Italy
4. Nazzareno Galiè, Bologna, Italy
5. Piotr Pruszczyk, Warsaw, Poland
6. Frank Bengel, Baltimore, USA
7. Adrian J.B. Brady, Glasgow, UK
8. Daniel Ferreira, Charneca De Caparica, Portugal
9. Uwe Janssens, Eschweiler, Germany
10. Walter Klepetko, Vienna, Austria
11. Eckhard Mayer, Mainz, Germany
12. Martine Remy-Jardin, Lille, France
13. Jean-Pierre Bassand, Besançon, France

ESC Staff:
1. Keith McGregor, Sophia Antipolis, France
2. Veronica Dean, Sophia Antipolis, France
3. Catherine Després, Sophia Antipolis, France

1. Introduction

Pulmonary embolism (PE) is a major health problem, and may present as a cardiovascular emergency. Occlusion of the pulmonary arterial bed by thrombus may lead to acute life-threatening, but potentially reversible, right ventricular failure in the most severe cases. Alternatively, the clinical presentation of PE may be non-specific, in cases where the pulmonary obstruction is less severe, or moderate.

The diagnosis of PE is difficult to establish, and may often go unrecognised, because of non-specific clinical presentations. However, early diagnosis is critical, since treatment is highly effective. Treatment strategy depends on the clinical presentation. In haemodynamically compromised patients it is primarily aimed at urgent restoration of the flow through occluded pulmonary arteries with potentially life-saving effects. In less severe cases, treatment aims at preventing the progression of the thrombotic process, and potentially fatal early recurrences.

In all patients, both initial and long term treatment should be justified by a certified diagnosis of PE using a validated diagnostic strategy.

Initial clinical assessment makes it possible to select optimal diagnostic and management strategies.

2. Predisposing factors, symptoms and signs of PE

Predisposing factors for VTE

Strong predisposing factors (OR > 10)
Fracture (hip or leg)
Hip or knee replacement
Major general surgery
Major trauma
Spinal cord injury
Moderate predisposing factors (OR 2 - 9)
Arthroscopic knee surgery
Central venous lines
Chemotherapy
Chronic heart or respiratory failure
Hormone replacement therapy
Malignancy
Oral contraceptive therapy
Paralytic stroke
Pregnancy/postpartum
Previous VTE
Thrombophilia
Weak predisposing factors (OR < 2)
Bed rest > 3 days
Immobility due to sitting (e.g. prolonged car or air travel)
Increasing age
Laparoscopic surgery (e.g. cholecystectomy)
Obesity
Pregnancy/antepartum
Varicose veins

OR = odds ratio

Adapted from: Anderson FA, Jr., Spencer FA. Risk factors for venous thromboembolism. Circulation 2003; 107(23 Suppl 1):I9-16

Note, that PE occurs in individuals without any predisposing factors (unprovoked or idiopathic PE) in around 30% of cases.

Symptoms and signs reported in confirmed PE

Symptoms	Approximate prevalence
Dyspnoea	80%
Chest pain (pleuritic)	52%
Chest pain (substernal)	12%
Cough	20%
Syncope	19%
Haemoptysis	11%
Signs	**Approximate prevalence**
Tachypnoea (≥ 20/min)	70%
Tachycardia (> 100/min)	26%
Signs of DVT	15%
Cyanosis	11%
Fever (> 38·5 °C)	7%

Adapted from Miniati M, Prediletto R, Formichi B, Marini C, Di Ricco G, Tonelli L et al., Am J Respir Crit Care Med 1999; 159(3):864-871 and Stein PD, Saltzman HA, Weg JG., Am J Cardiol 1991; 68(17):1723-1724

Results of routine laboratory tests (chest X-ray, electrocardiogram, arterial blood gas analysis) are often abnormal in PE. Similarly to clinical symptoms and signs, their negative and positive predictive value for diagnosis of PE is low.

Clinical symptoms, signs, predisposing factors and routine laboratory tests do not allow excluding or confirming acute PE, but may serve as components of diagnostic and management algorithms, which should be followed in each suspected case.

3. Initial risk stratification

Immediate bedside clinical assessment for the presence or absence of clinical haemodynamic compromise allows for stratification into "high-risk" and "non-high-risk" PE. This classification should be also applied to patients with suspected PE, helping to choose the optimal diagnostic strategy and initial management. High-risk PE is a life-threatening emergency requiring specific diagnostic and therapeutic strategy (short-term mortality above 15 %).

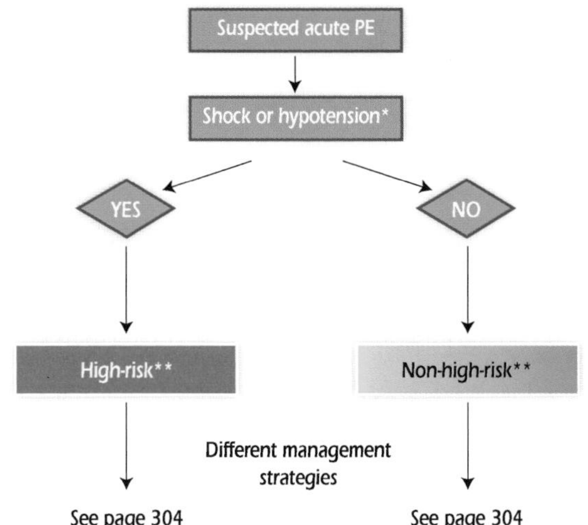

*** Defined as a systolic blood pressure < 90 mmHg or a pressure drop of ≥ 40 mmHg for > 15 minutes**

if not caused by new-onset arrhythmia, hypovolaemia or sepsis

**** Defined as risk of early (in-hospital or 30 day) PE-related mortality**

4. Assessment of clinical probability

In patients with suspected PE, initial clinical assessment is mandatory for concomitant:

- initial risk stratification (see above)
- assessment of clinical probability of PE

Assessment of "clinical probability" is based on predisposing factors, symptoms and signs identified at presentation.

Clinical probability can be estimated either by applying a validated score (e.g. Geneva or Wells score, see tabels on this page) or global clinical judgment. In any case it should be done prior to laboratory diagnostic evaluation.

Initial risk stratification is necessary for identifying high-risk patients who should be submitted to a specific diagnostic and management strategy (page 304). Clinical probability assessment is necessary to select the optimal diagnostic strategy and interpret diagnostic test results in patients with non high-risk suspected PE.

Revised Geneva score

Variables	Points
Predisposing factors	
Age > 65 years	+1
Previous DVT or PE	+3
Surgery or fracture within one month	+2
Active malignancy	+2
Symptoms	
Unilateral lower limb pain	+3
Haemoptysis	+2
Clinical signs	
Heart rate	
75 to 94 beats per minute	+3
≥ 95 beats per minute	+5
Pain on lower limb deep vein at palpation and unilateral oedema	+4
Clinical probability	Total
Low	0 to 3
Intermediate	4 to 10
High	≥ 11

Wells score

Variables	Points
Predisposing factors	
Previous DVT or PE	+1.5
Recent surgery or immobilization	+1.5
Cancer	+1
Symptoms	
Haemoptysis	+1
Clinical signs	
Heart rate > 100 beats per minute	+1.5
Clinical sign of DVT	+3
Clinical judgement	
Alternative diagnosis less likely than PE	+3
Clinical probability (3-level)	**Total**
Low	0 to 1
Intermediate	2 to 6
High	≥ 7
Clinical probability (2-level)	**Total**
PE unlikely	0-4
PE likely	> 4

5. Diagnostic assessment

Diagnostic algorithm for patients with suspected high-risk PE

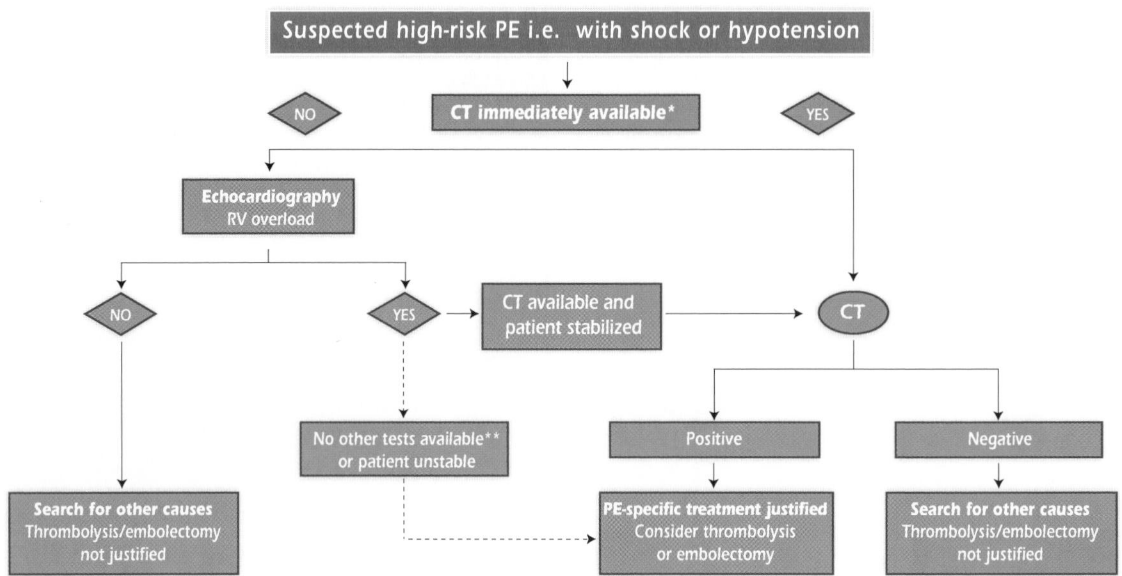

* CT is considered not immediately available also if critical condition of a patient allows only bedside diagnostic tests.

** Note that transesophageal echocardiography may detect thrombi in the pulmonary arteries in a significant proportion of patients with RV overload and PE ultimately confirmed at spiral CT and that confirmation of DVT with bedside CUS might also help in decision making.

Diagnostic algorithm for patients with suspected non-high-risk PE

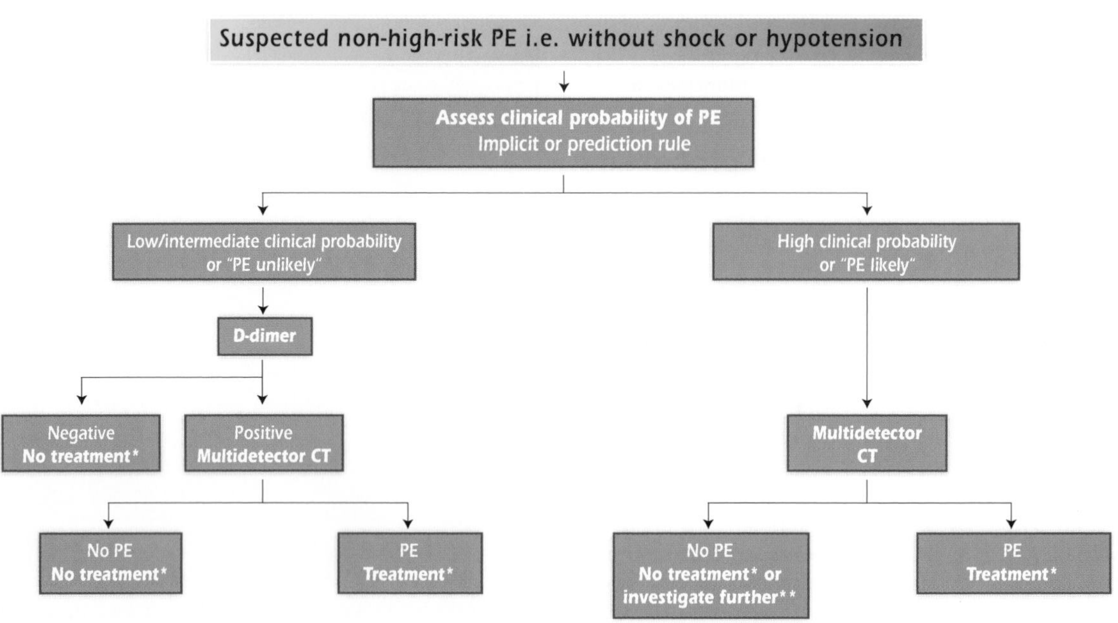

See page 303 for clinical probability assessment scores.

When using a moderately sensitive assay, decision to withhold anticoagulation based on negative D-dimer test result should be restricted to patients with a low clinical probability or a "PE unlikely" classification.

D-dimer measurement is of limited usefulness in suspected PE occurring in hospitalised patients, due to high number needed to test to obtain a negative result.

* Treatment refers to anticoagulant treatment for PE.

** In case of a negative multi-detector CT in patients with high clinical probability further investigation may be considered before withholding PE-specific treatment.

See page 305 for all validated diagnostic criteria for patients with non-high risk PE, which might be helpful in constructing alternative diagnostic algorithms, whenever needed.

Validated diagnostic criteria for patients without shock and hypotension according to clinical probability

Non-high-risk PE

Exclusion of pulmonary embolism			
Diagnostic criterion	Clinical probability of PE		
	Low	Intermediate	High
Normal pulmonary angiogram	+	+	+
D-dimer			
Negative result, highly sensitive assay	+	+	–
Negative result, moderately sensitive assay	+	–	–
V/Q scan			
Normal lung scan	+	+	+
Non-diagnostic lung scan*	+	–	–
Non-diagnostic lung scan* and negative proximal CUS	+	+	±
Chest CT angiography			
Normal single-detector CT and negative proximal CUS	+	+	±
Normal multi-detector CT alone	+	+	±

Valid criterion (no further testing required): +, color green.

Invalid criterion (further testing mandatory): –, color red.

Controversial criterion (further testing to be considered); ±, color orange.

* Non diagnostic lung scan: low or intermediate probability lung scan according to the PIOPED (Prospective Investigation On Pulmonary Embolism Diagnosis study) classification.

Validated diagnostic criteria for patients without shock and hypotension according to clinical probability

Non-high-risk PE

Confirmation of pulmonary embolism			
Diagnostic criterion	Clinical probability of PE		
	Low	Intermediate	High
Pulmonary angiogram showing PE	+	+	+
High probability V/Q scan	±	+	+
CUS showing a proximal DVT	+	+	–
Chest CT angiography			
Single or multi-detector helical CT scan showing PE (at least segmental)	±	+	+
Single or multi-detector helical CT scan showing sub-segmental PE	±	±	±

Valid criterion (no further testing required): +, color green.

Invalid criterion (further testing mandatory): –, color red.

Controversial criterion (further testing to be considered); ±, color orange.

6. Comprehensive risk stratification

Concurrently with the diagnosis of PE, prognostic assessment is required for risk stratification and therapeutic decision-making. Risk stratification of PE is performed in stages: it starts with clinical assessment of the haemodynamic status and continues with the help of laboratory tests.

Severity of PE should be understood as an individual estimate of PE-related early mortality risk, rather than anatomic burden, shape and distribution of intrapulmonary emboli. Therefore current guidelines suggest replacing potentially misleading terms such as "massive, sub-massive, non-massive" with the estimated levels of risk of PE-related early death.

Recommendations	Class [a]	Level [b]
• Initial risk stratification of suspected and/or confirmed PE based on the presence of shock and hypotension is recommended to distinguish between patients with high and non-high risk of PE related early mortality	I	B
• In non-high-risk PE patients, further stratification to an intermediate or low-risk PE subgroup based on the presence of imaging or biochemical markers of RV dysfunction and myocardial injury should be considered	IIa	B

[a] Class of recommendation, [b] Level of evidence

Principal markers useful for risk stratification

Clinical markers	Shock Hypotension*
Markers of RV dysfunction	RV dilatation, hypokinesis or pressure overload on echocardiography RV dilatation on spiral computed tomography BNP or NT-proBNP elevation Elevated right heart pressures at right heart catheterization
Markers of myocardial injury	Cardiac troponin T or I positive**

BNP - brain natruretic peptide, NT-proBNP - N-terminal proBNP

* Defined as a systolic blood pressure < 90 mmHg or a pressure drop of ≥ 40 mmHg for > 15 minutes if not caused by new-onset arrhythmia, hypovolaemia or sepsis.

** Heart-type fatty-acids binding protein (H-FABP) is an emerging marker in this category, but still requires confirmation.

Several variables collected during routine clinical and laboratory evaluation also have prognostic significance in PE. Many of them are related to the preexisting condition and comorbidities of the individual patient rather than to the severity of the index PE episode. Consideration of preexisting patient-related factors may be useful for final risk stratification and management decisions.

Risk stratification according to expected PE-related early mortality rate

PE-related early MORTALITY RISK		RISK MARKERS			Potential treatment implications
		CLINICAL (Shock or hypotension)	RV Dysfunction	Myocardial injury	
HIGH > 15%		+	(+)*	(+)*	Thrombolysis or Embolectomy
NON HIGH	Inter mediate 3 - 15%	–	+	+	Hospital Admission
			+	–	
			–	+	
	Low <1%	–	–	–	Early discharge or home treatment

* In the presence of shock or hypotension it is not mandatory to confirm RV dysfunction/injury to classify as high risk for PE-related early mortality.

It is likely that patients with intermediate-risk PE in whom markers of dysfunction and injury are both positive have increased risk compared to patients with discordant results.

The currently available data do not allow proposing specific cut-off levels of markers which could be used for therapeutic decision-making in patients with non-high-risk PE.

An ongoing multi-center randomized trial is evaluating the potential benefit of thrombolysis in normotensive patients with predefined echocardiographic signs of RVD and troponin levels.

7. Initial treatment

High-risk PE

Recommendations	Class [a]	Level [b]
• Anticoagulation with UFH should be initiated without delay in patients with high-risk PE	I	A
• Systemic hypotension should be corrected to prevent progression of RV failure and death due to PE	I	C
• Vasopressive drugs are recommended for hypotensive patients with PE	I	C
• Dobutamine and dopamine may be used in patients with PE, low cardiac output and normal blood pressure	IIa	B
• Aggressive fluid challenge is not recommended	III	B
• Oxygen should be administered to patients with hypoxaemia	I	C
• Thrombolytic therapy should be used in patients with high-risk PE presenting with cardiogenic shock and/or persistent arterial hypotension	I	A
• Surgical pulmonary embolectomy is a recommended therapeutic alternative in patients with high-risk PE in whom thrombolysis is absolutely contraindicated or has failed	I	C
• Catheter embolectomy or fragmentation of proximal pulmonary arterial clots may be considered as an alternative to surgical treatment in high-risk patients when thrombolysis is absolutely contraindicated or has failed	IIb	C

[a] Class of recommendation, [b] Level of evidence

Non-high-risk PE

Recommendations	Class [a]	Level [b]
• Anticoagulation should be initiated without delay in patients with high or intermediate clinical probability of PE while diagnostic work-up is still ongoing	I	C
• Use of LMWH or fondaparinux is the recommended form of initial treatment for most patients with non-high-risk PE	I	A
• In patients at high bleeding risk and in those with severe renal dysfunction UFH with an aPTT target range of 1.5 – 2.5 times normal is a recommended form of initial treatment	I	C
• Initial treatment with UFH, LMWH or fondaparinux should be continued for at least 5 days and may be replaced by Vit K antagonists only after achieving target INR levels for at least 2 consecutive days	I I	A C
• Routine use of thrombolysis in non–high-risk PE patients is not recommended, but it may be considered in selected patients with intermediate risk PE	IIb	B
• Thrombolytic therapy should not be used in patients with low-risk PE	III	B

[a] Class of recommendation, [b] Level of evidence

Approved thrombolytic regimens for pulmonary embolism

Streptokinase	250,000 IU as a loading dose over 30 min, followed by 100,000 IU/h over 12-24 h
	Accelerated regimen: 1.5 million IU over 2 h
Urokinase	4,400 IU/kg as a loading dose over 10 min, followed by 4,400 IU/Kg/h over 12-24 h
rtPA	Accelerated regimen: 3 million IU over 2 h 100 mg over 2 h; or 0.6 mg/kg over 15 min (maximum dose 50 mg)

Contra-indications to thrombolytic therapy

Absolute contra-indications*:
• Haemorrhagic stroke or stroke of unknown origin at any time • Ischaemic stroke in preceding 6 months • Central nervous system damage or neoplasms • Recent major trauma/surgery/head injury (within preceding 3 weeks) • Gastro-intestinal bleeding within the last month • Known bleeding
Relative contra-indications
• Transient ischaemic attack in preceding 6 months • Oral anticoagulant therapy • Pregnancy or within 1 week post partum • Non-compressible punctures • Traumatic resuscitation • Refractory hypertension (systolic blood pressure > 180 mm Hg) • Advanced liver disease • Infective endocarditis • Active peptic ulcer

* Contra-indications to thrombolysis which are considered absolute e.g. in acute myocardial infarction, might become relative in a patient with immediately life-threatening high-risk PE.

Adjustment of intravenous unfractionated heparin dosage based on the APTT

APTT	Change of Dosage
< 35 sec (< 1.2 times control)	80 U/kg bolus, increase infusion rate by 4 U/kg/h
35-45 sec (1.2-1.5 times control)	40 U/kg bolus, increase infusion rate by 2 U/kg /h
46-70 sec (1.5-2.3 times control)	no change
71-90 sec (2.3-3.0 times control)	reduce infusion rate by 2 U/kg /h
> 90 sec (> 3.0 times control)	stop infusion for 1 h, then reduce infusion rate by 3 U/kg/h

Table legend: aPTT = activated partial thromboplastin time

Subcutaneous regimens of low molecular-weight heparins and fondaparinux approved for the treatment of PE

	Dosage	Interval
Enoxaparin	1.0 mg/kg or 1.5 mg/kg*	Every 12 h Once daily*
Tinzaparin	175 U/kg	Once daily
Fondaparinux	5 mg (body weight < 50 kg); 7.5 mg (body weight 50-100 kg); 10 mg (body weight > 100 kg)	Once daily

* Once-daily injection of enoxaparin at the dosage of 1.5 mg/kg is approved for inpatient (hospital) treatment of PE in the United States and in some, but not all, European countries.

In patients with cancer Dalteparin is approved for extended treatment of symptomatic VTE (proximal DVT and/or PE), at an initial dose of 200 IU/kg s.c. once daily (see drug labeling for details). Other LMWH approved for the treatment of DVT are sometimes used also in PE.

8. Long term treatment

Recommendations	Class [a]	Level [b]
• For patients with PE secondary to a transient (reversible) risk factor, treatment with a VKA is recommended for 3 months	I	A
• For patients with unprovoked PE, treatment with a VKA is recommended for at least 3 months	I	A
• Patients with a first episode of unprovoked PE and low bleeding risk, and in whom stable anticoagulation can be achieved, may be considered for long-term oral anticoagulation	IIb	B
• For patients with a second episode of unprovoked PE, long-term treatment is recommended	I	A
• In patients who receive long-term anticoagulant treatment, the risk-benefit ratio of continuing such treatment should be reassessed at regular intervals	I	C
• For patients with PE and cancer, LMWH should be considered for the first 3 to 6 months	IIa	B
after this period, anticoagulant therapy with VKA or LMWH should be continued indefinitely, or until the cancer is considered cured	I	C
• In patients with PE, the dose of VKA should be adjusted to maintain a target INR of 2.5 (INR range, 2.0 to 3.0) regardless of treatment duration	I	A

[a] Class of recommendation, [b] Level of evidence

9. Venous filters

Recommendations	Class [a]	Level [b]
• IVC filters may be used when there are absolute contra-indications to anticoagulation and a high risk of VTE recurrence	IIb	B
• The routine use of IVC filters in patients with PE is not recommended	III	B

[a] Class of recommendation, [b] Level of evidence

Permanent inferior vena cava (IVC) filters may provide lifelong protection against PE; however, they are associated with complications and late sequelae including recurrent DVT episodes and development of the post-thrombotic syndrome.

10. Specific situations

PREGNANCY: in pregnant women with a clinical suspicion of PE, an accurate diagnosis is mandatory, as a prolonged course of heparin is required.

The amount of radiation absorbed by the foetus for different diagnostic tests is shown in the appendix (page 310). The upper limit with regard to danger of injury for the foetus is considered to be 50 mSv (50 000 μGy). Therefore, all diagnostic modalities may be used without a significant risk to the foetus. CT radiation dose delivered to the foetus seems lower than that of a perfusion lung scintigraphy in the 1st and 2nd trimester. However, perfusion lung scintigraphy has high diagnostic yield (75%) in pregnant women with less breast tissue radiation compared to CT. Ventilation phase does not appear to add enough information to warrant the additional radiation. In women left undiagnosed by perfusion lung scintigraphy, however, CT should be preferred over pulmonary angiography, which carries a significantly higher X-ray exposure for the foetus (2.2 to 3.7 mSv).

Low-molecular heparins are recommended in confirmed PE, while VKA are not recommended during the first and the third trimesters and may be considered with caution in the second trimester of pregnancy. Thrombolysis carries higher risk of bleeding in pregnant women but - similarly to embolectomy - it should be considered in life-threatening situations.

Anticoagulant treatment should be administered for at least 3 months after the delivery.

MALIGNANCY is a predisposing factor for development and recurrence of VTE. However, routine extensive screening for cancer in patients with first episode of unprovoked PE is not recommended. In cancer patients with confirmed PE, LMWH should be considered for the first 3 to 6 months of treatment and anticoagulant treatment should be continued indefinitely or until definitive cure of the cancer.

RIGHT HEART THROMBI, particularly when mobile, "in-transit" from the systemic veins, are associated with a significantly increased early mortality risk in patients with acute PE. Immediate therapy is mandatory, but optimal treatment is controversial in the absence of controlled trials. Thrombolysis and embolectomy are probably both effective while anticoagulation alone appears less effective.

HEPARIN INDUCED THROMBOCYTOPENIA (HIT) is a life-threatening immunological complication of heparin therapy. Monitoring of platelet counts in patients treated with heparin is important for early detection of HIT.

Treatment consists of discontinuation of heparin and alternative anticoagulant treatment, if still required.

CHRONIC THROMBOEMBOLIC PULMONARY HYPERTENSION (CTEPH) is a severe though rare consequence of PE. Pulmonary endarteriectomy provides excellent results, and should be considered as a first line treatment, whenever possible. Drugs targeting the pulmonary circulation in patients in whom surgery is not feasible or failed are currently being tested in clinical trials.

NON-THROMBOTIC PE does not represent a distinct clinical syndrome. It may be due to a variety of embolic materials and result in a wide spectrum of clinical presentations making the diagnosis difficult. With the exception of severe air and fat embolism, the haemodynamic consequences of non-thrombotic emboli are usually mild. Treatment is mostly supportive but may differ according to the type of embolic material and clinical severity.

11. Appendix

Estimated radiation absorbed by foetus in procedures for diagnosing PE

Test	Estimated radiation	
	μGy	mSv
Chest radiography	< 10	0.01
Perfusion lung scan with Technetium-99m labelled albumin (1–2mCi)	60 - 120	0.06 - 012
Ventilation lung scan	200	0.2
CT angiography		
1st trimester	3 - 20	0.003 - 0.02
2nd trimester	8 - 77	0.008 - 0.08
3rd trimester	51 - 130	0.051 - 0.13
Pulmonary angiography by femoral access	2210 - 3740	2.2 - 3.7
Pulmonary angiography by brachial access	< 500	< 0.5

Section XV: Heart Failure

1. Diagnosis and Treatment of Acute and Chronic Heart Failure

Chapter 1

Diagnosis and Treatment of Acute and Chronic Heart Failure*

2008

The Task Force on Heart Failure of the European Society of Cardiology (ESC) Developed in collaboration with the Heart Failure Association of the ESC (HFA)

Chairperson:
Kenneth Dickstein, MD, PhD, FESC
Cardiology Division
Stavanger University Hospital
University of Bergen
4011 Stavanger
Norway
Phone: +47 51 51 80 00
Fax: +47 51 51 99 21
Email: kenneth.dickstein@med.uib.no

Task Force Members:
1. Alain Cohen-Solal, Paris, France
2. Gerasimos Filippatos, Athens, Greece
3. John J. V. McMurray, Glasgow, UK
4. Piotr Ponikowski, Wroclaw, Poland
5. Philip Alexander Poole-Wilson, London, UK
6. Anna Stromberg, Linkoping, Sweden
7. Dirk J. van Veldhuisen, Groningen, The Netherlands
8. Dan Atar, Oslo, Norway
9. Arno W. Hoes, Utrecht, The Netherlands
10. Andre Keren, Jerusalem, Israel
11. Alexandre Mebazaa, Paris, France
12. Markku Nieminen, Hus, Finland
13. Silvia Giuliana Priori, Pavia, Italy
14. Karl Swedberg, Goteborg, Sweden

ESC Staff:
1. Keith McGregor, Sophia Antipolis, France
2. Veronica Dean, Sophia Antipolis, France
3. Catherine Després, Sophia Antipolis, France

Special thanks to Tessa Baak for her contribution.

1. Introduction

The aim of this document is to provide practical guidelines for the diagnosis, assessment, and treatment of acute and chronic heart failure (HF). National health policy as well as clinical judgement may dictate the order of priorities in implementation. An evidence-based approach has been used to generate the grade of any recommendation in the guidelines, with an additional assessment of the quality of the evidence. In Table 1 the language used to specify a recommendation is presented.

*Adapted from the ESC Guidelines on Diagnosis and Treatment of Acute and Chronic Heart Failure 2008 (European Heart Journal 2008)doi:10.1093/eurheartj/ehn309

Table 1: ESC Classes of Recommendations

Classes of Recommendations	Definition	Suggested wording to use
Class I	Evidence and/or general agreementthat a given treatment or procedure is beneficial,useful and effective	Is recommended/ is indicated
Class II	Conflicting evidence and/or a divergence of opinion about the use fulness/efficacy of the given treatment or procedure	
Class IIa	Weight of evidence/opinion is in favour of usefulness/ efficacy	Should be considered
Class IIb	Usefulness/efficacy is less well established by evidence/opinion	May be considered
Class III	Evidence or general agreement that the given treatment or procedure is not useful/effective, and in some cases may be harmful	Is not recommended

2. Definition & Diagnosis

Definition of heart failure

HF is a complex syndrome in which the patients should have the following features: symptoms of HF, typically shortness of breath at rest or during exertion, and/or fatigue; signs of fluid retention such as pulmonary congestion or ankle swelling; objective evidence of an abnormality of the structure or function of the heart at rest (Table 2).

A clinical response to treatment directed at HF alone is not sufficient for the diagnosis, but is helpful when the diagnosis remains unclear after appropriate diagnostic investigations.

Table 2: Definition of heart failure

HF is a clinical syndrome in which patients have the following features:

• Symptoms typical of HF (breathlessness at rest or on exercise, fatigue, tiredness, ankle swelling)
and
• Signs typical of HF (tachycardia, tachypnoea, pulmonary rales, pleural effusion, raised jugular venous pressure, peripheral oedema, hepatomegaly)
and
• Objective evidence of a structural or functional abnormality of the heart at rest (cardiomegaly, third heart sound, cardiac murmurs, abnormality on the echocardiogram, raised natriuretic peptide concentration)

Table 3: Common clinical manifestatons of heart failure

Dominant clinical feature	Symptoms	Signs
Peripheral oedema/ congestion	Breathlessness Tiredness, fatigue Anorexia	Peripheral oedema Raised jugular venous pressure Pulmonary oedema Hepatomegaly, ascites Fluid overload (congestion) Cachexia
Pulmonary oedema	Severe breathlessness at rest	Crackles or rales over lungs, effusion Tachycardia, tachypnoea
Cardiogenic shock (low output syndromes)	Confusion Weakness Cold periphery	Poor peripheral perfusion Systolic BP < 90 mmHg Anuria or oliguria
High blood pressure (hypertensive HF)	Breathlessness	Usually raised BP, LVH and preserved EF
Right HF	Breathlessness Fatigue	Evidence of RV dysfunction Raised JVP, peripheral oedema, hepatomegaly, gut congestion

Acute and chronic heart failure

A useful classification of HF based on the nature of the clinical presentation makes a distinction between new onset HF, transient HF and chronic HF. Transient HF refers to symptomatic HF over a limited time period although long-term treatment may be indicated.

Systolic versus diastolic heart failure

Most patients with HF have evidence of both systolic and diastolic dysfunction at rest or on exercise. Patients with diastolic HF have symptoms and/or signs of HF and a preserved left ventricular ejection fraction above 45-50%. We have elected to use the abbreviation HFPEF in this document.

Table 4: Classification of HF by structural abnormality (ACC/AHA) or by symptoms relating to functional capacity (NYHA)

ACC/AHA Stages of HF Stage of heart failure based on structure and damage to heart muscle		NYHA Functional Classification Severity based on symptoms and physical activity	
Stage A	At high risk for developing HF. No identified structural or functional abnormality; no signs or symptoms.	Class I	No limitation of physical activity. Ordinary physical activity does not cause undue fatigue, palpitation, or dyspnoea.
Stage B	Developed structural heart disease that is strongly associated with the development of HF, but without signs or symptoms.	Class II	Slight limitation of physical activity. Comfortable at rest, but ordinary physical activity results in fatigue, palpitation, or dyspnoea.
Stage C	Symptomatic HF associated with underlying structural heart disease.	Class III	Marked limitation of physical activity. Comfortable at rest, but less than ordinary activity results in fatigue, palpitation, or dyspnoea.
Stage D	Advanced structural heart disease and marked symptoms of HF at rest despite maximal medical therapy.	Class IV	Unable to carry on any physical activity without discomfort. Symptoms at rest. If any physical activity is undertaken, discomfort is increased.
ACC = American College of Cardiology; AHA, American Heart Association. Hunt SA et al. Circulation. 2005;112:1825-1852.		NYHA = New York Heart Association. The Criteria Committee of the New York Heart Association. Nomenclature and Criteria for Diagnosis of Diseases of the Heart and Great Vessels. 9th Ed. Boston. Mass: Little, Brown & Co; 1994:253-256	

Epidemiology

The prevalence of HF in the overall population is between 2 and 3%. The prevalence of asymptomatic ventricular dysfunction is similar so that HF, or asymptomatic ventricular dysfunction, is evident in about 4% of the population. The prevalence rises sharply around 75 years of age so the prevalence in 70 to 80 year old people is between 10 and 20%.

Overall 50% of patients are dead at four years. Forty percent of patients admitted to hospital with HF are dead or readmitted within one year.

HFPEF (ejection fraction > 45-50%) is present in half the patients with HF. The prognosis in more recent studies has been shown to be essentially similar to systolic HF.

Aetiology of heart failure

The most common causes of functional deterioration of the heart are damage or loss of heart muscle acute or chronic ischaemia, increased vascular resistance with hypertension or the development of a tachyarrhythmia such as atrial fibrillation. Coronary heart disease is by far the commonest cause of myocardial disease being the initiating cause in about 70% of patients with HF. Valve disease accounts for 10% and cardiomyopathies for another 10%.

3. Diagnostic Techniques

Algorithm for the diagnosis of heart failure

An algorithm for the diagnosis of HF or left ventricular dysfunction is shown in Figure 1. The diagnosis of HF is not sufficient alone. Although the general treatment of HF is common to most patients some causes require specific treatments and may be correctable.

Diagnostic tests in heart failure

Diagnostic tests are usually most sensitive for the detection of patients with HF and reduced ejection fraction. Diagnostic findings are often less pronounced in patients with HFPEF. Echocardiography is the most useful method for evaluating systolic and diastolic dysfunction.

Electrocardiogram

An electrocardiogram (ECG) should be performed in every patient with suspected HF (Table 5).

Figure 1: Flow-chart for the diagnosis of HF in untreated patients with symptoms suggestive of HF using natriuretic peptides

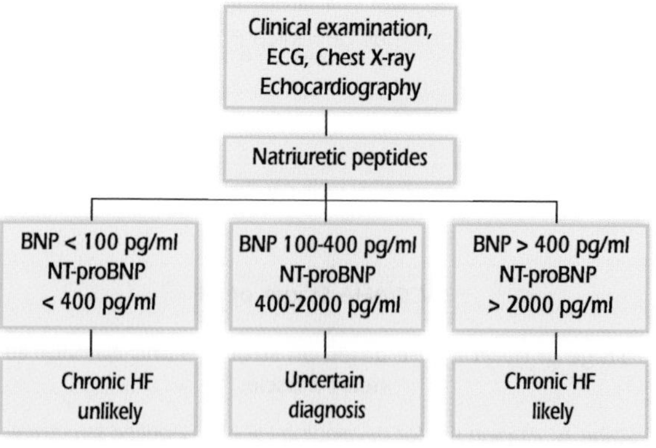

Table 5: Common ECG abnormalities in HF

Abnormality	Causes	Clinical Implications
Sinus tachycardia	Decompensated HF, anaemia, fever, hyperthyroidism	Clinical assessment Laboratory investigation
Sinus bradycardia	Beta-blockade, anti-arrhythmics, hypothyroidism, sick sinus syndrome	Evaluate drug therapy Laboratory investigation
Atrial tachycardia/flutter/ fibrillation	Hyperthyroidism, infection, decompensated HF, infarction	Slow AV conduction, medical conversion, electroversion, catheter ablation, anticoagulation
Ventricular arrhythmias	Ischaemia, infarction, cardiomyopathy, myocarditis hypokalaemia, hypomagnesaemia, digitalis overdose	Laboratory investigation, exercise test, perfusion studies, coronary angiography, electrophysiology testing, ICD
Ischaemia/Infarction	Coronary artery disease	Echo, troponins, coronary angiography, revascularization
Q waves	Infarction, hypertrophic cardiomyopathy, LBBB, pre-excitation	Echo, coronary angiography
LV hypertrophy	Hypertension, aortic valve disease, hypertrophic cardiomyopathy	Echo/Doppler
AV block	Infarction, drug toxicity, myocarditis, sarcoidosis, Lyme disease	Evaluate drug therapy, pacemaker, systemic disease
Microvoltage	Obesity, emphysema, pericardial effusion, amyloidosis	Echo, chest X-ray
QRS length >120 msec of LBBB morphology	Electrical dyssynchrony	Echo, CRT-P, CRT-D

Chest X-ray

Chest X-ray is an essential component of the diagnostic work-up in HF. It permits assessment of pulmonary congestion and may demonstrate important pulmonary or thoracic causes of dyspnoea (Table 6).

Table 6: Common chest X-ray abnormalities in heart failure

Abnormality	Causes	Clinical Implications
Cardiomegaly	Dilated LV, RV, atria Pericardial effusion	Echo/Doppler
Ventricular hypertrophy	Hypertension, aortic stenosis, hypertrophic cardiomyopathy	Echo/Doppler
Normal pulmonary findings	Pulmonary congestion unlikely	Reconsider diagnosis (if untreated) Serious lung disease unlikely
Pulmonary venous congestion	Elevated LV filling pressure	Left heart failure confirmed
Interstitial oedema	Elevated LV filling pressure	Left heart failure confirmed
Pleural effusions	Elevated filling pressures HF likely if bilateral Pulmonary infection, surgery or malignant effusion	Consider non-cardiac aetiology If abundant, consider diagnostic or therapeutic centesis
Kerley B lines	Increased lymphatic pressures	Mitral stenosis or chronic HF
Hyperlucent lung fields	Emphysema or pulmonary embolism	Spiral CT, spirometry, Echo
Pulmonary infection	Pneumonia may be secondary to pulmonary congestion	Treat both infection and HF
Pulmonary infiltration	Systemic disease	Diagnostic work-up

Laboratory tests

Marked haematological or electrolyte abnormalities are uncommon in untreated mild to moderate HF, although mild anaemia, hyponatraemia, hyperkalaemia and reduced renal function are frequently seen, especially in patients treated with a diuretic and/or ACEI, ARB, or an aldosterone antagonist (Table 7).

Table 7: Common laboratory test abnormalities in heart failure

Abnormality	Causes	Clinical Implications
Increased serum creatinine (> 150 μmol/l)	Renal disease, ACEI/ARB, aldosterone blockade	Calculate GFR, consider reducing ACEI/ARB, or aldosterone blockers dose, check potassium and BUN
Anaemia (13g/dl in men, 12 in women)	Chronic HF, haemodilution, iron loss or poor utilisation, renal failure, chronic disease	Diagnostic work-up, consider treatment
Hyponatraemia (< 135 mmol/l)	Chronic HF, haemodilution, AVP release, diuretics	Consider water restriction, reducing diuretic dosage, ultrafiltration, vasopressin antagonis
Hypernatraemia (> 150 mmol/l)	Hyperglycaemia, dehydratation	Assess water intake, diagnostic work-up
Hypokalaemia (< 3.5 mmol/l)	Diuretics, secondary hyperaldosteronism	Risk of arrhythmia, consider potassium supplements, ACEI/ARB, aldosterone blockers
Hyperkalaemia (> 5.5 mmol/l)	Renal failure, potassium supplement, renin-angiotensin-aldosterone system blockers	Stop potassium sparing treatment (ACEI/ARB, aldosterone blockers), assess renal function and pH, risk of bradycardia
Hyperglycaemia (> 6.5 mmol/l)	Diabetes, insulin resistance	Evaluate hydration, treat glucose intolerance
Hyperuricaemia (> 500 μmol/l)	Diuretic treatment, gout, malignancy	Allopurinol, reduce diuretic dose
BNP > 400 pg/ml, NT proBNP > 2000 pg/ml	Increased ventricular wall stress	HF likely, indication for echo, consider treatment
BNP < 100 pg/ml, NT proBNP < 400 pg/ml	Normal wall stress	Re-evaluate diagnosis, HF unlikely if untreated
Albumin high (> 45 g/l)	Dehydratation, myeloma	Rehydrate
Albumin low (< 30 g/l)	Poor nutrition, renal loss	Diagnostic work-up
Transaminase increase	Liver dysfunction, right HF , drug toxicity	Diagnostic work-up, liver congestion, reconsider therapy
Elevated troponins	Myocyte necrosis, prolonged ischaemia, severe HF, myocarditis, sepsis, renal failure, pulmonary embolism	Evaluate pattern of increase (mild increases common in severe HF), coronary angiography, evaluation for revascularization
Abnormal thyroid tests	Hyper/hypothyroidism, amiodarone	Treat thyroid abnormality
Urinalysis	Proteinuria, glycosuria, bacteria	Diagnostic work-up, rule out infection
INR > 2.5	Anticoagulant overdose, liver congestion	Evaluate anticoagulant dosage, assess liver function, assess anticoagulant dose
CRP > 10 mg/l, neutrophilic leucocytosis	Infection, inflammation	Diagnostic work-up

Natriuretic peptides

Evidence exists supporting the use of plasma concentrations of natriuretic peptides for diagnosing, staging, making hospitalisation/discharge decisions and identifying patients at risk for clinical events. A normal concentration in an untreated patient has a high negative predictive value and makes HF an unlikely cause of symptoms (Figure 1).

Troponin I or T

Troponin should be sampled in suspected HF when the clinical picture suggests an acute coronary syndrome. Mild increases in cardiac troponin are frequently seen in severe HF or during episodes of HF decompensation in patients without evidence of myocardial ischaemia.

Echocardiography*

Confirmation by echocardiography of the diagnosis of HF and/or cardiac dysfunction is mandatory and should be performed shortly following suspicion of the diagnosis of HF. Tables 8 and 9 present the most common echocardiographic and Doppler abnormalities in HF.

* The term echocardiography is used to refer to all cardiac ultrasound imaging techniques, including pulsed and continuous wave Doppler, colour Doppler and Tissue Doppler Imaging (TDI).

Table 8: Common echocardiographic abnormalities in heart failure

Measurement	Abnormality	Clinical Implications
LV ejection fraction	Reduced (< 45-50%)	Systolic dysfunction
Left ventricular function, global and focal	Akinesis, hypokinesis, dyskinesis	Myocardial infarction/ischaemia Cardiomyopathy, myocarditis
End diastolic diameter	Increased (> 55-60 mm)	Volume overload - HF likely
End systolic diameter	Increased (> 45 mm)	Volume overload Systolic dysfunction likely
Fractional shortening	Reduced (< 25%)	Systolic dysfunction
Left atrial size	Increased (> 40 mm)	Increased filling pressures Mitral valve dysfunction Atrial fibrillation
Left ventricular thickness	Hypertrophy (> 11-12 mm)	Hypertension, aortic stenosis, hypertrophic cardiomyopathy
Valvular structure and function	Valvular stenosis or regurgitation (especially aortic stenosis and mitral insufficiency)	May be primary cause of HF or complicating factor Assess gradients and regurgitant fraction - Assess haemodynamic consequences Consider surgery
Mitral diastolic flow profile	Abnormalities of the early and late diastolic filling patterns	Indicates diastolic dysfunction and suggests mechanism
Tricuspid regurgitation peak velocity	Increased (> 3 m/sec)	Increased right ventricular systolic pressure - suspect pulmonary hypertension
Pericardium	Effusion, haemopericardium, thickening	Consider tamponade, uraemia, malignancy, systemic disease, acute or chronic pericarditis, constrictive pericarditis
Aortic outflow velocity time integral	Reduced (< 15 cm)	Reduced low stroke volume
Inferior vena cava	Dilated retrograde flow	Increased right atrial pressures Right ventricular dysfunction Hepatic congestion

Table 9: Doppler-echocardiographic indices and ventricular filling

Doppler indices	Pattern	Consequence
E/A waves ratio	Restrictive (> 2, short deceleration time < 115 to 150 msec)	High filling pressures Volume overload
	Slowed relaxation (< 1)	Normal filling pressures Poor compliance
	Normal (> 1)	Inconclusive as may be pseudo-normal
E/Ea	Increased (> 15)	High filling pressures
	Reduced (< 8)	Low filling pressures
	Intermediate (8 - 15)	Inconclusive
(A mitral - A pulm) duration	> 30 msec	Normal filling pressures
	< 30 msec	High filling pressures
Pulmonary S wave	> D wave	Low filling pressures
Vp	< 45 cm/sec	Slow relaxation
E/Vp	> 2.5	High filling pressures
	< 2	Low filling pressures
Valsalva manoeuver	Change of the pseudonormal to abnormal filling pattern	Unmasks high filling pressure in the setting of systolic and diastolic dysfunction

The diagnosis of HFPEF requires three conditions to be satisfied:

(1) presence of signs or symptoms of CHF,

(2) presence of normal or only mildly abnormal left ventricular systolic function (LVEF ≥ 45-50%),

(3) evidence of diastolic dysfunction (abnormal left ventricular relaxation or diastolic stiffness).

Stress echocardiography

Stress echocardiography (dobutamine or exercise echo) is used to detect ventricular dysfunction caused by ischaemia and to assess myocardial viability in the presence of marked hypokinesis or akinesis.

Further non-invasive imaging may include cardiac magnetic resonance imaging (CMR) or radionuclide imaging.

Cardiac magnetic resonance imaging (CMR)

CMR is a versatile, highly accurate, reproducible, non-invasive imaging technique for the assessment of left and right ventricular volumes, global function, regional wall motion, myocardial viability, myocardial thickness, thickening, myocardial mass and tumours, cardiac valves, congenital defects, and pericardial disease.

CT Scan

CT angiography may be considered in patients with a low or intermediate pre-test probability of CAD and an equivocal exercise or imaging stress test.

Radionuclide ventriculography

Radionuclide ventriculography is recognised as a relatively accurate method of determining LVEF and is most often performed in the context of a myocardial perfusion scan providing information on viability and ischaemia.

Pulmonary function tests

These tests are useful in demonstrating or excluding respiratory causes of breathlessness and assessing the potential contribution of lung disease to the patient's dyspnoea.

Exercise testing

Exercise testing is useful for the objective evaluation of exercise capacity and exertional symptoms, such as dyspnoea and fatigue. The 6 minute walk test is a simple, reproducible, readily available tool frequently employed to assess submaximal functional capacity and evaluate the response to intervention.

Cardiac catheterisation

Cardiac catheterisation is unnecessary for the routine diagnosis and management of patients with HF but may be indicated to elucidate aetiology, to obtain important prognostic information and if revascularization is being considered.

Coronary angiography

Coronary angiography should be considered in HF patients with a history of exertional angina or suspected ischaemic LV dysfunction. Coronary angiography is also indicated in patients with refractory HF of unknown aetiology and in patients with evidence of severe mitral regurgitation or aortic valve disease potentially correctable by surgery.

Right heart catheterisation

Right heart catheterisation provides valuable haemodynamic information regarding filling pressures, vascular resistance and cardiac output. Monitoring of haemodynamic variables may be considered to monitor treatment in patients with severe HF not responding to appropriate treatment.

Ambulatory ECG monitoring (Holter)

Ambulatory ECG monitoring is valuable in the assessment of patients with symptoms suggestive of an arrhythmia (e.g. palpitations or syncope) and in monitoring ventricular rate control in patients with atrial fibrillation.

Prognosis

Determining prognosis in HF is complex. The variables most consistently cited as independent outcome predictors are reported in Table 10.

Table 10: Conditions associated with a poor prognosis in HF

Demographics	Clinical	Electrophysiological	Functional/ Exertional	Laboratory	Imaging
Advanced age* Ischaemic aetiology* Resuscitated sudden death*	**Hypotension* NYHA Functional Class III-IV* Recent HF hospitalization***	**Tachycardia Q Waves Wide QRS* LV hypertrophy Complex ventricular arrhythmias***	**Reduced work, Low peak VO2***	**Marked elevation of BNP/NT pro-BNP* Hyponatraemia* Elevated troponin* Elevated biomarkers, neurohumoral activation***	**Low LVEF***
Poor compliance Renal dysfunction Diabetes Anaemia COPD Depression	Tachycardia Pulmonary rales Aortic stenosis Low body mass index Sleep related breathing disorders	Low heart rate variability T-wave alternans Atrial fibrillation	Poor 6 min walk distance High VE/VCO2 slope Periodic breathing	Elevated creatinine/BUN Elevated bilirubin Anaemia Elevated uric acid	Increased LV volumes Low cardiac index High left ventricular filling pressure Restrictive mitral filling pattern, pulmonary hypertension Impaired right ventricular function

* = powerful predictors

4. Non-pharmacological Management

Self-care management

Self-care management is a part of successful HF treatment and can significantly impact on symptoms, functional capacity, well being, morbidity and prognosis.

Self-care can be defined as actions aimed at maintaining physical stability, avoidance of behaviour that can worsen the condition and detection of the early symptoms of deterioration. The essential topics and self-care behaviours are presented in Table 11.

Table 11: Essential topics in patient education with associated skills and appropriate self care behaviours

Educational topics	Skills and Self-care Behaviours
Definition and aetiology of heart failure	Understand the cause of heart failure and why symptoms occur
Symptoms and signs of heart failure	Monitor and recognise signs and symptoms Record daily weight and recognise rapid weight gain Know how and when to notify health care provider Use flexible diuretic therapy if appropriate and recommended
Pharmacological treatment	Understand indications, dosing and effects of drugs Recognise the common side-effects of each drug prescribed
Risk factor modification	Understand the importance of smoking cessation Monitor blood pressure if hypertensive Maintain good glucose control if diabetic Avoid obesity
Diet recommendation	Sodium restriction if prescribed - Avoid of excessive fluid intake Modest intake of alcohol - Monitor and prevent malnutrition
Exercise recommendations	Be reassured and comfortable about physical activity Understand the benefits of exercise Perform exercise training regularly
Sexual activity	Be reassured about engaging in sex and discuss problems with health care professionals Understand specific sexual problems and various coping strategies
Immunisation	Receive immunisation against infections such as influenza and pneumococcal disease
Sleep and breathing disorders	Recognise preventive behaviour such as weight loss if obese, smoking cession and abstinence from alcohol Learn about treatment options if appropriate
Adherence	Understand the importance of following treatment recommendations and maintaining motivation to follow treatment plan
Psychosocial aspects	Understand that depressive symptom and cognitive dysfunction are common in patients with heart failure and the importance of social support - Learn about treatment options if appropriate
Prognosis	Understand important prognostic factors and make realistic decisions - Seek psychosocial support if appropriate

The Web Site **heartfailurematters.org** represents an internet tool provided by the Heart Failure Association of the ESC that permits patients, their next of kin and caregivers to obtain useful, practical information in a user-friendly format.

5. Pharmacological Therapy

The objectives of the treatment of HF are summarised in Table 12.

Figure 2 provides a treatment strategy for the use of drugs and devices in patients with symptomatic HF and systolic dysfunction. It is essential to detect and consider treatment of the common cardiovascular and non-cardiovascular comorbidities.

Table 12: Objectives of treatment in chronic heart failure

1. Prognosis	Reduce mortality
2. Morbidity	Relieve symptoms and signs Improve quality of life Eliminate oedema and fluid retention Increase exercise capacity Reduce fatigue and breathlessness Reduce need for hospitalisation Provide for end of life care
3. Prevention	Occurrence of myocardial damage Progression of myocardial damage Remodelling of the myocardium Reoccurrence of symptoms and fluid accumulation Hospitalisation

Figure 2: Treatment strategy for the use of drugs and devices in patients with symptomatic HF and systolic dysfunction

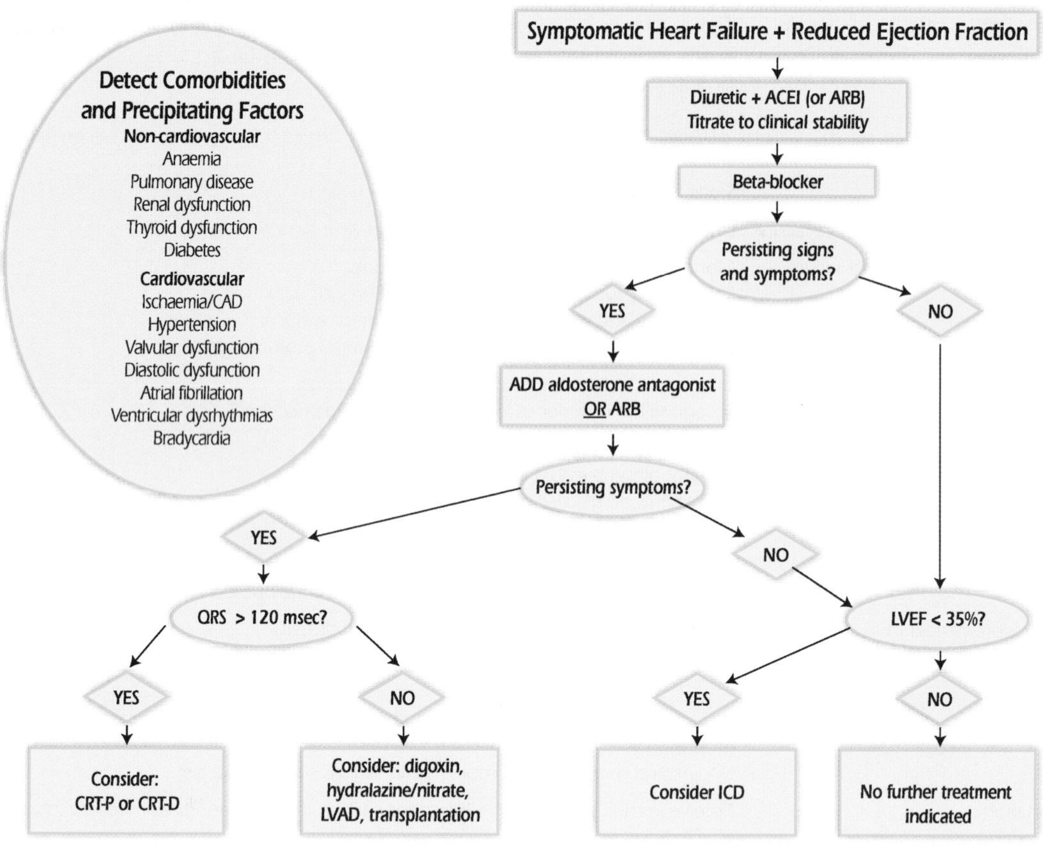

Table 13: Dosages of commonly used drugs in HF

	Starting dose (mg)		Target dose (mg)	
ACEI				
captopril	6.25	t.i.d.	50 - 100	t.i.d.
enalapril	2.5	b.i.d.	10 - 20	b.i.d.
lisinopril	2.5 - 5.0	o.d.	20 - 35	o.d.
ramipril	2.5	o.d.	5	b.i.d.
trandolapril	0.5	o.d.	4	o.d.
ARB				
candesartan	4 or 8	o.d.	32	o.d.
valsartan	40	b.i.d.	160	b.i.d.
Aldosterone antagonist				
eplerenone	25	o.d.	50	o.d.
spironolactone	25	o.d.	25 - 50	o.d.
Beta-blocker				
bisoprolol	1.25	o.d.	10	o.d.
carvedilol	3.125	b.i.d.	25 - 50	b.i.d.
metoprolol succinate	12.5/25	o.d.	200	o.d.
nebivolol	1.25	o.d.	10	o.d.
Hydralazine-ISDN				
Hydralazine-ISDN	37.5/20	t.i.d.	75/40	t.i.d.

Angiotensin converting enzyme inhibitors (ACEI)

Treatment with an ACEI improves ventricular function and patient well-being, reduces hospital admission for worsening HF and increases survival.

Patients who should get an ACEI

- LVEF ≤ 40%, irrespective of symptoms

Initiation of an ACEI:

- Check renal function and serum electrolytes.
- Consider dose up-titration after 2-4 weeks.
- Do not increase dose if worsening renal function or hyperkalaemia.
- It is common to up-titrate slowly but more rapid titration is possible in closely monitored patients.

Angiotensin receptor blockers (ARBs)

Treatment with an ARB improves ventricular function and patient well being and reduces hospital admission for worsening HF. An ARB is recommended as an alternative in patients intolerant of an ACEI.

Patients who should get an an ARB

- LVEF ≤ 40% and either:
- As an alternative in patients with mild to severe symptoms (NYHA functional class II-IV) who are intolerant of an ACEI.
- or in patients with persistent symptoms (NYHA functional class II-IV) despite treatment with an ACEI and beta-blocker.

Initiation of an ARB:

- Check renal function and serum electrolytes.
- Consider dose up-titration after 2-4 weeks.
- Do not increase dose if worsening renal function or hyperkalaemia.
- It is common to up-titrate slowly but more rapid titration is possible in closely monitored patients.

Beta-blockers

Beta-blockade improves ventricular function and patient well-being, reduces hospital admission for worsening HF and increases survival.

Patients who should get a beta-blocker

- LVEF ≤ 40%.
- Mild to severe symptoms (NYHA functional class II-IV).
- Optimal dose level of an ACEI or/and ARB.
- Patients should be clinically stable (e.g. no recent change in dose of diuretic).

Initiation of a beta-blocker:

- Beta-blockers may be initiated prior to hospital discharge in recently decompensated patients with caution.
- Visits every 2-4 weeks to up-titrate the dose of beta-blocker (slower dose up-titration may be needed in some patients). Do not increase dose if signs of worsening HF, symptomatic hypotension (e.g. dizziness) or excessive bradycardia (pulse rate < 50/minute) at each visit.

Diuretics

Diuretics are recommended in patients with HF and clinical signs or symptoms of congestion. Dosages of commonly used diuretics in HF are provided in Table 14.

Table 14: Diuretic dosages

Diuretics	Initial dose (mg)		Usual daily dose (mg)	
Loop diuretics*				
• furosemide	20 - 40		40 - 240	
• bumetanide	0.5 - 1.0		1 - 5	
• torasemide	5 - 10		10 - 20	
Thiaides**				
• bendroflumethiazide	2.5		2.5 - 10	
• hydrochlorothiazide	25		12.5 - 100	
• metolazone	2.5		2.5 - 10	
• indapamide	2.5		2.5 - 5	
Potassium-sparing diuretics***				
	+ ACEI/ ARB	– ACEI/ ARB	+ ACEI/ ARB	– ACEI/ ARB
• spironolactone/ eplerenone	12.5 - 25	50	50	100-200
• amiloride	2.5	5	20	40
• triamterene	25	50	100	200

* Dose might need to be adjusted according to volume status/weight; excessive doses may cause renal impairment and ototoxicity.

*** Do not use thiazides if eGFR < 30 mL/min, except when prescribed synergistically with loop diuretics.

*** Aldosterone antagonists should always be preferred to other potassium sparing diuretics.

Volume depletion and hyponatraemia from excessive diuresis may increase the risk of hypotension and renal dysfunction with ACEI/ARB therapy (Table 15).

Table 15: Practical considerations in treatment with loop diuretics:

Problems	Suggested actions
Hypokalaemia/ hypomagnesaemia	• increase ACEI/ARB dosage • add aldosterone antagonist • potassium supplements • magnesium supplements
Hyponatraemia	• water restriction • stop thiazide diuretic or switch to loop diuretic, if possible • reduce dosage/stop loop diuretics if possible • consider AVP antagonist e.g. tolvaptan if available • i.v. inotropic support • consider ultrafiltration
Hyperuricaemia/ gout	• consider allopurinol • for symptomatic gout use colchicine for pain relief • avoid NSAIDs
Hypovolaemia/ dehydration	• assess volume status • consider diuretic dosage reduction
Insufficient response or diuretic resistance	• check compliance and fluid intake • increase dose of diuretic • consider switching from furosemide to bumetanide or torasemide • add aldosterone antagonist • combine loop diuretic and thiazide • administer loop diuretic twice daily or on empty stomach • consider short-term i.v. infusion of loop diuretic
Renal failure (excessive rise in urea/BUN and/or creatinine)	• check for hypovolaemia/dehydration • exclude use of other nephrotoxic agents e.g. NSAIDs, trimethoprim • withhold aldosterone antagonist • if using concomitant loop and thiazide diuretic stop thiazide diuretic • consider reducing dose of ACEI/ARB • consider ultrafiltration

Initiation of diuretic therapy:

- Check renal function and serum electrolytes.
- Most patients are prescribed loop diuretics rather than thiazides due to the higher efficiency of induced diuresis and natriuresis.
- Self-adjustment of diuretic dose based on daily weight-measurements and other clinical signs of fluid retention should be encouraged in HF outpatient care. Patient education is required.

Aldosterone antagonists

Aldosterone antagonists reduce hospital admission for worsening HF and increase survival when added to existing therapy, including an ACEI.

Patients who should get an aldosterone antagonist

- LVEF ≤ 35%
- Moderate to severe symptoms (NYHA functional class III-IV).
- Optimal dose of a beta-blocker and an ACEI or an ARB (but not an ACEI and an ARB).

Initiation of spironolactone (eplerenone):

- Check renal function and serum electrolytes.
- Consider dose up-titration after 4-8 weeks. Do not increase dose if worsening renal function or hyperkalaemia.

Hydralazine and isosorbide dinitrate (H-ISDN)

Treatment with H-ISDN may be considered to reduce the risk of death and hospital admission for worsening HF.

Patients who should get H-ISDN

- An alternative to an ACEI/ARB where both of the latter are not tolerated.
- As add-on, therapy to an ACEI if an ARB or aldosterone antagonist is not tolerated or if significant symptoms persist despite therapy with an ACEI, ARB, beta-blocker, and aldosterone antagonist.

Initiation of H-ISDN:

- Consider dose up-titration after 2-4 weeks. Do not increase dose with symptomatic hypotension.

Digoxin

In patients in sinus rhythm with symptomatic HF and a LVEF ≤ 40%, treatment with digoxin may improve patient well-being and reduce hospital admission for worsening HF, but has no effect on survival.

- Patients in atrial fibrillation with ventricular rate at rest > 80, and at exercise > 110-120 beats/minute should get digoxin.
- In patients with sinus rhythm and left ventricular systolic dysfunction (LVEF ≤ 40%) receiving optimal doses of diuretic, ACEI or/and ARB, beta-blocker and

aldosterone antagonist if indicated, who are still symptomatic, digoxin may be considered.

Anticoagulants (vitamin K antagonists)

- Warfarin (or an alternative oral anticoagulant) is recommended in patients with HF and permanent, persistent or paroxysmal atrial fibrillation without contra-indications.

Pharmacologic management of patients with HF and Coronary Artery Disease

ACEI

- are recommended in patients with atherosclerotic arterial disease and symptoms of HF with impaired LVEF (≤ 40%). Should also be considered in patients with CAD and HFPEF.

ARBs

- are recommended in patients following MI with symptoms of HF or impaired LVEF intolerant to ACEI.

Beta-blockers

- are recommended for CAD patients with symptoms of HF and impaired LVEF (≤ 40%).
- are recommended for all patients following MI with preserved LVEF.

Aldosterone antagonists

- are recommended in patients following MI with impaired LVEF and/or signs and symptoms of HF.

Nitrates

- may be considered to control anginal symptoms.

Calcium channel blockers

- may be considered to control anginal symptoms. In patients with reduced LVEF, amlodipine or felodipine are preferable.

Statins

- may be considered for all patients with HF and CAD. There is no evidence that statins improve survival in patients in these patients, but they may reduce the risk of hospital admissions.

Management of patients with HF and preserved left ventricular ejection fraction (HFPEF)

No treatment has yet been shown, convincingly, to reduce morbidity and mortality in patients with HFPEF. Diuretics are used to control sodium and water retention and relieve breathlessness and oedema. Adequate treatment of hypertension and myocardial ischaemia is also important, as is control of the ventricular rate.

6. Devices & Surgery

Revascularization procedures, valvular and ventricular surgery

- If clinical symptoms of HF with present, surgically correctable conditions should be detected and corrected if indicated.

Revascularization in patients with HF

CABG or PCI should be considered in selected HF patients with CAD. Decisions regarding the choice of the method of revascularization should be based on a careful evaluation of comorbidities, procedural risk, coronary anatomy and evidence of the extent of viable myocardium in the area to be revascularised, LV function and the presence of haemodynamically significant valvular disease.

Valvular surgery

- Valvular heart disease (VHD) may be the underlying aetiology for HF or an important aggravating factor.
- Although impaired LVEF is an important risk factor for higher peri- and postoperative mortality, surgery may be considered in symptomatic patients with poor LV function.
- Optimal medical management of both HF and comorbid conditions prior to surgery is imperative. Emergency surgery should be avoided if possible.

Aortic stenosis (AS)

Surgery:

- is recommended in eligible patients with HF symptoms and severe AS.
- is recommended in asymptomatic patients with severe AS and impaired LVEF (< 50%).
- may be considered in patients with severely reduced valve area and LV dysfunction.

Aortic regurgitation (AR)

Surgery:

- is recommended in all eligible patients with severe AR who have symptoms of HF.
- is recommended in asymptomatic patients with severe AR and moderately impaired LVEF (LVEF ≤ 50%).

Mitral regurgitation (MR)

- Surgery should be considered in patients with severe MR whenever coronary revascularization is an option. Surgical repair of the valve may be an attractive option in carefully selected patients.

Organic MR

Surgery:

- is recommended for patients with LVEF > 30% (valve repair if possible).

Functional MR

Surgery:

- may be considered in selected patients with severe functional MR and severely depressed LV function, who remain symptomatic despite optimal medical therapy.
- Cardiac Resynchronization Therapy should be considered in eligible patients as it may improve LV geometry,papillary muscle dyssynchrony and may reduce MR.

Ischaemic MR

Surgery:

- is recommended in patients with severe MR and LVEF > 30% when CABG is planned.
- should be considered in patients with moderate MR undergoing CABG if repair if feasible.

Tricuspid regurgitation (TR)

- Functional TR is extremely common in HF patients with biventricular dilatation, systolic dysfunction and pulmonary hypertension. Surgery for isolated functional TR is not indicated.

LV aneurysmectomy

- LV aneurysmectomy may be considered in symptomatic patients with large, discrete left ventricular aneurysms.

Pacemakers

- The conventional indications for patients with normal LV function also apply to patients with HF.
- Physiologic pacing to maintain an adequate chronotropic response and maintain atrial-ventricular coordination with a DDD system is preferable to VVI pacing in patients with HF.
- The indications for an ICD, CRT-P or CRT-D device should be detected and evaluated in patients with HF prior to implantation of a pacemaker for an AV conduction defect.
- Right ventricular pacing may induce dyssynchrony and worsen symptoms.
- Pacing, in order to permit initiation or titration of beta-blocker therapy in the absence of conventional indications, is not recommended.

Cardiac Resynchronization Therapy (CRT)

- CRT-P is recommended to reduce morbidity and mortality in patients in NYHA III–IV class who are symptomatic despite optimal medical therapy, and who have a reduced ejection fraction (LVEF ≤ 35%) and QRS prolongation (QRS width ≥ 120 ms).
- CRT with defibrillator function (CRT-D) is recommended to reduce morbidity and mortality in patients in NYHA III–IV class who are symptomatic despite optimal medical therapy, and who have a reduced ejection fraction(LVEF ≤ 35%) and QRS prolongation (QRS width ≥ 120 ms).

Implantable cardioverter defibrillator (ICD)

- ICD therapy for *secondary prevention* is recommended for survivors of VF and also for patients with documented haemodynamically unstable VT and/ or VT with syncope, an LVEF ≤ 40%, on optimal medical therapy and with an expectation of survival with good functional status for more than 1 year.
- ICD therapy for *primary prevention* is recommended to reduce mortality in patients with LV dysfunction due to prior MI who are at least 40 days post-MI, have an LVEF ≤ 35%, in NYHA functional class II or III, receiving optimal medical therapy, and who have a reasonable expectation of survival with good functional status for more than 1 year.
- ICD therapy for *primary prevention* is recommended to reduce mortality in patients with non-ischaemic

cardiomyopathy with a LVEF ≤ 35%, in NYHA functional class II or III, receiving optimal medical therapy, and who have a reasonable expectation of survival with good functional status for more than 1 year.

Heart transplantation, ventricular assist devices, and artificial hearts

Heart transplantation

- Heart transplantation is an accepted treatment for end stage HF. There is consensus that transplantation, provided proper selection criteria are applied, significantly increases survival, exercise capacity, return to work and quality of life compared with conventional treatment.

Left ventricular assist devices (LVAD) and artificial heart

- There has been rapid progress in the development of LVAD technology and artificial hearts. Current indications for LVADs and artificial hearts include bridging to transplantation and managing patients with acute, severe myocarditis. Although experience is limited, these devices may be considered for long-term use when no definitive procedure is planned.

Ultrafiltration

- Ultrafiltration should be considered to reduce fluid overload (pulmonary and/or peripheral oedema) in selected patients and to correct hyponatraemia in symptomatic patients refractory to diuretics.

Remote monitoring

- Remote monitoring can be summarised as the continuous collection of patient information and the capability to review this information without the patient present.

- Continuous analysis of these trends can activate notification mechanisms when clinical relevant changes are detected and therefore facilitate patient management. Remote monitoring may decrease health care utilization through fewer hospital admissions for chronic HF, fewer HF related re-admissions, and more efficient device management.

7. Arrhythmias in Heart Failure

Atrial fibrillation

- A beta-blocker or digoxin is recommended to control the heart rate at rest in patients with HF and LV dysfunction.

- A combination of digoxin and a beta-blocker may be considered to control the heart rate at rest and during exercise.

- In LV systolic dysfunction, digoxin is the recommended initial treatment if the patient is haemodynamically unstable.

- IV administration of digoxin or amiodarone is recommended to control the heart rate in patients with AF and HF, who do not have an accessory pathway.

- Atrio-ventricular node ablation and pacing should be considered to control the heart rate when other measures are unsuccessful or contra-indicated.

Prevention of thromboembolism

- Antithrombotic therapy to prevent thromboembolism is recommended for all patients with AF, unless contra-indicated.

- In patients with AF at highest risk of stroke/ thromboembolism, chronic oral anticoagulant therapy with a vitamin K antagonist is recommended, unless contra-indicated.

Rhythm control

- Electrical cardioversion is recommended when the rapid ventricular response does not respond promptly to appropriate pharmacological measures, especially in patients with AF causing myocardial ischaemia, symptomatic hypotension or symptoms of pulmonary congestion. Precipitating factors should be detected and treated. Patients should be anticoagulated.

Ventricular arrhythmias (VA)

- It is essential to detect, and if possible, correct all potential factors precipitating VA. Neurohumoral blockade with optimal doses of beta-blockers, ACEI, ARBs and/or aldosterone blockers is recommended.

- Routine, prophylactic use of antiarrhythmic agents in patients with asymptomatic, non-sustained VA is not recommended. In HF patients, Class Ic agents should not be used.

Patients with HF and symptomatic VA:

- In patients who survived VF or had a history of haemodynamically unstable VT or VT with syncope, with reduced LVEF (< 40%), receiving optimal pharmacological treatment and with a life expectancy of > 1 year, ICD implantation is recommended.

- Amiodarone is recommended in patients with an implanted ICD, otherwise optimally treated, who continue to have symptomatic VA.

- Catheter ablation is recommended as a adjunct therapy in patients with ICD implanted who have recurrent symptomatic VT with frequent shocks that is not curable by device reprogramming and drug therapy.

- Amiodarone may be considered in HF patients with an ICD implanted with frequent ICD shocks despite optimal therapy to prevent discharge.

Bradycardia

The conventional indications for pacing in patients with normal LV function also apply to patients with HF.

8. Comorbidities & Special Populations

Arterial hypertension

- Treatment of hypertension substantially reduces the risk of developing HF (Table 16).

Table 16: Management of arterial hypertension in HF

In hypertensive patients with evidence of LV dysfunction:
• systolic and diastolic blood pressure should be carefully controlled with a therapeutic target of ≤ 140/90 and ≤ 130/80 mmHg in diabetics and high risk patients. • anti-hypertensive regimens based on renin-angiotensin system antagonists (ACEI or ARBs) are preferable.
In hypertensive patients with HFPEF:
• aggressive treatment (often with several drugs with complementary mechanisms of action) is recommended. • ACEI and/or ARBs should be considered the first-line agents.

Non-cardiovascular comorbidities

Diabetes mellitus (DM)

- DM is a major risk factor for the development of cardiovascular disease and HF.

- ACEI and ARBs can be useful in patients with DM to decrease the risk of end-organ damage and subsequently the risk of HF.

- All patients should receive life-style recommendations.

- Elevated blood glucose should be treated with tight glycaemic control.

- Oral antidiabetic therapy should be individualised.

- *Metformin* should be considered as a first-line agent in overweight patients with type II DM without significant renal dysfunction.

- *Thiazolidinediones* have been associated with increased peripheral oedema and symptomatic HF. They are contraindicated in HF patients with NYHA functional class III-IV, but may be considered in patients with NYHA functional class I-II with careful monitoring for fluid retention.

- Early initiation of insulin may be considered if glucose target cannot be achieved.

- Agents with documented effects on morbidity and mortality such as ACEI, beta-blockers, ARBs and diuretics confer benefit at least comparable to that demonstrated in non-diabetic HF patients.

- Evaluation of the potential for revascularization may be particularly important in patients with ischaemic cardiomyopathy and DM.

Renal dysfunction

- Renal dysfunction is common in HF and the prevalence increases with HF severity, age, a history of hypertension or diabetes mellitus.

- In HF renal dysfunction is strongly linked to increased morbidity and mortality.

- The cause of renal dysfunction should always be sought in order to detect potentially reversible causes such as hypotension, dehydration, deterioration in renal function due to ACEI, ARBs or other concomitant medications [e.g. NSAIDs] and renal artery stenosis.

Chronic Obstructive Pulmonary Disease (COPD)

- COPD is a frequent comorbidity in HF. Restrictive and obstructive pulmonary abnormalities are common.

- There is a significant overlap in the signs and symptoms with a relatively lower sensitivity of diagnostic tests such as chest X-ray, ECG, echocardiography and spirometry.

- It is essential to detect and treat pulmonary congestion.

- Agents with documented effects on morbidity and mortality such as ACEI, beta-blockers and ARBs are recommended in patients with co existing pulmonary disease.

- The majority of patients with HF and COPD can safely tolerate beta-blocker therapy. Mild deterioration in pulmonary function and symptoms should not lead to prompt discontinuation.

- A history of asthma should be considered a contra-indication to the use of any beta-blocker.

Anaemia

- The prevalence of anaemia increases with HF severity, advanced age, female gender, renal disease and other coexisting comorbidities.

- Anaemia may aggravate the pathophysiology of HF by adversely affecting myocardial function, activating neurohormonal systems, compromising renal function and contributing to circulatory failure.

- Correction of anaemia has not been established as routine therapy in HF. Simple blood transfusion is not recommended to treat the anaemia of chronic disease in HF.

Cachexia

- Body wasting is a serious complication of HF. This is a generalized process that encompasses loss in all body compartments. Cachexia can be defined as involuntary non-oedematous weight loss of ≥ 6% of total body weight within the last 6-12 months.
  It has not yet been established whether prevention and treatment of cachexia complicating HF should be a treatment goal.

Gout

- Patients with HF are prone to develop hyperuricaemia as a result of loop diuretic therapy use and renal dysfunction. In acute gout, a short course of colchicine to suppress pain and inflammation may be considered. NSAIDs should be avoided if possible in symptomatic patients. Prophylactic therapy with a xanthine oxidase inhibitor (allopurinol) is recommended to prevent recurrence.

Special Populations

Adults with congenital heart disease

- In children, HF is most often related to high-output situations due to intracardiac shunting. This is less frequently observed in adults. Complex lesions associated with cyanosis secondary to impaired pulmonary perfusion may make the diagnosis of HF difficult. Many of these patients benefit from afterload reduction even before significant HF symptoms are clinically manifest.

The Elderly

- HF in the elderly is frequently underdiagnosed, as cardinal symptoms of exercise intolerance are often attributed to ageing, coexisting comorbidities and poor health status. Common comorbidities, may have an impact on management.

- HF with a preserved ejection fraction is more common in the elderly and in females.

- Polypharmacy increases the risk of adverse interactions and side-effects which may reduce compliance. Altered pharmacokinetic and pharmacodynamic properties of drugs must be considered.

- For elderly HF patients suffering from cognitive impairment, individually structured multidisciplinary HF programmes may be particularly useful and improve adherence to therapy and prevent hospitalisation.

- Relative contra-indications to diagnostic procedures and interventions should be carefully evaluated and weighed against the indications.

9. Acute Heart Failure

Definition

Acute HF (AHF) is defined as a rapid onset or change in the signs and symptoms of HF, resulting in the need of urgent therapy. It may present as new HF or worsening HF in the presence of chronic HF. It may be associated with worsening symptoms or signs or as a medical emergency such as acute pulmonary oedema. Multiple cardiovascular and non-cardiovascular morbidities may precipitate AHF (Table 17).

Table 17: Causes and precipitating factors of AHF

Ischaemic heart disease	Circulatory failure
• Acute coronary syndromes • Mechanical complications of acute MI • Right ventricular infarction	• Septicaemia • Thyrotoxicosis • Anaemia • Shunts • Tamponade • Pulmonary embolism
Valvular	
• Valve stenosis • Valvular regurgitation • Endocarditis • Aortic dissection	**Decompensation of preexisting chronic HF**
Myopathies	• Lack of adherence • Volume overload • Infections, especially pneumonia • Cerebrovascular insult • Surgery • Renal dysfunction • Asthma, COPD • Drug abuse • Alcohol abuse
• Postpartum cardiomyopathy • Acute myocarditis	
Hypertension/arrhythmia	
• Hypertension • Acute arrhythmia	

The patient with AHF will usually present in one of 6 clinical categories:

- **Worsening or decompensated chronic HF:** There is usually a history of progressive worsening of known chronic HF on treatment and evidence of systemic and pulmonary congestion.

- **Pulmonary oedema:** patients present with severe respiratory distress, tachypnoea and orthopnoea with rales over the lung fields. Arterial O_2 saturation is usually < 90% on room air prior to treatment with oxygen.

- **Hypertensive HF:** Signs and symptoms of HF accompanied by high blood pressure and usually relatively preserved left ventricular systolic function. There is evidence of increased sympathetic tone with tachycardia and vasoconstriction. The response to appropriate therapy is rapid and hospital mortality is low.

- **Cardiogenic shock:** Cardiogenic shock is defined as evidence of tissue hypoperfusion induced by HF after adequate correction of preload and major arrhythmia. Evidence of organ hypoperfusion and pulmonary congestion develop rapidly.

- **Isolated right HF:** is characterised by a low output syndrome in the absence of pulmonary congestion.

- **ACS and HF:** Many patients with AHF present with a clinical picture and laboratory evidence of an ACS. Approximately 15% of patients with an ACS have signs and symptoms of HF.
  Episodes of acute HF are frequently associated with or precipitated by an arrhythmia (bradycardia, atrial fibrillation, ventricular tachycardia).

Diagnosis of AHF

The assessment of patients with AHF is based on the presenting symptoms and clinical findings (Figure 3). The diagnostic algorithm is similar for AHF developing de novo or as an episode as decompensation in chronic HF (Figure 4).

Figure 3: A clinical assessment of patients with AHF

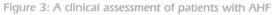

Clinical classifications

Tissue perfusion ↑		
	Dry and warm	Wet and warm
	Dry and cold	Wet and cold

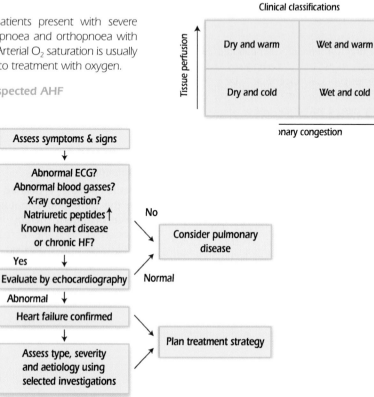

→ nary congestion

Figure 4: Diagnosis of suspected AHF

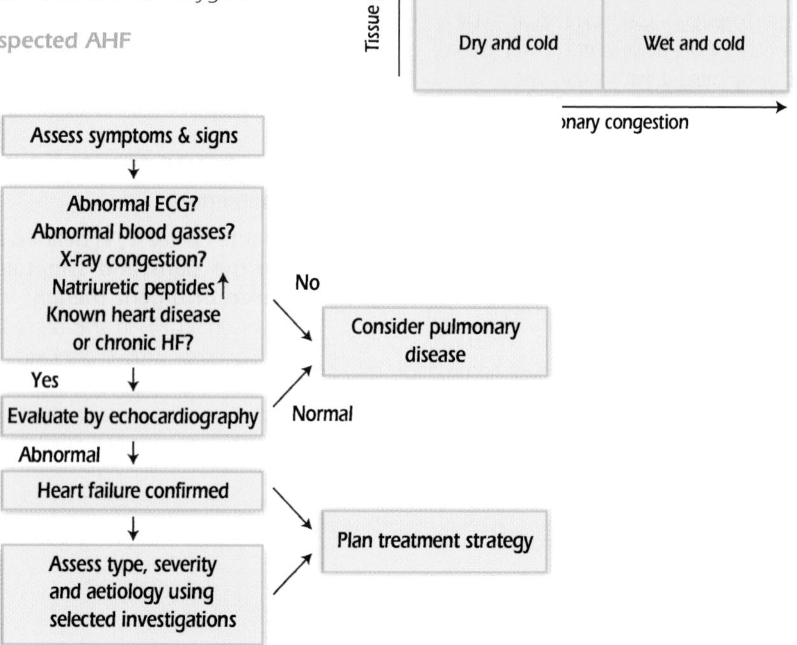

The following investigations are considered appropriate in patients with AHF:

Electrocardiogram (ECG)

- The ECG provides essential information regarding heart rate, rhythm, conduction and frequently aetiology. The ECG may indicate ischaemic ST segment changes suggestive of STEMI or non-STEMI.

Chest X-ray

- Chest X-ray should be performed as soon as possible at admission for all patients with AHF to assess the degree of pulmonary congestion and to evaluate other pulmonary or cardiac conditions.

Arterial blood gas analysis

- Arterial blood gas analysis enables assessment of oxygenation (pO_2), respiratory function (pCO_2) and acid–base balance (pH), and should be assessed in all patients with severe respiratory distress.

Laboratory tests

- Initial diagnostic evaluation of patients with AHF includes full blood count, sodium, potassium, urea, creatinine, glucose, albumin, hepatic enzymes and INR. A small elevation in cardiac troponins may be seen in patients with AHF without ACS.

Natriuretic peptides

- B-type natriuretic peptides (BNP, NT-proBNP) taken in the acute phase have a reasonable negative predictive value for excluding HF. There is no consensus regarding BNP or NT-proBNP reference values in AHF. During 'flash' pulmonary oedema or acute mitral regurgitation, natriuretic peptide levels may remain normal at the time of admission.

Echocardiography

- Echocardiography with Doppler is an essential tool for the evaluation of the functional and structural changes underlying or associated with AHF. The findings will frequently direct treatment strategy.

Instrumentation and monitoring of patients in AHF

- Monitoring of the patient with AHF should be started as soon as possible after the arrival at the emergency unit, concurrent with ongoing diagnostic measures focused on determining the primary aetiology as well as the response to the initial treatment strategy.

Non-invasive Monitoring

- In all critically ill patients, monitoring the routine basic observations of temperature, respiratory rate, heart rate, blood pressure, oxygenation, urine output and the electrocardiogram is mandatory. A pulse oximeter should be used continuously in any unstable patient who is being treated with a fraction of inspired oxygen (FiO_2) that is greater than air.

Arterial line

- The indications for the insertion of an arterial catheter are the need for either continuous analysis of arterial blood pressure due to haemodynamic instability, or the requirement for frequent arterial blood samples.

Central venous lines

- Central venous lines provide access to the central circulation and are therefore useful for the delivery of fluids, drugs and monitoring of the CVP and venous oxygen saturation (SVO_2).

Pulmonary artery catheter

- A PAC may be useful in haemodynamically unstable patients who are not responding as expected to traditional treatments. It is critical to have clear objectives prior to insertion of the catheter.

Coronary Angiography

- In cases of AHF and evidence of ischaemia such as unstable angina or ACS, coronary angiography is indicated in patients without strong contra-indications.

Organisation of AHF treatment

The immediate goals are to improve symptoms and to stabilize the haemodynamic condition (Figure 5). Treatment of hospitalised patients with AHF requires a well-developed treatment strategy with realistic objectives and a plan for follow-up that should be initiated prior to discharge (Table 18).

Figure 5: Initial treatment algorithm in AHF

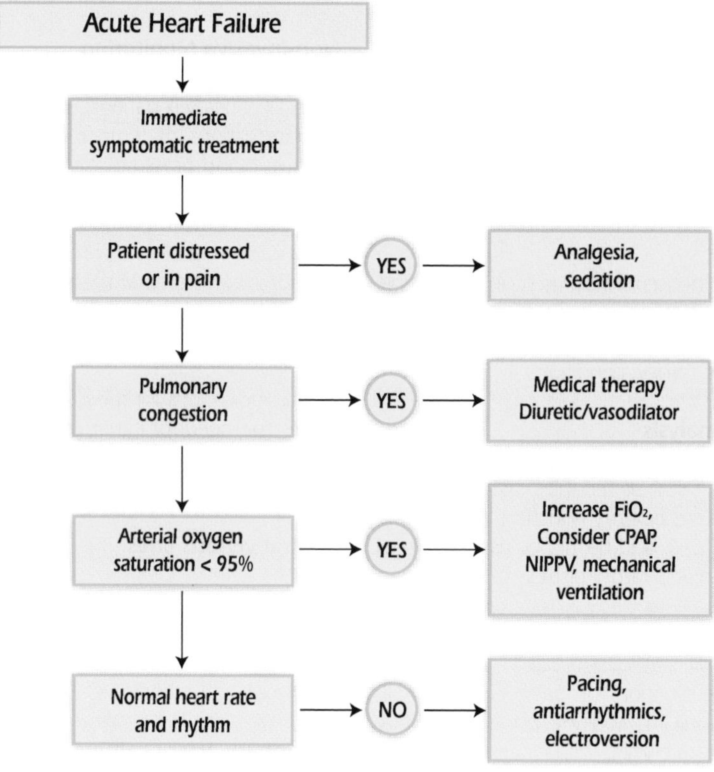

Table 18: Golas of treatment in AHF

• **Immediate (ED/ICU/CCU)**
Improve symptoms Restore oxygenation Improve organ perfusion and haemodynamics Limit cardiac/renal damage Minimize ICU length of stay
• **Intermediate (in hospital)**
Stabilise patient and optimise treatment strategy Initiate appropriate (life-saving) pharmacological therapy Consider device therapy in appropriate patients Minimise hospital length of stay
• **Long-term and predischarge management**
Plan follow-up strategy Educate and initiate appropriate lifestyle adjustments Provide adequate secondary prophylaxis Prevent early readmission Improve quality of life and survival

The following management options are considered appropriate in patients with AHF

Oxygen

- It is recommended to administer oxygen as early as possible in hypoxaemic patients to achieve an arterial oxygen saturation = > 95% (> 90% in COPD patients).

Non-invasive ventilation (NIV)

- Non-invasive ventilation refers to all modalities that assist ventilation without the use of an endotracheal tube but rather with a sealed face-mask.

- Non-invasive ventilation with positive end-expiratory pressure (PEEP) should be considered as early as possible in every patient with acute cardiogenic pulmonary oedema and hypertensive acute HF. NIV should be used with caution in cardiogenic shock and right ventricular failure.

- Intubation and mechanical ventilation should be restricted to patients in whom oxygen delivery is not adequate by oxygen mask or NIV, and in patients with increasing respiratory failure or exhaustion as assessed by hypercapnia.

How to use NIV

- A PEEP of 5-7.5 cm H_2O should be applied first and titrated to clinical response up to 10 cm H_2O; FiO_2 delivery should be ≥ 0.40.

- Usually 30 min/hour until patient's dyspnoea and oxygen saturation remain improved without continuous positive airway pressure (CPAP).

Morphine and its analogues in AHF

Morphine should be considered in the early stage of the treatment of patients admitted with severe AHF especially if they present with restlessness, dyspnoea, anxiety or chest pain. Morphine relieves dyspnoea and other symptoms in patients with AHF and may improve cooperation for the application of NIV.

- IV boluses of morphine 2.5-5 mg may be administered as soon as the IV line is inserted in AHF patients.

- Respiration should be monitored.

- Nausea is common and anti-emetic therapy may be required.

Loop diuretics

Administration of i.v. diuretics is recommended in AHF patients in the presence of symptoms secondary to congestion and volume overload.

- Excessive treatment with diuretics may lead to hypovolaemia and hyponatraemia, and increase the likelihood of hypotension on initiation of ACEI or ARBs. (Table 19).

Table 19: Indications and dosing of diuretics in AHF

Fluid retention	Diuretic	Daily Dose (mg)	Comments
Moderate	furosemide or bumetanide or torasemide	20 - 40 0.5 - 1 10 - 20	Oral or i.v. according to clinical symptoms Titrate dose according to clinical response - Monitor K, Na, creatinine, blood pressure
Severe	furosemide furosemide infusion bumetanide torasemide	40 - 100 (5 - 40 mg/h) 1 - 4 20 - 100	i.v. Increase dose. better than very high bolus doses oral or i.v. oral
Refractory to loop diuretic	add hydrochlorothiazide or metolazone or spironolactone	50 - 100 2.5 - 10 25 - 50	Combination better than very high dose of loop diuretics MTZ more potent if creatinine clr < 30ml/min Spironolactone best choice if no renal failure and normal or low serum potassium
With alkalosis	acetazolamide	0.5 mg	i.v.
Refractory to loop diuretics and thiazides	add dopamine (renal vasodilation) or dobutamine		Consider ultrafiltration or haemodialysis if coexisting renal failure Hyponatraemia

Vasodilators

Vasodilators are recommended at an early stage for AHF patients without symptomatic hypotension, systolic BP <90 mmHg or serious obstructive valvular disease. The recommended dosage of vasodilators is presented in Table 20.

- Vasodilators relieve pulmonary congestion usually without compromising stroke volume or increasing myocardial oxygen demand in acute HF, particularly in patients with ACS.

- Hypotension (systolic BP <90 mmHg) should be avoided, especially in patients with renal dysfunction.

Table 20: Indications and dosing of IV vasodilators in AHF

Vasodilator	Indication	Dosing	Main side effects	Other
Nitroglycerine	pulmonary congestion/oedema BP > 90 mmHg	start 10 - 20 μg/min, increase up to 200 μg/min	hypotension, headache	tolerance on continuous use
Isosorbide dinitrate	pulmonary congestion/oedema BP > 90 mmHg	start with 1mg/h, increase up to 10 μg/h	hypotension, headache	tolerance on continuous use
Nitroprusside	hypertensive HF congestion/oedema BP > 90 mmHg	start with 0.3 μg/kg/min and increase up to 5 μg/kg/min	hypotension, isocyanate toxicity	light sensitive
Nesiritide*	pulmonary congestion/oedema BP > 90 mmHg	bolus 2 μg/kg + infusion 0.015 - 0.03 μg/kg/min	hypotension	

* Not available in many ESC countries

Inotropic agents

The recommended dosage of inotropic agents is reported in Table 21.

- Inotropic agents should be considered in patients with low output states, in the presence of signs of hypoperfusion or congestion despite the use of vasodilators and/or diuretics.

Table 21: Dosing of positive inotropic agents in AHF

	Bolus	Infusion rate
Dobutamine	No	2 to 20 μg/kg/min (ß+)
Dopamine	No	< 3 μg/kg/min: renal effect (δ+) 3 - 5 μg/kg/min: inotropic (ß+) > 5 μg/kg/min: (ß+), vasopressor (α+)
Milrinone	25 - 75 μg/kg over 10 - 20 min	0.375 - 0.75 μg/kg/min
Enoximone	0.25 - 0.75 mg/kg	1.25 - 7.5 μg/kg/min
Levosimendan*	12 μg/kg over 10 min (optional)**	0.1 μg/kg/min which can be decreased to 0.05 or increased to 0.2 μg/kg/min
Norepinephrine	No	0.2 - 1.0 μg/kg/min
Epinephrine	Bolus: 1 mg can be given i.v. during resuscitation, repeated every 3 - 5 min	0.05 - 0.5 μg/kg/min

* This agent also has vasodilator properties.
** In hypotensive patients, (SBP < 100 mmHg) initiation of therapy without a bolus is recommended.

- Infusion of most inotropes is accompanied by an increased incidence of both atrial and ventricular arrhythmias. Continuous clinical monitoring and ECG telemetry is required.

Dobutamine

- Dobutamine, a positive inotropic agent acting through stimulationof ß1-receptors to produce dose-dependent positive inotropic and chronotropic effects.

Dopamine

- Dopamine, also stimulate ß-adrenergic receptors. Infusion of low doses of dopamine stimulates dopaminergic receptors but has been shown to have limited effects on diuresis.

- Higher doses of dopamine may be used to maintain blood pressure but with an increasing risk of tachycardia, arrhythmia and alpha-adrenergic stimulation with vasoconstriction. Low dose dopamine is frequently combined with higher doses of dobutamine.

Milrinone and enoximone

- Milrinone and enoximone are the two type III phosphodiesterase inhibitors (PDEI) used in clinical practice. The agents have inotropic and peripheral vasodilating effects with an increase in cardiac output and stroke volume, and reductions in systemic and pulmonary vascular resistance.

Levosimendan

- Levosimendan improves cardiac contractility and exerts significant vasodilatation mediated through ATP-sensitive potassium channels. Levosimendan infusion in patients with acutely decompensated HF increases cardiac output and stroke volume and reduces systemic and pulmonary vascular resistance.
- The haemodynamic response to levosimendan is maintained over several days. In that the inotropic effect is independent of beta-adrenergic stimulation, it represents an alternative for patients on beta-blocker therapy.

Vasopressors

- Vasopressors (norepinephrine) are not recommended as first-line agents and are only indicated in cardiogenic shock when the combination of an inotropic agent and fluid challenge fails to restore adequate blood pressure with inadequate organ perfusion. Patients with sepsis complicating AHF may require a vasopressor. Since cardiogenic shock is usually associated with high vascular resistances, all vasopressors should be used with caution and discontinued as soon as possible.

Cardiac glycosides

- In AHF, cardiac glycosides produce a small increase in cardiac output and a reduction of filling pressures. It may be useful to slow ventricular rate in rapid atrial fibrillation.

Algorithm for AHF Management

The goal of treatment in the prehospital setting or at the emergency room is to improve tissue oxygenation and optimise haemodynamics in order to improve symptoms and permit interventions.

Figure 6 describes a treatment algorithm based on the level of systolic blood pressure and Figure 7 describes the treatment algorithm based on a clinical assessment of patients filling pressures and perfusion.

Figure 6: Treatment strategy in AHF according to systolic blood pressure

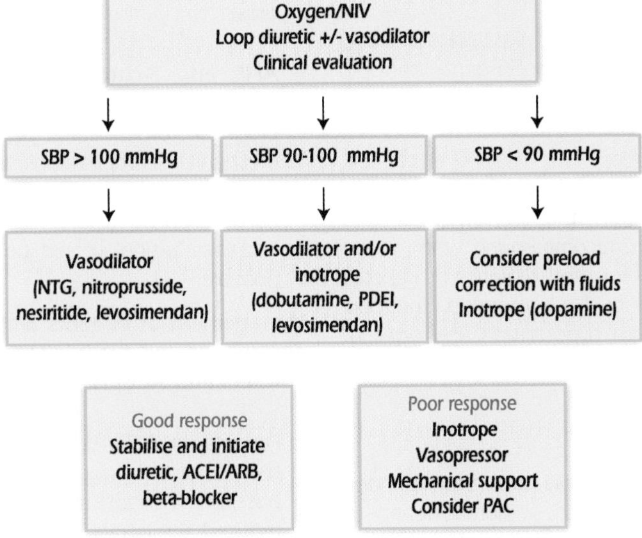

Figure 7: Treatment strategy in AHF according to LV filling pressure

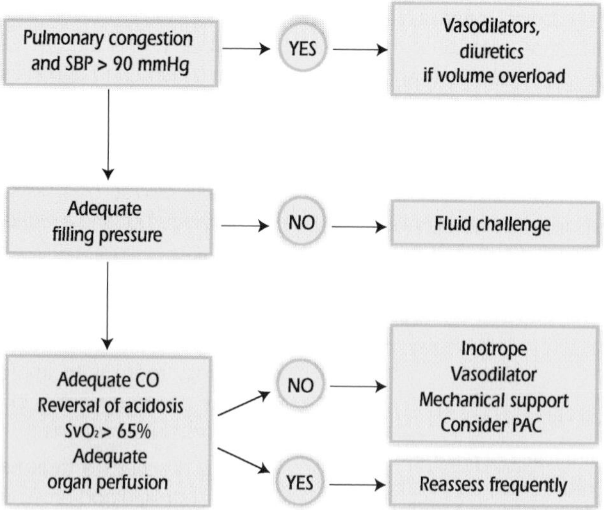

Treatment should be tailored to the clinical presentation:

- **Decompensated chronic HF:** Vasodilators along with loop diuretics are recommended. Inotropic agents are required with hypotension and signs of organ hypoperfusion.
- **Pulmonary oedema:** Morphine is usually indicated especially when dyspnoea is accompanied by pain and anxiety. Vasodilators are recommended when blood pressure is normal or high and diuretics in patients with volume overload or fluid retention. Inotropic agents are required with hypotension and signs of organ hypoperfusion. Intubation and mechanical ventilation may be required to achieve adequate oxygenation.
- **Hypertensive HF:** Vasodilators are recommended with close monitoring and low dose diuretic treatment in patients with volume overload or pulmonary oedema.
- **Cardiogenic shock:** A fluid challenge if clinically indicated followed by an inotrope if SBP remains < 90 mmHg is recommended. An intra-aortic balloon pump (IABP) and intubation should be considered. LVADs may be considered for potentially reversible causes of acute HF as a bridge to treatment response (i.e. surgery or recovery).
- **Right HF:** A fluid challenge is usually ineffective. Inotropic agents are required when there are signs of organ hypoperfusion.
- **AHF and Acute Coronary Syndromes:** In ACS complicated by AHF early reperfusion may improve prognosis. Urgent surgery is indicated in patients with mechanical complications after AMI. In cardiogenic shock caused by ACS, insertion of an intra-aortic balloon pump (IABP), coronary angiography and revascularization should be considered as soon as possible.

Management of patients with acutely decompensated chronic HF treated with beta-blockers and ACEI/ARBs.

- Patients on ACEI/ARBs admitted with worsening HF should be continued on this treatment whenever possible. The dose of beta-blocker may need to be reduced temporarily or omitted. Treatment may be interrupted or reduced in the presence of complications (bradycardia, advanced AV block, severe bronchospasm or cardiogenic shock) or in cases of severe AHF and an inadequate response to initial therapy.
- In patients admitted with AHF, beta-blockers should be considered when the patient has been stabilised on an ACEI or ARB and preferably initiated before hospital discharge.

10. Implementation & Delivery of Care

Management programmes are designed to improve outcomes through structured follow-up with patient education, optimisation of medical treatment, psychosocial support, and access to care. Table 22 summarises the goals and measures involved during potential phases of this transition.

Table 22: Treatment goals and strategies during the course of the patient's journey

Phase	Diagnostic Strategy	Action	Goals	Players
Acute	Assess clinical status Identify cause of symptoms	Treat and stabilise Initiate monitoring Plan required interventions	Stabilise, admit and triage to appropriate department	Primary care services/ Paramedics/ER physicians/ Intensivists Nurses Cardiologists
Subacute	Assess cardiac function Identify aetiology and comorbidities	Initiate chronic medical treatment Perform additional diagnostics Perform indicated procedures	Shorten hospitalisation Plan post-discharge follow-up	Hospital physicians Cardiologists CV nurses HF Management team
Chronic	Target symptoms, adherence and prognosis Identify decompensation early	Optimise pharmacological and device treatment Support self-care behaviour Remote monitoring	Reduced morbidity and mortality	Primary care physicians HF Management team Cardiologists
End of life	Identify patient concerns and symptoms	Symptomatic treatment Plan for long-term care	Palliation Provide support for patients and family	Palliative care team

Heart Failure Management Programmes

- HF management programmes are recommended for patients with HF recently hospitalised and for other high-risk patients.
- Many programmes focus on symptomatic, hospitalised patients with HF since they have a poorer prognosis and are at a higher risk for readmissions. An outpatient visit, early after discharge, is recommended to assess clinical status, identify objectives and design an effective treatment strategy. It is recommended that HF management programmes include the components shown in Table 23.
- Remote management is an emerging field within the broader context of HF management programmes and extends the reach of individualised care to the large group of individuals unable to access traditional programmes of care.

Table 23: Recommended Components of HF Management Programmes

• Multidisciplinary approach frequently led by HF nurses in collaboration with physicians and other related services
• First contact during hospitalisation, early follow-up after discharge through clinic and home-based visits, telephone support and remote monitoring
• Target high-risk, symptomatic patients
• Increased access to health care (telephone, remote monitoring and follow-up)
• Facilitate access during episodes of decompensation
• Optimised medical management
• Access to advanced treatment options
• Adequate patient education with special emphasis on adherence and self-care management
• Patient involvement in symptom monitoring and flexible diuretic use
• Psychosocial support to patients and family and/or caregiver

Palliative care for patients with heart failure

Features that should trigger such consideration and the proposed steps in the process of providing palliative care are presented in Table 24.

- Patients with clinical features of advanced HF who continue to experience symptoms refractory to optimal evidence-based therapy have a poor short-term prognosis and should be considered appropriate for a structured palliative care approach.

Table 24: Steps in the process of providing palliative care

Patient features	> 1 episode of decompensation/6 months Need for frequent or continual i.v. support Chronic poor quality of life with NYHA IV symptoms Signs of cardiac cachexia Clinically judged to be close to the end of life
Confirm diagnosis	Essential to ensure optimal treatment.
Patient education	Principles of self-care maintenance and management of HF.
Establish an advanced care plan	Designed with the patient and a family member. Reviewed regularly and includes the patients' preferences for future treatment options.
Services should be organised	The patients' care within the multidisciplinary team, to ensure optimal pharmacological treatment, self-care management and to facilitate access to supportive services.
Symptom management	Requires frequent assessment of patients' physical, psychological, social and spiritual needs. Patients frequently have multiple co-morbidities that need to be identified.
Identifying end-stage HF	Confirmation of end-stage HF is advisable to ensure that all appropriate treatment options have been explored a plan for the terminal stage of illness should be agreed upon.
Breaking bad news to the patient and family	Explaining disease progression and a change in treatment emphasis is a sensitive issue and must be approached with care.
Establishing new goals of care	End of life care should include avoidance of circumstances which may detract from a peaceful death. All current pharmacological treatment and device programmes should be considered. Resuscitation orders should be clear.

Glossary

6MWT	Six Minute Walk Test
A	Atrial
AA	Antiarrhythmic
AAD	Antiarrhythmic Drugs
AAIR	Rate responsive single chamber pacemaker that senses/paces in the atrium and is inhibited by intrinsic rhythm
ACC	American College of Cardiology
ACE	Angiotensin Converting Enzyme
ACEI or ACE-I	ACE-Inhibitors
ACS	Acute Coronary Syndrome
ACT	Activated Clotting Time
ADA	Adenosine Deaminase
ADH	Antidiuretic Hormone
ADP	Adenosine Diphosphate
AED	Automated External Defibrillator
AF	Atrial Fibrillation
AF CL	Atrial Fibrillation Cycle Length
AFP	Alpha-Feto Protein
AHA	American Heart Association
AHF	Acute Heart Failure
ALS	Advanced Life Support
ALTE	Apparent Life-Threatening Events
AMI	Acute Myocardial Infarction
ANA	Antinuclear Antibodies
ant.	anterior
ant. RP	anterograde Refractory Period
ANTITACHY	Antitachycardia algorithms in pacemaker
AP	Antero-Posterior
AP	Accessory Pathway
ApoA	Apolipoprotein A
ApoB	Apolipoprotein B
aPTT	activated Partial Thromboplastin Time
AR	Aortic Regurgitation
ARB	Angiotensin Receptor Blocker
ARR	Absolute Risk Reduction
ARVC	Arrhythmogenic Right Ventricular Cardiomyopathy
AS	Aortic Stenosis
ASA	Acetylsalicyclic Acid
ASA	Alcohol Septal Ablation
ASD	Atrial Septal Defect
ASVD	Arteriosclerotic Vascular Disease
asympt. pts.	symptomatic patients
AT	Atrial Tachycardia
ATP	Adenosine Triphosphate
ATT	Antithrombotic Trialist
AV or A-V	AtrioVentricular
AVB	Atrioventricular Block
AVNRT	AtrioVentricular Nodal Reciprocating Tachycardia
AVP	Arginine Vasopressin
AVR	Aortic Valve Replacement
AVRT	AtrioVentricular Reciprocating Tachycardia
BB	Beta Blocker
BBB	Bundle Branch Block
BC	Blood Culture
BE	Bacterial Endocarditis
b.i.d	bis in die – two times a day - twice a day
BLS	Basic Life Support
BMI	Body Mass Index
BMS	Bare Metal Stent
BNP	Brain Natriuretic Peptide
BNP	B-type Natriuretic Peptide
BP	Blood Pressure
bpm	beat per minute
BRS	Baroreflex Sensitivity
BS	Brugada Syndrome
BSA	Body Surface Area
BUN	Blood Urea Nitrogen
BV	Biventricular
CA	Calcium Antagonists
CA	Carbohydrate Antigen
CA	Cardiac Arrest
CABG	Coronary Artery Bypass Graft
CAD	Coronary Artery Disease
cath	Cathether or Catheterization
cAVSD	complete Atrio-Ventricular Septal Defect

CCB	Calcium Channel Blocker
CCD	Congenital Cyanotic Disease
CCU	Coronary Care Unit
CD	Carbohydrate Dehydratase
CE	Cardiac Event
CEA	CarcinoEmbryonic Antigen
cGMP	cyclic Guanosine 3′- 5′ Monophosphate
CHB	Complete Heart Block
CHD	Coronary Heart Disease
CHF	Congestive Heart Failure
CHF	Chronic Heart Failure
CI	Confidence Interval
CI	Cardiac Index
CIN	Contrast-Induced Nephropathy
CK	Creatinine Kinase
CKD	Chronic Kidney Disease
CK-MB	Creatinine Kinase Myocardial Brand
CKMB	Creatinine Kinase Myocardial Band
Class 1c	Vaughan Williams antiarrhythmic classification
cm	Centimeter
CMR	Cardiac Magnetic Resonance
CMV	Cytomegalovirus
CNE	Culture-Negative Endocarditis
CNS	Central Nervous System
CO	Cardiac Output
CoA	Coarctation of the Aorta
CoNS	Coagulase-Negative Staphylococci
COPD	Chronic Obstructive Pulmonary Disease
COX	Cyclo-Oxygenase
CPAP	Continuous Positive Airway Pressure
CPET	Cardiopulmonary Exercise Testing
CPR	Cardiopulmonary Resuscitation
CPVT	Catecholaminergic Polymorphic Ventricular Tachycardia
CrCl	Creatinine Clearance
CRP	C-Reactive Protein
CRT	Cardiac Resynchronisation Therapy
CRT-D	Cardiac Resynchronization Therapy – Defibrillator
CRT-P	Cardiac Resynchronization Therapy – Pacemaker
CSNRT	Corrected Sinus Node Recovery Time
CT	Computed Tomography
CT	Computerised Tomography/ Computed Tomography
CTD	Connective Tissue Diseases
CTEPH	Chronic Thromboembolic Pulmonary Hypertension
CTI	Cavotricuspid Isthmus
cTnI	Cardiac Troponin I
cTnT	Cardiac Troponin T
CTO	Chronic Total Occlusion
CUS	Compression Ultrasonography
CV	Cardiovascular
CVA	Cardiovascular Accident
CVD	Cardiovascular Disease
CW	Continuous Wave
CXR	Chest X ray
DBP	Diastolic Blood Pressure
DC	Direct Current
DCA	Directional Coronary Atherectomy
DCM	Dilated Cardiomyopathy (Nonischaemic)
DDD	Dual chamber pacemaker that senses/ paces in the atrium/ventricle and is inhibited/triggered by intrinsic rhythm
DDDR	Rate responsive dual chamber pacemaker that senses/paces in the atrium/ventricle and is inhibited/ triggered by intrinsic rhythm
DES	Drug-Eluting Stents
DHA	Docosahexaenoic Acid
dL/dl	decilitre
DLco	Diffusion Capacity for Carbon Monoxide
DM	Diabetes Mellitus
DMF	Diabetes determined by fasting plasma glucose 7.0 mmol/L and 2-h plasma glucose ,<11.1 mmol/L
DMP	Diabetes determined by 2-h plasma glucose 11.1 mmol/L and fasting plasma glucose, <7.0 mmol/L
DNA	Deoxyribonucleic Acid
DPG	Diphosphoglyceric
DTI	Direct Thrombin Inhibitor
DTS	Duke Treadmill Score
DVT	Deep Vein Thrombosis
e.g.	for example
EB-CT	Electron Beam Computer Tomography
ECG	Electrocardiogram
ECHO	Echocardiogram
ECHO	Echocardiography
ED	Emergency Department
EDTA	Ethylenediamine Triacetic Acid
EF	Ejection Fraction
EGM	Electrogram
EHRA	European Heart Rhythm Association
EMB	Endomyocardial Biopsy
EMS	Emergency Medical System
EP	Electrophysiological
EPA	Eicosaperntaenoic Acid
EPS	Electrophysiologic Study
ER	Emergency Room
ERO	Effective Regurgitant Orifice Area
ESD	End Systolic Dimension
ESR	Erythrocyte Sedimentation Rate
ET	Endothelin
ET	Exercice Testing
f/u	follow-up
Factor-Xa	Activated factor-X
Fam. hist.	Familial history
FAT	Focal Atrial Tachycardia
FDG	Fluorodeoxyglucose

FiO2	Fraction of Inspired Oxygen
FPG	Fasting Plasma Glucose
g	gram
GFR	Glomerular Filtration Rate
GI	Gastrointestinal
GOT	Glutamine-Oxaloacetic Transaminase
GPI	Glycoprotein Inhibitor
GPIIb/IIIa inhibitors	Glycoprotein IIb/IIIa inhibitors
GUCH	Grown-up Congenital Heart Disease
h	hour
HB	Heart Block
HbA1c	Glycated Haemoglobin
HbCT	Helical Biphasic Contrast Enhanced CT
HCM	Hypertrophic Cardiomyopathy
Hct	Hematocrit
HCTZ	Hydrochlorothiazide
HD	Heart Disease
HDL	High Density Lipoprotein
HDL-C	High Density Lipoprotein Cholesterol
HF	Heart Failure
HFPEF	Heart Failure with Preserved Ejection Fraction
H-ISDN	Hydralazine and Isosorbide Dinitrate
HIT	Heparin-Induced Thrombocytopenia
HIV	Human Immunodeficiency Virus
HMG-CoA	beta-Hydroxy-Beta-Methylglutaryl-Coenzyme A
HOCM	Hypertrophic Obstructive Cardiomyopathy
Hosp.	Hospitalisation
HR	Hazard Ratio
HR	Heart Rate
HRCT	High Resolution Computerised Tomography
HRT	Heart Rate Turbulence
HRV	Heart Rate Variability
hs	at bed time (Hora Somni)
hsCRP	High sensitive-C-Reactive Protein
HT	Hypertension
HV	Hyperventilation
Hx	Family History
Hypot. EST	Hypotensive response during Exercise Stress Test
i.e.	that is (id est)
IABP	Intra-Aortic Balloon Pump
ICD	Implantable Cardioverter Defibrillator
ICU	Intensive Care Unit
IDCM	Ischaemic Dilated Cardiomyopathy
IE	Infective Endocarditis
IFG	Impaired Fasting Glucose
IGH	Impaired Glucose Homeostasis
IgM	Immunoglobulin M
IGT	Impaired Glucose Tolerance
IMD	Interventricular Electromechanical Delay
IMT	Intima-Media Thickness
Inf. H	Infra-Hissian
INR	International Normalized Ratio
IPAH	Idiopathic Pulmonary Arterial Hypertension
IRAF	Immediate Recurrence of Atrial Fibrillation
ISDN	Isosorbide Dinitrate
ISH	Isolated Systolic Hypertension
IU	International Units
IV or i.v.	intravenous
IVC	Inferior Vena Cava
IVDA	Intravenous Drug Abuser
IVRT	Isovolumic Relaxation Time
IVS	Interventricular Septum
IVUS	Intra-Vascular Ultrasound
JLN	Jervell and Lange Nielsen
JVP	Jugular Venous Pressure
kg	kilogram
L	Litre
LA	Left Atrial
LA	Left Atrium
LAD	Left Anterior Descending (Coronary Artery)
LAO	Left Anterior Oblique
LBBB	Left Bundle-Branch block
LCSD	Left Cardiac Sympathetic Denervation
LD	Lactate Dehydrogenase
LDH	Lactate Dehydrogenase
LDL	Low Density Lipoprotein
LDL-C	Low Density Lipoprotein Cholesterol
LIPS	Lescol Intervention Prevention Study
LM	Left Main
LMWH	Low Molecular Weight Heparin
LOE	Level of Evidence
LP	Late Potentials
Lpa	Lipoprotein a
LQTS	Long QT Syndrome
LV	Left Ventricle
LV	Left Ventricular
LVAD	Left Ventricular Assist Device
LVD d/t MI	Left Ventricular Dysfunction due to prior Myocardial Infarction
LVEDD	Left Ventricular End Diastolic Diameter
LVEDP	Left Ventricular End Diastolic Pressure
LVEF	Left Ventricular Ejection Fraction
LVESV	Left Ventricular End-Systolic Volume
LVH	Left Ventricular Hypertrophy
LVMI	Left Ventricular Mass Index
LVOT	Left Ventricular Outflow Tract
LVOTG	Left Ventricular Outflow Tract Gradient
LVOTO	Left Ventricular Tract obstruction
LVV	Left Ventricular Volume
MACE	Major Adverse Cardiac Event
MAT	Multifocal Atrial Tachycardia
MB	Myocardial Band
MB	Myocardial Bridging
MBC	Minimum Bactericidal Concentration
MDRD	Modification of Diet in Renal Disease
MET	Metabolic Equivalent
mg	milligram

MI Myocardial Infarction
MIC Minimal Inhibitory Concentration
min minute
mL millilitre
MLVWT Maximal Left Ventricular Wall Thickness
mm millimetre
mmHg Millimetres of Mercury
mmol millimole
mmol/L or mmol.l millimole per litre
MPO Myeloperoxidase
MPS Myocardial Perfusion Scintigraphy
MPV Minimisation of Pacing in the Ventricles
MR Mitral Regurgitation
MRA Magnetic Resonance Arteriography
MRI Magnetic Resonance Imaging
MRSA Methicillin-Resistant Staphylococcus Aureus
ms millisecond
MS Metabolic Syndrome
MS Mitral Stenosis
MSSA Methicillin-Sensitive Staphylococcus Aureus
MUGA Multigated Angiogram
mV millivolt
MV Mitral Valve
MVA Malignant Ventricular Arrhythmias
MVP Mitral Valve Prolapse
NA Not Applicable
NA Not Addressed
NaCl Sodium Chloride
NGR Normal Glucose Regulation
NICM Non-Ischaemic Cardiomyopathy
NIDCM Non-Ischaemic Dilated Cardiomyopathy
NIPPV Noninvasive Positive Pressure Ventilation
NIV Non-Invasive Ventilation
NNT Numbers Needed to Treat
NSAID Non-Steroidal Anti-Inflammatory Drug
NSTE-ACS Non-ST-segment Elevation Acute Coronary Syndrome
NSTEMI Non-ST-segment Elevation Myocardial Infarction
NSVT Nonsustained Ventricular Tachycardia
NTG Nitroglycerine
NT-proBNP N-terminal Pro-Hormone Brain Natriuretic Peptide
NVE Native Valve Endocarditis
NYHA New York Heart Association
O2 Oxygen
OB/Gyn Obstetrician-Gynecologist
o.d. once a day
OD Organ Damage
OGTT Oral Glucose Tolerance Test
op. operative
OPT Optimal Pharmacological Treatment
OR Odds Ratio
OTFP Opinion of the Task Force Panel
PA Peripheral Artery
PAB Premature Atrial Beat
PAC Pulmonary Artery Catheterisation
PaCO2 Arterial Carbon Dioxide Pressure (Tension)
PAH Pulmonary Arterial Hypertension
PaO2 Arterial Oxygen Pressure (Tension)
PAP Pulmonary Arterial Pressure
pASVD partial Atrio-Ventricular Septal Defect
PAV Percutaneous Aortic Valvuloplasty
PCH Pulmonary Capillary Haemangiomatosis
PCI Percutaneous Coronary Intervention
PCR Polymerase Chain Reaction
PCWP Pulmonary Capillary Wedge Pressure
PDA Personal Digital Assistant
PDA Patent Ductus Anteriosus
PDE Phosphodiesterase
PDEI Phosphodiesterase Inhibitors
PE Pulmonary Embolism
PEEP Positive End-Expiratory Pressure
PES Programmed Electrical Stimulation
PET Positron Emission Tomography
PF4 Platelet Factor 4
PFO Patent Foramen Ovale
PG Plasma Glucose
PH Pulmonary Hypertension
PHT Pulmonary Hypertension
PJRT Permanent Form of Junctional Reciprocating Tachycardia
PLE Panlobular Emphysema
PLVEF Preserved Left Ventricular Ejection Fraction
PM PaceMaker
PMC Percutaneous Mitral Commissurotomy
Post-MI Post Myocardial Infarction
POTS Postural Orthostatic Tachycardia Syndrome
PPCM Peripartum Cardiomyopathy
PPH Primary Pulmonary Hypertension
PS Pulmonary Stenosis
PSVT Paroxysmal SupraVentricular Tachycardia
PTFE Polytetrafluoroethylene
pts. patients
PUFA Polyunsaturated Fatty Acids
PVB Premature Ventricular Beat
PVC Premature Ventricular Contraction
PVD Pulmonary Valve Dysplasia
PVE Prosthetic Valve Endocarditis
PVL ParaValvular Leak
pVO2 peak Oxygen Consumption
PVOD Pulmonary Veno-Occlusive Disease
PVR Pulmonary Vascular Resistance
PWP Pulmonary Wedge Pressure
Q-Ao QRS onset to onset of aortic flow
Q-Mit QRS onset to onset of mitral annulus systolic wave
QOL Quality Of Life
Q-Pulm QRS onset to onset of Pulmonary flow
QRS Electrocardiographic wave (complex or interval)
QRS Ventricular Activation on ECG

QT	Electrocardiographic Interval from the beginning of QRS complex to end of the T wave
Q-Tri	QRS onset to onset of tricuspid annulus systolic wave
R vol	Regurgitant volume
RA	Right Atrial
RAAS	Renin Angiotensin Aldosterone System
RAO	Right Anterior Oblique
RA-RV	Right Atrium - Right Ventricle
RBBB	Right Bundle Branch Block
RCT	Randomized Clinical Study
rec.	receptor(s)
RF	Radio Frequency
RF	Regurgitant Fraction
RFA	Radio Frequency ablation
RHC	Right Heart Catheterization
R-L	Right-Left
r-PA	Reteplase
RR	Risk Ratio
RRR	Relative Risk Reduction
rtPA	recombinant tissue Plasminogen Activator
RV	Right Ventricular
RV	Right Ventricle
RVEDP	Right Ventricular Ejection Diastolic Pressure
RVH	Right Ventricular Hypertrophy
RVOT	Right Ventricular Outflow Tract
RVSP	Right Ventricular Systolic Pressure
Rx	Treatment
S/D (ratio)	Systolic/Diastolic (ratio)
SAM	Systolic Anterior Motion
SAS	Subaortic Stenosis
SBP	Systolic Blood Pressure
SCD	Sudden Cardiac Death
SCN5A	Cardiac Sodium Channel Gene
SD	Sudden Death
SES	Socio-Economic Status
SK	Streptokinase
SPECT	Single Photon Emission Computed Tomography
SpO2	Oxygen Saturation via Pulse Oxymetry
spp	Plural of "species"
SR	Sinus Rhythm
SR	Segment
SRAF	Subacute Recurrence of Atrial Fibrillation
SSR	Stable Sinus Rhythm
STE-ACS	ST-Elevation Acute Coronary Syndrome
STEMI	ST-Elevation Acute Myocardial Infarction
Sv02	Mixed Venous Oxygen Saturation
SVA	SupraVentricular Arrhythmias
Sympt. VT	Symptomatic Ventricular Tachycardia
Synd	Syndactyly
TC	Total Cholesterol
TCPC	Total Cavo Pulmonary Connection
TdP	Torsades de Pointe
TEE	Trans-oesophageal Echocardiography
TG	Triglyceride
TGA	Transposition of Great Artery
TIA	Transient Ischaemic Attack
t.i.d.	three times a day
TNK-tPA	Tenecteplase
TOE	Tracheoesophageal
TOF	Tetralogy of Fallot
tPA	Alteplase
t-PA	Tissue Plasminogen Activator
TR	Tricuspid Regurgitation
TS	Tricuspid Stenosis
TTE	TransThoracic Echocardiography
TVR	Target Vessel Revascularization
TWA	T Wave Alternans
TX	Thromboxane
U	Unit
UA	Unstable Angina
UAP	Unstable Angina Pectoris
UFH	Unfractioned Heparin
ULN	Upper Limits of Normal
URL	Upper Reference Limit
V	Ventricular
V/Q	Ventilation/Perfusion
VA	Ventricular Arrhythmias
VAD	Ventricular Assist Device
VE/CO2	Minute Ventilation/Carbon Dioxide Production
VF	Ventricular Fibrillation
VHD	Valvular Heart Disease
VKA	Vitamin K Antagonist
VO2	Oxygen Consumption
vs.	Against
VSD	Ventricular Septal Defect
VSR	Ventricular Septal Rupture
VT	Ventricular Tachyarrhythmias
VT	Ventricular Tachycardia
VTE	Venous Thrombo-Embolism
VTns	non sustained Ventricular Tachycardia
VTs	sustained Ventricular Tachycardia
VVD	Pacemaker that senses in the atrium/ventricle paces in the ventricle and is inhibited/triggered by intrinsic rhythm
V/Q Scan	Ventilation/Perfusion Scintigraphy
VVI	Single chamber pacemaker that senses/paces in the ventricle and is inhibited by intrinsic rhythm.
VVIR	Rate-responsible single chamber pacemaker that senses/paces in the ventricle and is inhibited by intrinsic rhythm.
WHF	World Heart Foundation
WPW	Wolff-Parkinson-White Syndrome
µg	microgram
µmol	micromole

Index

Please visit the ESC website to view the guidelines at www.escardio.org/guidelines

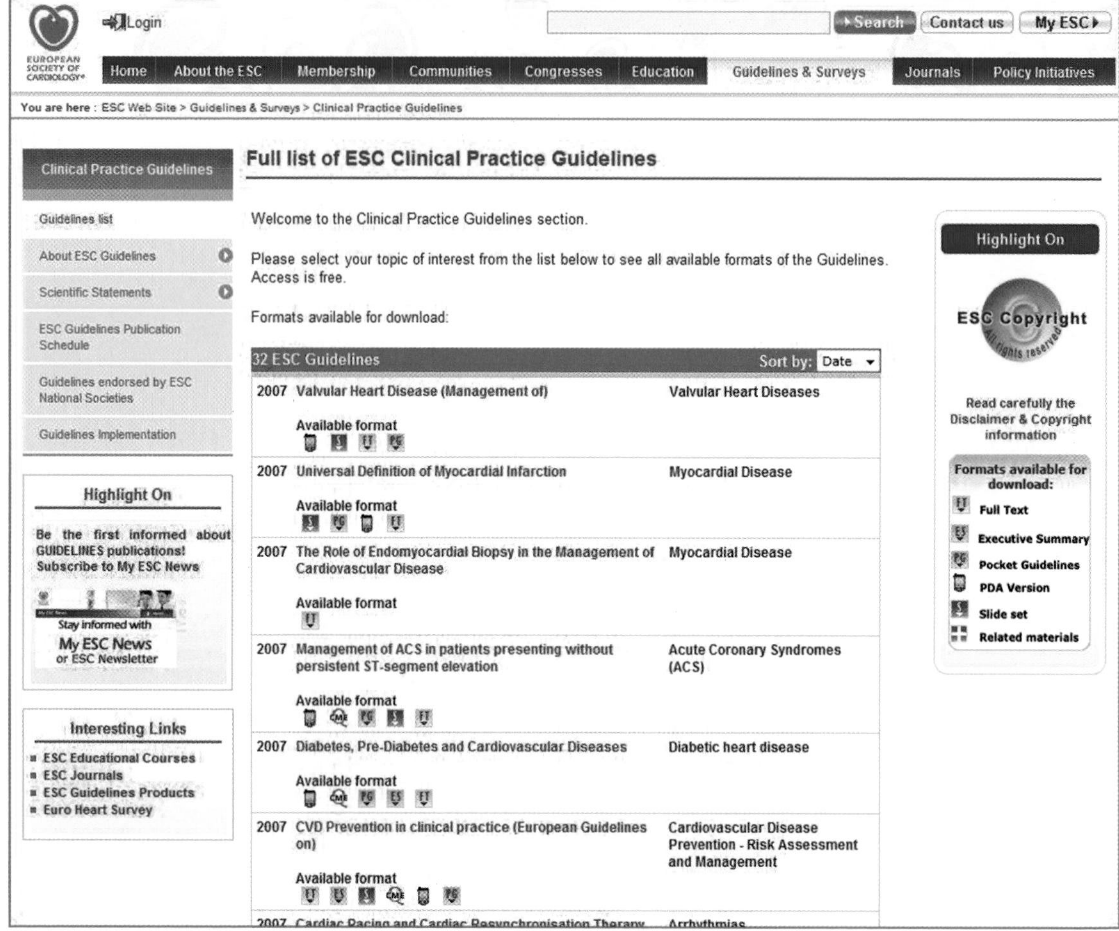